Cluster Randomization Trials
Statistical Design and Analysis

Sin-Ho Jung

CRC Press
Taylor & Francis Group
Boca Raton London New York

CRC Press is an imprint of the
Taylor & Francis Group, an **informa** business
A CHAPMAN & HALL BOOK

Designed cover image: © Sin-Ho Jung

First edition published 2025
by CRC Press
2385 NW Executive Center Drive, Suite 320, Boca Raton FL 33431

and by CRC Press
4 Park Square, Milton Park, Abingdon, Oxon, OX14 4RN

CRC Press is an imprint of Taylor & Francis Group, LLC

Library of Congress Cataloging-in-Publication Data
Names: Jung, Sin-Ho, author.
Title: Cluster randomization trials : statistical design and analysis /
Sin-Ho Jung. Description: First edition. |
Boca Raton, FL : CRC Press, 2025. |
Series: Chapman & Hall/CRC biostatistics series |
Includes bibliographical references and index.
Identifiers: LCCN 2024024655 (print) | LCCN 2024024656 (ebook) |
ISBN 9781032110806 (hbk) | ISBN 9781032118727 (pbk) |
ISBN 9781003221951 (ebk)
Subjects: LCSH: Group-randomized trials. |
Clinical trials–Statistical methods.
Classification: LCC R853.G76 J86 2025 (print) |
LCC R853.G76 (ebook) | DDC 610.72/7–dc23/eng/20240912
LC record available at https://lccn.loc.gov/2024024655
LC ebook record available at https://lccn.loc.gov/2024024656

ISBN: 9781032110806 (hbk)
ISBN: 9781032118727 (pbk)
ISBN: 9781003221951 (ebk)

DOI: 10.1201/9781003221951

Typeset in Palatino
by Newgen Publishing UK

Contents

Preface

Design and analysis of experiments, including clinical trials, involving clustered data cast statistical challenges to account for the dependency of data within each cluster. The author has been publishing methods tackling these problems. This book combines these publications of the author and related literatures published by other statisticians to fully cover the topics on clustered data. The topics of the book are selected to assist statisticians or investigators who want to design and analyze real projects rather than theoretical statisticians. Pure theoretical methods are avoided unless they can be used directly for real projects, possibly with some minor modifications.

The author wants to thank coauthors of the chapters that are reviewed in this book, especially Dr. Jianghao Li who developed the sample size calculation methods for time-to-event endpoints for his PhD thesis.

1

Introduction

Depending on the units of randomization and outcome data collection, there are various types of clinical trials. In a traditional randomized trial, patients are randomized between a control and an experimental arm and individually treated. In this case, their outcome data are independent so that standard test statistics are used to compare the resulting outcome data between two treatment arms. Their sample size methods are well developed for most types of outcome variables.

Oftentimes, small groups of individuals, called clusters, are randomized between treatment arms. Typically, clusters are families, classes, communities, surgeons operating patients, and so on. Such trials are called cluster randomization trials (CRTs). The subjects, called subunits, in each cluster share common frailties so that their outcomes tend to be positively correlated. Since clusters are independent, the data in two arms are independent in CRTs.

In a clinical trial, more than one site (such as teeth or ears) from each subject may be randomized into different treatment arms. In this case, the sites (subunits) of each subject (cluster) share common genetic, physiological, or environmental characteristics so that their observations tend to be positively correlated. This kind of trials are called subunit randomization trials (SRTs). In SRTs, dependency exists both within and between treatment arms.

Individually randomized group treatment (IRGT) trials are composite of traditional independent subject randomization and cluster randomization trials. In an IRGT trial, the control arm is to treat patients individually, whereas the experimental arm is to treat patients using a group training, education, or treatment to increase the treatment effect by close interactions among patients. As a result, the outcome data of the control arm are independent as in traditional trials, but those in the experimental arm are correlated within each group (cluster) as in CRTs. Hence, two arms in IRGT trials have different dependency structures. Unlike standard CRTs, clusters of IRGT trials are usually organized after randomization. But statistically, they have identical statistical issues between the two types of trials, i.e., accounting for the dependency within each cluster.

Although this book is entitled *Cluster Randomization Trials*, it covers all three types of trials resulting in clustered data. For outcome variables of

DOI: 10.1201/9781003221951-1

binary, continuous, and time-to-event types, we investigate generalized estimating equation (Liang and Zeger 1986) type statistical tests and their sample size formulas. Also presented are random number generation algorithms for different types of outcome variables and randomization methods. The methods are discussed in terms of clinical trials in this book, but can be used to design and analyze any types of experiments involving clustered data.

Chapters 2–7 cover CRTs and SRTs with binary or discrete data, Chapter 8 with continuous data, Chapters 9–15 with time-to-event data, and Chapter 16 for IRGT trials with different outcome variable types. Random number generation algorithms for clustered data are discussed in Chapter 6 for binary data and in Chapter 14 for time-to-event data. These chapters deal with K-sample (mostly two sample) testing methods, but Chapter 13 discusses group sequential tests for CRTs with time-to-event outcomes, and Chapter 15 reviews the extension of Cox's proportional hazards regression by Lee, Wei, and Amato (1992). Chapters 17 and 18 discuss statistical methods for various types of biomarker studies, including ROC methods.

References

Lee EW, Wei LJ, Amato DA. Cox-type regression analysis for large numbers of small groups of correlated failure time observations. In JP Klein and PK Goel (eds), Survival Analysis: State of the Art. Dordrecht: Kluwer; 1992. p. 237–247.

Liang KY, Zeger SL. Longitudinal data analysis using generalized linear models. Biometrika 1986; 73(1): 13–22.

2

One-Sample Binary Data

Correlated binary data arise frequently in various fields of applications. Examples include the presence of arthritic pain in one or more joints, and the occurrence of regional lymph node metastases in cancer patients. For site-specific observations, the fundamental unit for statistical analysis is the site rather than the subject. In periodontal diagnostic tests, site often refers to a tooth surface within a subject's mouth. The observations for sites from the same subject can be highly correlated. In these examples, cites are called subunits and subjects are called clusters.

For clustered binary data, the standard variance estimator of sample proportions based on binomial distribution estimator is inappropriate since the observations from subunits tend to be positively correlated within each cluster. Ignoring the correlation between subunits of each cluster, called intracluster correlation, tends to underestimate the true variance of a sample proportion. To avoid this problem, clustered data should be analyzed using a statistical method accounting for possible intracluster correlation.

In this chapter, we will discuss the estimation of response probability and a sample size calculation method for clustered one-sample binary data. For estimation methods, we investigate different weighting systems for subunits. Among the estimators, the optimal estimator uses weights minimizing the variance of the response probability by incorporating cluster size distribution and intracluster correlation. The sample size method is used when designing studies that will collect clustered binomial data.

Estimation of Binomial Proportions

Let n denote the total number of clusters, and m_i $(i = 1, ..., n)$ the number of dependent subunits in the ith cluster, called cluster size. For subunit j $(j = 1, ..., m_i)$ of cluster i, x_{ij} denotes a binary random variable taking the value 1 for response and 0 for no response with expected value $E(x_{ij}) = p$ and $\text{var}(x_i) = p(1 - p)$. For clustered data, subunits belonging to different clusters are independent, while those in the same cluster $(x_{i1}, ..., x_{i,n_i})$ share a common frailty so that they tend to have a positive intracluster correlation

DOI: 10.1201/9781003221951-2

coefficient (ICC) $\rho = \text{corr}(x_{ij}, x_{ij'})$ for $j \neq j'$. We assume that the number of clusters n is large for asymptotic theory and $\max m_i \leq \bar{M}(< \infty)$.

Weighted Estimators

Let $y_i = \sum_{j=1}^{m_i} x_{ij}$ denote the total number of responses among the subunits of cluster i and $\hat{p}_i = y_i/m_i$ an unbiased estimator of p from cluster i. Let $(w_1, ..., w_n)$ be a set of weights such that $w_i > 0$ and $\sum_{i=1}^{n} w_i = 1$. Note that $w_i = O_p(1/n)$ by the assumption of $\sum_{i=1}^{n} w_i = 1$. Since $\text{E}(\hat{p}_i) = p$, we consider an estimator of p given as

$$\hat{p} = \sum_{i=1}^{n} w_i \hat{p}_i \tag{2.1}$$

refer to Jung and Ahn (2000). We use $w_i = m_i / \sum_{i'=1}^{n} m_{i'}$ to assign equal weights to subunits and $w_i = 1/n$ to assign equal weights to clusters. If weights are constants as in these two weighting methods, then $\hat{p}$ is an unbiased estimator of p. As in the optimal estimator that will be discussed below, the weights may include some unknown parameters. In this case, we replace the parameters with their consistent estimators. In this case, the resulting weighted estimator $\hat{p}$ will be consistent, but may be biased.

To derive the asymptotic distribution of $\hat{p}$, we assume that the weights are free of any unknown parameters or they use their true values in this section. Even when the parameters in the weights are replaced by their consistent estimators, however, we can show that the limiting distribution of $\hat{p}$ is unchanged by using Slutsky's theorem.

Since $\sqrt{n}(\hat{p} - p) = \sqrt{n} \sum_{i=1}^{n} w_i(\hat{p}_i - p)$ and $\epsilon_i = w_i(\hat{p}_i - p)$ are independent random variables with mean 0, for large n, $\sqrt{n}(\hat{p} - p)$ is asymptotically normal with mean 0 and variance σ^2 that can be estimated by

$$\hat{\sigma}^2 = n \sum_{i=1}^{n} w_i^2 (\hat{p}_i - \hat{p})^2.$$

Hence, $100(1 - \alpha)\%$ confidence interval (CI) for p can be calculated by $\hat{p} \pm z_{1-\alpha/2}\hat{\sigma}/\sqrt{n}$, where $z_{1-\alpha/2}$ denotes the $100(1-\alpha/2)$ percentile of the standard normal distribution. For testing $H_0 : p = p_0$, we may estimate σ^2 under H_0 by

$$\hat{\sigma}_0^2 = n \sum_{i=1}^{n} w_i^2 (\hat{p}_i - p_0)^2. \tag{2.2}$$

If the cluster sizes, m_i, are constant, then the two weighting methods of equal weights to units and equal weights to clusters will be identical. If the cluster sizes are varying cluster by cluster and ICC is so low that subunits within each cluster behave independently, then the estimator using equal weights to subunits will be more reasonable as in the standard independent binary data case. On the other hand, if subunits in each cluster are highly dependent, then having more subunits in each cluster will not add much information to the resulting data. In this case, the estimator assigning equal weights to clusters will be more efficient. In the following section, we investigate an efficient estimator of p that will always minimize the variance of estimator.

Optimal Estimator

We have $\text{var}(\hat{p}_i) = p(1-p)\{1+(m_i-1)\rho\}/m_i$ since

$$\begin{aligned}
\text{var}(y_i) &= \text{var}(x_{i1} + \cdots + x_{i,m_i}) \\
&= \sum_{j=1}^{m_i} \text{var}(x_{ij}) + \sum\sum_{j \neq j'} \text{cov}(x_{ij}, x_{ij'}) \\
&= m_i \text{var}(x_{ij}) + m_i(m_i - 1)\text{cov}(x_{ij}, x_{ij'}) \\
&= m_i p(1-p) + m_i(m_i-1)p(1-p)\rho \\
&= m_i p(1-p)\{1 + (m_i - 1)\rho\}.
\end{aligned}$$

It is well known that weights that are inversely proportional to the variances minimize the variance of a weighted estimator. Hence, we can optimize $\hat{p}$ by using weights

$$w_i = \frac{m_i\{1+(m_i-1)\rho\}^{-1}}{\sum_{i'=1}^{n} m_{i'}\{1+(m_{i'}-1)\rho\}^{-1}}. \tag{2.3}$$

Note that the optimal weights reduce to equal weights to subunits if $\rho = 0$ and to equal weights to clusters if $\rho = 1$.

Since the optimal weights (2.3) include an unknown parameter ρ, we have to replace it with a consistent estimator for $\hat{p}$ and its variance estimator. One of most popular is the ANOVA estimator (Donner and Donald 1987, Donner and Klar 1993) that is given as

$$\hat{\rho} = \frac{\text{msc} - \text{mse}}{\text{msc} + (n_A - 1)\text{mse}},$$

where $\text{msc} = \sum_{i=1}^{n} m_i(\hat{p}_i - \hat{p})^2/(n-1)$, $\text{mse} = \sum_{i=1}^{n} y_i(1-\hat{p}_i)/(M-n)$, $M = \sum_{i=1}^{n} m_i$ denotes the total number of subunits, and $n_A = (M - \sum_{i=1}^{n} m_i^2/M)/(n-1)$.

Example

The data of Hujoel et al. (1990) are used to illustrate our estimation methods for the sensitivity and the specificity of an enzymatic diagnostic test. An

TABLE 2.1

Estimates of the sensitivity and the specificity of an enzymatic diagnostic test

	Sensitivity			Specificity		
Method	$\hat{p}$	SE	95% CI	$\hat{p}$	SE	95% CI
$\hat{p}_u$	66.2%	5.3%	(55.8%, 76.6%)	81.3%	6.2%	(69.2%, 93.3%)
$\hat{p}_c$	64.9%	5.6%	(54.1%, 75.8%)	75.4%	8.1%	(59.5%, 91.3%)
$\hat{p}_o$	65.9%	5.2%	(55.6%, 76.2%)	80.0%	6.2%	(67.8%, 92.2%)

enzymatic diagnostic test was used to determine whether a site is infected by two specific organisms, treponema denticola and bacteroides gingivalis, or not. Each subject (cluster) has a different number of infected sites (subunits), as determined by an antibody assay against the two organisms as a gold standard.

From $n = 29$ subjects, the number of true positive test results divided by the number of infected sites (sensitivity data), y_i/m_i, for each subject is

$3/6, 2/6, 2/4, 5/6, 4/5, 5/5, 4/6, 3/4, 2/4, 3/4, 5/5, 4/4, 6/6, 3/3, 5/6, 1/2, 4/6, 0/4, 5/6, 4/5, 4/6, 0/6, 4/5, 3/5, 0/2, 2/6, 2/4, 5/5, 4/6.$

And, from $n = 21$ subjects, the number of true negative test results divided by the number of non-infected sites (specificity data) y_i/m_i for each subject is

$0/1, 3/3, 1/2, 3/3, 1/1, 2/3, 3/3, 1/1, 0/1, 2/3, 2/3, 1/1, 0/1, 1/3, 1/1, 2/2, 4/4, 3/3, 5/5, 1/1, 3/3.$

In the enzymatic diagnostic test data, the ANOVA estimates of the ICCs are $\hat{\rho} = 0.20$ and 0.25 for the sensitivity and specificity data sets, respectively. Note that cluster sizes, m_i, are distributed between 2 and 6 for the sensitivity data and between 1 and 5 for the specificity data.

Table 2.1 displays comparisons of the estimates, $\hat{p}$, of the sensitivity and the specificity, and their standard errors, $\text{SE}(\hat{p}) = \hat{\sigma}/\sqrt{n}$, and 95% CIs for the three different weighting systems. Let $\hat{p}_u$, $\hat{p}_c$, and $\hat{p}_o$ denote estimators using equal weights to subunits, equal weights for clusters, and optimal weights, respectively. We observe that there are negligible differences in the estimates of sensitivity, but the estimate with optimal weights has the smallest SE and the shortest CI. For specificity, the estimate using equal weights to clusters is smaller than those based on the other two weighting methods. Optimal estimate and the estimate using equal weights to subunits have smaller SE than that using equal weights to clusters.

Simulation Studies

Simulations are conducted to evaluate the small sample property of the estimators. We set the number of clusters at $n = 10, 30$, or 50. For cluster i, its size m_i is generated from the discrete uniform distribution taking an integer value between 1 and 10. Once m_i is generated, a random variable y_i is generated from a beta-binomial distribution with the true success probability $p = 0.5$ or 0.8 and ICC $\rho = 0.0, 0.2, 0.4$, or 0.6. The probability mass function (PMF) of beta-binomial random variable y_i with cluster size m_i, marginal response rate p, and ICC ρ is given as

$$g(y_i|m_i, p, \rho) = \binom{m_i}{y_i} \frac{B(\alpha + y_i, \beta + m_i - y_i)}{B(\alpha, \beta)}$$

for $y_i = 0, 1, ..., m_i$, where $\alpha = p(1-\rho)/\rho$, $\beta = (1-p)(1-\rho)/\rho$, $B(a, b) = \Gamma(a)\Gamma(b)/\Gamma(a+b)$, and $\Gamma(a) = \int_0^\infty t^{a-1} \exp(-t)dt$.

We repeat 5,000 simulations for each combination of parameter values. From each simulation sample, p is estimated using one of the three weighting systems. For each of these estimators, SE and 95% CI are calculated. The ICC for the optimal weights is estimated using Donner and Klar (1993) formula.

Bias and SE of each estimator are estimated by their averages over 5,000 simulations. Empirical coverage probability (ECP) of an estimator is obtained as the proportion of the 95% CIs covering p.

Simulation results are reported in Table 2.2. We observe that all three estimators have negligible bias. As expected, as ρ increases, SE of $\hat{p}_u$ increases and that of $\hat{p}_c$ decreases. However, $\hat{p}_o$ always has the smallest SE among the three. More specifically, we have SE($\hat{p}_o$) $\approx$ SE($\hat{p}_u$) $<$ SE($\hat{p}_c$) for $\rho = 0$ and SE($\hat{p}_o$) $\approx$ SE($\hat{p}_c$) $<$ SE($\hat{p}_u$) for a large ρ, such as 0.6.

When $p = 0.5$, all three estimators have small ECPs for small sample size and positive ρ. We observe that $\hat{p}_c$ has a small ECP even when $\rho = 0$. When $p = 0.8$, all three estimators tend to have small ECP in most cases reported here. This may be resulted from the fact that, when p is close to 0 or 1, asymptotic CIs estimated from data with small or moderate size can include a range out of $(0, 1)$ so that the true coverage probability becomes smaller than the nominal one.

Jung and Ahn (2000) show that a transformation, such as arcsine or logit, of $\bar{p}$ may improve the performance of the CIs for small sample sizes.

Modified McNemar's Test for Clustered Paired Binary Data

Matched pairs of data often arise in medical statistics for comparing two diagnostic tests. Usually, measurements of two diagnostic tests are collected from each subject, and their diagnostic accuracy is compared using McNemar's (1947) test. In this case, although the outcomes of two diagnostic tests are paired and correlated, the pairs from different subjects are independent.

The independence assumption is violated in some biomedical studies by having multiple sites or repeated measurements for diagnosis from each subject. In these cases, the paired measurements (subunits) from the same subject

TABLE 2.2
Simulation results

			$p = 0.5$			$p = 0.8$		
ρ	n		Bias	SE	ECP	Bias	SE	ECP
0.0	10	$\hat{p}_u$	0.001	0.074	0.957	−0.003	0.059	0.950
		$\hat{p}_c$	−0.001	0.079	0.906	−0.002	0.061	0.878
		$\hat{p}_o$	−0.001	0.073	0.955	−0.004	0.058	0.950
	30	$\hat{p}_u$	−0.001	0.041	0.959	0.000	0.033	0.953
		$\hat{p}_c$	0.000	0.048	0.939	0.001	0.038	0.919
		$\hat{p}_o$	−0.001	0.041	0.960	−0.001	0.033	0.952
	50	$\hat{p}_u$	0.000	0.031	0.954	−0.001	0.025	0.953
		$\hat{p}_c$	0.000	0.038	0.944	0.001	0.030	0.931
		$\hat{p}_o$	0.000	0.031	0.954	−0.001	0.025	0.954
0.2	10	$\hat{p}_u$	−0.002	0.099	0.912	−0.003	0.077	0.890
		$\hat{p}_c$	−0.001	0.097	0.896	0.000	0.075	0.871
		$\hat{p}_o$	−0.002	0.093	0.909	−0.005	0.073	0.890
	30	$\hat{p}_u$	0.000	0.057	0.937	0.000	0.046	0.930
		$\hat{p}_c$	0.001	0.059	0.938	0.001	0.047	0.924
		$\hat{p}_o$	0.000	0.055	0.935	−0.001	0.044	0.934
	50	$\hat{p}_u$	0.000	0.045	0.943	−0.001	0.035	0.931
		$\hat{p}_c$	0.001	0.046	0.941	0.001	0.037	0.933
		$\hat{p}_o$	0.000	0.043	0.942	−0.001	0.034	0.936
0.4	10	$\hat{p}_u$	−0.003	0.122	0.899	−0.003	0.094	0.860
		$\hat{p}_c$	−0.001	0.112	0.894	0.000	0.086	0.854
		$\hat{p}_o$	−0.002	0.111	0.897	−0.006	0.086	0.869
	30	$\hat{p}_u$	0.000	0.072	0.943	0.000	0.057	0.922
		$\hat{p}_c$	0.001	0.068	0.940	0.001	0.054	0.922
		$\hat{p}_o$	0.000	0.067	0.943	−0.001	0.053	0.922
	50	$\hat{p}_u$	−0.001	0.056	0.946	−0.001	0.044	0.933
		$\hat{p}_c$	0.001	0.053	0.949	0.001	0.042	0.935
		$\hat{p}_o$	0.000	0.052	0.948	−0.001	0.041	0.934
0.6	10	$\hat{p}_u$	−0.003	0.142	0.899	−0.004	0.108	0.847
		$\hat{p}_c$	−0.002	0.126	0.897	−0.002	0.096	0.853
		$\hat{p}_o$	−0.002	0.126	0.897	−0.006	0.097	0.863
	30	$\hat{p}_u$	0.000	0.083	0.941	−0.001	0.066	0.927
		$\hat{p}_c$	0.001	0.076	0.943	0.000	0.060	0.922
		$\hat{p}_o$	0.000	0.076	0.943	−0.001	0.060	0.924
	50	$\hat{p}_u$	−0.001	0.065	0.949	−0.001	0.051	0.928
		$\hat{p}_c$	0.000	0.059	0.952	0.001	0.047	0.927
		$\hat{p}_o$	0.000	0.059	0.952	−0.001	0.047	0.925

(cluster) result in clustered paired data. Adjusted McNemar's tests for clustered data have been proposed by many statisticians, including Eliasziw and Donner (1991), Obuchowski (1998), Durkalski et al. (2003), and Wu (2021).

We discuss a simple adjustment of McNemar's test for clustered test by using the estimation method discussed in the previous section. In this section, we consider assigning equal weights to subunits or equal weights to clusters to avoid estimation of the ICC for the weights. Contrary to these other methods, ours does not require complicated computations for estimation of

TABLE 2.3

Frequencies of measurements from clustered pairs by two diagnostic tests

		Diagnosis 2	
		Benign	Malignant
Diagnosis 1	Benign	X_{00}	X_{01}
	Malignant	X_{10}	X_{11}

ICCs between pairs or among subunits within each cluster. It can be easily extended to the modification of McNemar's test using optimal estimators.

Clustered McNemar's Test

For site $j(=1,...,\tilde{m}_i)$ of subject $i(=1,...,\tilde{n})$, let t_{kij} denote the measurement of diagnostic test $(k=1,2)$ taking value 0 if benign and 1 if malignant. Let $X_{l_1,l_2}=\sum_{i=1}^{\tilde{n}}\sum_{j=1}^{\tilde{m}_i}I(t_{1ij}=l_1,t_{2ij}=l_2)$ for $l_1,l_2=0,1$, where $I(\cdot)$ is the indicator function. The frequencies of measurements from all $\sum_{i=1}^{\tilde{n}}\tilde{m}_i$ can be summarized in Table 2.3.

The McNemar's test is to determine if one diagnostic test tends to have more malignancy readings than the other. If all the sites included in data analysis are proven to be malignant by a gold standard, then we are testing if one diagnostic test is more sensitive than the other or not. On the other hand, if all the sites are proven to be benign by a gold standard, then this is to test if one diagnostic test is more specific than the other. To this end, we test if $p=P(t_{1ij}=1,t_{2ij}=0|t_{1ij}\neq t_{2ij})$ equals $1/2$ or not. By the conditioning in this probability, the sites with concordant pairs between two diagnostic tests are excluded in a McNemar testing so that only X_{01} and X_{10} contribute to the testing. We will have $p>1/2$ if diagnostic test 1 is more sensitive and all sites are malignant, and $p<1/2$ if diagnostic test 1 is more specific and all sites are benign.

Suppose that X_{01} and X_{10} include paired measurements from n clusters, which have at least one discordant sites. Let m_i denote the number of sites with discordant measurements for subject $i(=1,...,n)$. By sorting out the pairs with discordant measurements only, n may be smaller than $\tilde{n}$ and m_i may be smaller than $\tilde{m}_i$ for some clusters. Among the discordant pairs, let $x_{ij}=I(t_{1ij}=1,t_{2ij}=0)$ for cluster i with at least one discordant site. Then, we have $p=P(x_{ij}=1)$ since concordant pairs are all excluded. McNemar's test is to test $H_0:p=1/2$ against $H_1:p\neq 1/2$.

From the data set $\{(x_{i1},...,x_{im_i}),i=1,...,n\}$, we estimate $\hat{p}$ and $\hat{\sigma}_0^2$ using (2.1) and (2.2), respectively, with $p_0=1/2$. We will reject H_0 if $\sqrt{n}|\hat{p}-1/2|/\hat{\sigma}_0>z_{1-\alpha/2}$.

In summary, we use (i) only discordant pairs between two diagnostic test as in the standard McNemar's test, (ii) estimate p by using two weighting methods for which weights are free of any unknown parameters, and (iii) estimate the variance using a generalized estimating equation type method (Liang and Zeger 1986). By using these approaches, our statistical testing becomes very simple, almost as simple as the standard McNemar's test for independent subjects because it does not require complicated computations for estimating the ICCs between paired measurements or within clusters.

Real Data Example

Two diagnostic tests in radiology, positron emission tomography (PET, $k = 1$) and single photon emission tomography (SPECT, $k = 2$), are compared for the detection of hyperparathyroidism (Neumann et al. 1996). The study's aim was to compare the two tests in terms of the sensitivity and specificity using measurement from multiple glands (subunits) of each patient (clusters). For illustration of our statistical method, however, we consider comparing the specificities of the prognostic tests here. The specificity data, displayed in Table IV of Obuchowski (1998), consist of $\sum_{i=1}^{\tilde{n}} \tilde{m}_i = 51$ glands with no hyperparathyroidism (as confirmed by surgery) from $\tilde{n} = 21$ patients.

Among these patients, only $n = 6$ patients have glands with discordant measurements between the two diagnostic tests. For these patients, we have $y_i/m_i = 0/2, 0/1, 0/1, 1/1, 0/2$, and $0/1$. Note that there are $M = 8$ glands in this data set. We have $\hat{p} = 0.1250$, $\hat{\sigma}_0^2 = 0.2813$, and a p-value of 0.0833 using equal weights to subunits, and $\hat{p} = 0.1667$, $\hat{\sigma}_0^2 = 0.2500$, and a p-value of 0.1025 using equal weights to clusters. Although it is not significant, probably due to the small sample size, PET seems to have a higher specificity than SPECT because the estimators of p is much smaller than $1/2$.

Ignoring the intracluster correlation, the variance estimator of $\hat{p}$ using equal weights to the subunits is given as $\hat{\sigma}_I^2 = np_0(1 - p_0)/M = 0.1875$ so that the standard McNemar's test gives a p-value of 0.0339. Note that the significance is erroneously amplified by ignoring the intracluster dependency

Sample Size Calculations for Clustered Binary Data

When conducting a study collecting clustered binary data, we need to calculate the number of clusters n required for a statistical testing. In this section, we discuss the sample size (i.e., number of clusters) method to test $H_0 : p = p_0$ that was presented by Jung et al. (2001).

For a sample size calculation under $H_1 : p = p_1 (\neq p_0)$, we need to specify following input parameters.

1. Type I error rate α and power $1 - \beta$

2. Response rates, p_0 and p_1
3. ICC ρ
4. Distribution of cluster sizes

If we have pilot data, we may use the observed relative frequency of cluster sizes as the PMF of a specified cluster size distribution. Otherwise, investigators may have a good knowledge of the distribution for the target population.

We derive the distribution of the test statistic under $H_1 : p = p_1$. For the purpose of sample size calculation, we assume the nearby alternative hypothesis assumption, i.e., $|p_1 - p_0| = o_p(n^{-1/2})$. Under this assumption, the limit of σ_0^2 and variance of $\sqrt{n}(\hat{p} - p_0)$ are commonly expressed as

$$\sigma^2 = \lim_{n\to\infty} n \sum_{i=1}^{n} w_i^2 \mathrm{var}(\hat{p}_i).$$

Since $\mathrm{var}(\hat{p}_i) = p_1(1 - p_1)\{1 + (m_i - 1)\rho\}/m_i$ under H_1, we have

$$\sigma^2 = d_w p_1(1 - p_1),$$

where

$$d_w = \lim_{n\to\infty} n \sum_{i=1}^{n} \frac{w_i^2\{1 + (m_i - 1)\rho\}}{m_i}.$$

In the absence of clustering effect, the variance of $\sqrt{M}(\hat{p} - p_1)$ is $p_1(1 - p_1)$ so that $D = d/\bar{m}$ is called the inflation factor, where $\bar{m} = E(m)$, the mean cluster size. Note that d depends on the weights used for $\hat{p}$. For example, with equal weights to subunits $w_i = m_i/M$, we have $d_w = d_u$, where

$$d_u = \bar{m}^{-1}\{1 + (\bar{\bar{m}}/\bar{m} - 1)\rho\},$$

and $\bar{\bar{m}} = E(m^2)$, the second moment of the distribution of cluster sizes.

Similarly, with equal weights to clusters $w_i = 1/n$, we have $d_w = d_c$, where

$$d_c = E(1/m) + \{1 - E(1/m)\}\rho$$

and the expectation is taken with respect to the distribution of cluster sizes m.

For the optimal estimator with

$$w_i = \frac{m_i\{1 + (m_i - 1)\rho\}^{-1}}{\sum_{i'=1}^{n} m_{i'}\{1 + (m_{i'} - 1)\rho\}^{-1}}$$

we have $d_w = d_o$, where

$$d_o = 1/E\left\{\frac{m}{1 + (m - 1)\rho}\right\}.$$

Given a sample size n, the power is given as

$$\begin{aligned}1-\beta =&P\left(\frac{\sqrt{n}|\hat{p}-p_0|}{\hat{\sigma}_0} > z_{1-\alpha/2}\Big|H_1\right)\\ \approx&P\left(\frac{\sqrt{n}|\hat{p}-p_0|}{\sigma} > z_{1-\alpha/2}\Big|H_1\right)\\ =&P\left\{\frac{\sqrt{n}(\hat{p}-p_1)}{\sigma} > z_{1-\alpha/2} - \frac{\sqrt{n}(p_1-p_0)}{\sigma}\Big|H_1\right\}.\end{aligned}$$

Since $\sqrt{n}(\hat{p}-p_1)/\sigma \sim N(0,1)$ under H_1, we have

$$-z_{1-\beta} = z_{1-\alpha/2} - \frac{\sqrt{n}(p_1-p_0)}{\sigma}. \tag{2.4}$$

By solving (2.4), with respect to n, we obtain the required sample size

$$n = \frac{\sigma^2(z_{1-\alpha/2}+z_{1-\beta})^2}{(p_1-p_0)^2} = \frac{d_w p_1(1-p_1)(z_{1-\alpha/2}+z_{1-\beta})^2}{(p_1-p_0)^2}.$$

Note that $n_0 = n/d_w$ is the required number of subunits by the sample size formula for independent dichotomous data. The required number of subunits is given as $M = n\bar{m}$. Furthermore, since d increases in ρ for any weights, the required sample size increases in ρ.

Example

Suppose that we want to investigate the sensitivity of an enzymatic diagnostic test that is used to determine if a site is infected by two specific organisms, treponema denticola and bacteroides gingivitis. For sample size estimation, we use the data of Hujoel et al. (1990) as pilot data. In a sample of 29 subjects, the number of true positive test results (y_i) and the number of infected sites (m_i) are given in Table 2.4.

Suppose that testing hypotheses are $H_0 : p_0 = 0.6$ and $H_1 : p_1 = 0.7$. From the data, ANOVA method gives the estimate of ICC $\hat{\rho} = 0.19$ so that we assume $\rho = 0.2$. Based on the observed frequency of cluster sizes, we may specify the distribution of m as in Table 2.4. Using the specified PMF $f(m)$,

TABLE 2.4

Distribution of cluster sizes, m

	$m = 2$	3	4	5	6
Relative frequency	2/29	1/29	7/29	7/29	12/29
Specified PMF, $f(m)$	0.05	0.05	0.25	0.25	0.4

we have $\bar{m} = E(m) = 4.9$ and $\bar{\bar{m}} = E(m^2) = 25.3$. Furthermore, we have $d_u = 0.374$, $d_c = 0.377$, and $d_o = 0.369$.

The required sample size for 90% of power is given as $n_u = 83$ using equal weights to subunits, $n_c = 84$ using equal weights to clusters, and $n_o = 82$ using the optimal weights. Although the differences are small, the test statistic using optimal estimator requires the smallest sample size. If $\rho = 0$, the required number of clusters (sample size) is only $n_0 = 46$ or the required number of subunits is $M_0 = \bar{m} \times n_0 = 226$.

Numerical Studies

Since the sample size calculation is based on asymptotic normality, we conduct simulations to investigate its finite sample performance. Suppose that the true distribution of cluster size has one of the following PMFs:

$$\begin{aligned}
f_1 &=(f(2), f(3), f(4), f(5), f(6)) = (0, 0, 1, 0, 0),\\
f_2 &=(f(2), f(3), f(4), f(5), f(6)) = (1/5, 1/5, 1/5, 1/5, 1/5),\\
f_3 &=(f(2), f(3), f(4), f(5), f(6)) = (1/2, 0, 0, 0, 1/2),
\end{aligned}$$

and that the true ICC is $\rho = 0.1, 0.3$, or 0.5. Note that $E(m) = 4$ for all three PMFs and $\text{var}(m) = 0, 2, 4$ for f_1, f_2, and f_3, respectively. We want to test and calculate the sample size for hypotheses $H_0 : p = p_0$ vs. $H_1 : p = p_1$ with $(\alpha, 1-\beta) = (0.05, 0.8)$ and $(p_0, p_1) = (.5, .6)$, (0.5,0.7), (0.7,0.8), or (0.7,0.9). Based on the prespecified $(\alpha, 1-\beta, p_0, p_1, \rho, f(\cdot))$, we calculate sample size n using the three weighted estimators.

Now, we generate random samples of size n from the specified distributions. That is, cluster size m_i $(i = 1, ..., n)$ is generated from the true distribution $f(\cdot)$, and then number of responses y_i is generated from a beta-binomial distribution with $p = p_0$ or p_1, and ICC ρ. Using the generated data, we conduct the testing for $H_0 : p = p_0$. We generate 5,000 simulation samples. The empirical type I error rate, $\hat{\alpha}$, and power, $1-\hat{\beta}$, are calculated as the proportion of samples rejecting H_0 from the simulated data sets under $p = p_0$ and $p = p_1$, respectively. We use ANOVA $\hat{\rho}$ in calculating the test statistic. We conclude that the estimated sample size is correct if the empirical power $1-\hat{\beta}$ is close to the nominal level $1-\beta = 0.8$, while we conclude that the test statistic maintains the type I error accurately at the estimated sample size n if the empirical type I error rate $\hat{\alpha}$ is close to the nominal level $\alpha = 0.05$.

Table 2.5 reports sample size n, empirical type I error $\hat{\alpha}$, and empirical power $1-\hat{\beta}$ under the various combinations of input parameter values. The unit for $\hat{\alpha}$ and $1-\hat{\beta}$ is percent. As ρ increases, sample sizes increase for all three estimators due to clustering effect. Sample sizes for all three estimators have similar finite sample performance although n_o is always smaller than or equal to n_u and n_c. If ρ is small, n_c is similar to n_o. Note that n_u is similar to n_o if ρ is small, while n_c is similar to n_o if ρ is large. For f_1, cluster sizes are constant, i.e., $m_i = 4$ so that all three estimators are identical

TABLE 2.5

For nominal $(\alpha, 1-\beta) = (5\%, 80\%)$, $n/\hat{\alpha}(\%)/1-\hat{\beta}(\%)$ of test statistics using weighted estimators with equal weights to subunits, $\hat{p}_u$, equal weights to clusters, $\hat{p}_c$, and optimal weights, $\hat{p}_o$

		$(p_0, p_1) = (0.5, 0.7)$			$(p_0, p_1) = (0.5, 0.6)$		
f	ρ	$\hat{p}_o$	$\hat{p}_u$	$\hat{p}_c$	$\hat{p}_o$	$\hat{p}_u$	$\hat{p}_c$
f_1	0.1	14/5.6/78.0	14/5.6/78.0	14/5.6/78.0	62/5.0/79.6	62/5.0/79.6	62/5.0/79.6
	0.3	20/6.4/76.6	20/6.4/76.6	20/6.4/76.6	90/5.1/79.7	90/5.1/79.7	90/5.1/79.7
	0.5	26/6.4/77.6	26/6.4/77.6	26/6.4/77.6	118/6.1/79.8	118/6.1/79.8	118/6.1/79.8
f_2	0.1	14/6.6/77.2	14/6.6/76.5	15/6.4/76.7	63/5.0/79.9	64/4.9/80.3	69/4.9/79.9
	0.3	21/6.5/77.4	22/6.4/78.2	21/6.8/76.6	93/5.4/79.2	97/5.4/79.5	95/5.4/79.5
	0.5	27/6.0/77.7	29/6.0/77.9	27/5.8/77.6	121/4.9/79.9	130/4.9/80.3	122/5.0/80.0
f_3	0.1	15/6.7/77.4	15/6.7/77.0	17/6.4/77.3	65/5.6/79.0	66/5.6/79.3	76/5.1/79.2
	0.3	21/6.9/77.0	23/6.5/77.0	22/6.5/76.7	96/4.9/79.4	104/4.8/79.4	101/5.0/79.6
	0.5	28/5.8/79.2	31/6.2/77.4	28/5.7/78.9	124/5.0/78.9	142/5.3/79.7	126/5.0/78.9
		$(p_0, p_1) = (0.7, 0.9)$			$(p_0, p_1) = (0.7, 0.8)$		
f_1	0.1	6/8.4/64.9	6/8.4/64.9	6/8.4/64.9	41/6.1/77.5	41/6.1/77.5	41/6.1/77.5
	0.3	9/10.5/65.9	9/10.5/65.9	9/10.5/65.9	60/5.4/77.2	60/5.4/77.2	60/5.4/77.2
	0.5	12/9.3/67.8	12/9.3/67.8	12/9.3/75.5	79/5.2/76.6	79/5.2/76.6	79/5.2/76.6
f_2	0.1	6/8.7/59.7	6/8.8/60.5	7/8.2/67.2	42/5.9/76.4	43/6.2/77.3	46/5.7/77.8
	0.3	9/10.2/63.9	10/10.2/69.5	9/9.8/63.5	62/6.3/78.1	65/6.0/77.3	64/5.7/78.4
	0.5	12/9.6/66.6	13/9.3/68.3	12/9.4/73.7	81/6.0/77.1	87/6.3/78.1	82/5.9/77.1
f_3	0.1	7/9.5/66.7	7/9.3/66.7	8/7.8/67.7	44/5.8/76.9	44/5.8/77.0	51/5.6/77.5
	0.3	9/9.4/60.4	10/10.4/67.3	10/8.8/66.6	64/5.5/76.6	70/5.8/76.7	67/5.5/76.6
	0.5	12/9.6/67.3	14/8.8/69.8	12/9.2/74.6	83/5.9/76.4	95/6.3/77.1	84/5.5/76.3

and have the same sample sizes and simulation performance. The sample size increases as the variance of cluster sizes increases, i.e., in the order of $f_1 < f_2 < f_3$. Since all three distributions have the same mean $\bar{m} = 4$, their variances, $\text{var}(m) = \bar{\bar{m}} - \bar{m}^2$, are determined by the second moments $\bar{\bar{m}}$ of the distributions. As a result, the impact of variance of cluster size distribution in sample size is larger for $\hat{p}_u$ than that for $\hat{p}_c$ and $\hat{p}_o$ since d_u (hence, its sample size) is proportional to $\bar{\bar{m}}$. When the required sample size is large, as in $(p_0, p_1) = (0.5, 0.6)$, all three test statistics have $(\hat{\alpha}, 1-\hat{\beta})$ that are very close to their nominal level $(\alpha, 1-\beta) = (5\%, 80\%)$. If the required sample size is small, however, the test statistics tend to be anticonservative and underpowered. Especially, when $(p_0, p_1) = (0.7, 0.9)$, the required sample size is very small and the discrepancy in $(\hat{\alpha}, 1-\hat{\beta})$ from their nominal correspondents is very large.

References

Donner A, Donald A. Analysis of data from a stratified design with the cluster; as unit of randomization. Statistics in Medicine 1987; 6: 43–52.

Donner A, Klar N. Confidence interval construction for effect measures arising from cluster randomization trials. Journal of Clinical Epidemiology 1993; 46: 123–131.

Durkalski VL, Palesch YY, Lipsitz SR, Rust PF. Analysis of clustered matched-pair data. Statistics in Medicine 2003; 22: 2417-2428.

Eliasziw M, Donner A. Application of the McNemar test to non-independent matched pair data. Statistics in Medicine 1991; 10(12): 1981-1991.

Hujoel P, Moulton L, Loesche W. Estimation of sensitivity and specificity of site-specific diagnostic tests. Journal of Periodontal Research 1990; 25: 193–196.

Jung SH, Ahn C. Estimation of response probability in correlated binary data: A new approach. Drug Information Journal 2000; 34: 599–604.

Jung SH, Kang SH, Ahn C. Sample size calculations for clustered binary data. Statistics in Medicine 2001; 20: 1971–1982.

Liang KY, Zeger SL. Longitudinal data analysis using generalized linear models. Biometrika 1986; 73: 13–22.

McNemar Q. Note on the sampling error of the difference between correlated proportions or percentages. Psychometrika 1947; 12: 153–157.

Neumann DR, Esselstyn CB, MacIntyre WJ, Go RT, Obuchowski NA, Chen EQ, Licata AA. Comparison of FDG-PET and Sestamibi-SPECT in primary hyperparathyroidism. Journal of Nuclear Medicine 1996; 37: 1809–1815.

Obuchowski NA. On the comparison of correlated proportions for clustered data. Statistics in Medicine 1998; 17: 1495–1507.

Wu W. A robust adjustment to McNemar test when the data are clustered. Communications in Statistics – Theory and Methods 2021; 50(6): 1515–1529.

3

Chi-Square Test for Two-Sample Clustered Binary Data (I)

Donner's Adjustment

In Chapter 2, we have investigated inference of one-sample binary probability with clustered data. In this and next chapters, we investigate how to adjust the chi-square test of 2×2 tables for two-sample clustered binary data. In this chapter, we consider an adjustment based on ANOVA method that was proposed by Donner and his colleagues. This method has been widely used for clustered binary data.

We assume that all subunits in each cluster belong to the same group as in cluster randomization trials. Suppose that n_k clusters are assigned to treatment group $k(=1,2)$. Cluster $i(=1,...,n_k)$ in group k has m_{ki} subunits. For subunit j $(j = 1,...,m_{ki})$ of cluster i in group k, we assume that x_{kij} is a binary variable taking value 1 with probability of success p_k. We further assume that subunits in each cluster have exchangeable dependency structure with intracluster correlation coefficient (ICC) $\rho_k = \text{corr}(y_{kij}, y_{kij'})$ for $j \neq j'$, while two subunits belonging to different clusters are independent.

Let $y_{ki} = \sum_{j=1}^{m_{ki}} x_{kij}$, $y_k = \sum_{i=1}^{n_k} y_{ki} = \sum_{i=1}^{n_k}\sum_{j=1}^{m_{ki}} x_{kij}$, $M_k = \sum_{i=1}^{n_k} m_{ki}$, $M = M_1 + M_2$ and $n = n_1 + n_2$. We assume that the number of clusters n is large compared to the cluster sizes so that asymptotic theories are based on large n. We want to test $H_0 : p_1 = p_2$ against $H_1 : p_1 \neq p_2$.

Donner's Test Statistic

Extending the method of Brier (1980), Donner (1989) and Donner and Banting (1988) propose the statistic, called the adjusted chi-square statistic hereafter,

$$X_D^2 = X_1^2/C_1^0 + X_2^2/C_2^0,$$

where

$$X_k^2 = (y_k - M_k\hat{p})^2/M_k\hat{p} + (M_k - y_k - M_k\hat{q})^2/M_k\hat{q}$$

$$C_k^0 = 1 + \left(\sum_{i=1}^{n_k} m_{ki}^2/M_k - 1\right)\hat{\rho},$$

 DOI: 10.1201/9781003221951-3

$\hat{p} = (y_1 + y_2)/M$, and $\hat{q} = 1 - \hat{p}$. Here, $\hat{\rho}$ is called the ANOVA-type estimator of the ICC ρ that is given by

$$\hat{\rho} = \frac{\text{msc} - \text{mse}}{\text{msc} + (\tilde{m} - 1)\text{mse}},$$

where

$$\begin{aligned}\text{msc} =&(n-2)^2 \sum_{k=1}^{2}\sum_{i=1}^{n_k} m_{ki}(\hat{p}_{ki} - \hat{p}_k)^2 \\ \text{mse} =&(M-n)^{-1}\sum_{k=1}^{2}\sum_{i=1}^{n_k} y_{ki}(1-\hat{p}_{ki})\end{aligned}$$

$\tilde{m} = (M - \sum_{k=1}^{2} M_k^{-1} \sum_{i=1}^{n_k} m_{ki}^2)/(n-2)$, $\hat{p}_{ki} = y_{ki}/m_{ki}$, and $\hat{p}_k = y_k/M_k$.

It is easy to show that X_D^2 can be expressed as

$$X_D^2 = (\hat{p}_1 - \hat{p}_2)^2 \frac{M_1^2 M_2^2}{M^2\hat{\sigma}^2}\left(\frac{1}{M_1 C_1^0} + \frac{1}{M_2 C_2^0}\right), \tag{3.1}$$

where $\hat{\sigma}^2 = \hat{p}(1-\hat{p})$. Thus, X_D^2 is based on an estimator of p_k assigning equal weights to subunits (refer to Chapter 2).

If subunits are independent,

$$X_0^2 = \frac{(\hat{p}_1 - \hat{p}_2)^2}{\hat{\sigma}^2(1/M_1 + 1/M_2)} = \frac{M_1 M_2 (1-\hat{p}_2)^2}{M\hat{\sigma}^2}$$

is the standard chi-square test statistic for two-sample independent binary data that has χ^2 distribution with degree of freedom 1 under H_0. Note that $X_D^2 = \text{AF} \times X_0^2$, where

$$\text{AF} = \frac{M_1 M_2}{M}\left(\frac{1}{M_1 C_1^0} + \frac{1}{M_2 C_2^0}\right) = \frac{1/M_1 C_1^0 + 1/M_2 C_2^0}{1/M_1 + 1/M_2}.$$

Hence, AF is an adjustment factor of the chi-square test statistic accounting for clustering effect.

Validation of Donner's Test

Jung et al. (2001) show that X_D^2 converges to the χ^2 distribution with 1 degree of freedom under some assumptions on the number of clusters, the distribution of cluster sizes, and the values of the ICCs ρ_1 and ρ_2 in two groups. This procedure has been evaluated in the context of randomization studies by some statisticians, including Donner et al. (1994), but its validity has not been assessed in the context of observational studies, where there could be systematic difference between ρ_1 and ρ_2. This is in contrast to experimental studies, where randomization assures the assumption of a common ICC, at least under the null hypothesis.

The simulation results in Donner et al. (1994) show that methods of testing the null hypothesis which exploit this assumption perform better than methods which separately estimate design effects in each group. Furthermore, Brier (1980) suggests that methods assuming a common ICC may still provide adequate results if the ICCs are only moderately different between two groups.

We show here that, even when $\rho_1 \neq \rho_2$, X_D^2 is still valid with some additional assumptions. We also investigate the conditions under which X_D^2 is strictly valid, i.e., conditions under which the null distribution of X_D^2 converges to χ_1^2 distribution.

Distribution of Donner's Test Statistic

Before investigating the validity of the statistic X_D^2, in the following lemma we derive the limit of the ANOVA estimator of the ICC under various conditions. These results will be used to investigate the validity of X_D^2.

Lemma: Let $\bar{m}_k = \lim_{n\to\infty} M_k/n_k$ for $k = 1, 2$, and $r_k = n_k/n$ denote the allocation proportion. As $n \to \infty$, the limit ρ^* of the common estimator of ICC $\hat{\rho}$ is given as follows.

Case 1. When $\rho_1 = \rho_2 (= \rho_0$, say):

1. Under H_0, $\rho^* = \rho_0$.
2. Under H_1, $\rho^* = \rho_0$ if $\bar{m}_1 = \bar{m}_2$.

Case 2. When $\rho_1 \neq \rho_2$ and $\bar{m}_1 = \bar{m}_2$:

1. Under H_0, $\rho^* = r_1\rho_1 + r_2\rho_2$, which is reduced to $\rho^* = (\rho_1 + \rho_2)/2$ in a balanced allocation.
2. Under H_1,

$$\rho^* = \frac{r_1\sigma_1^2\rho_1 + r_2\sigma_2^2\rho_2}{r_1\sigma_1^2 + r_2\sigma_2^2},$$

where $\sigma_k^2 = p_k(1 - p_k)$.

Proof: From Chapter 2, $\hat{p}_{ki}$ are independent random variables with mean p_k and variance $m_{ki}^{-1}\sigma_k^2\{1 + (m_{ki} - 1)\rho_k\}$. Further, $\hat{p}_k$ is an unbiased and consistent estimator of p_k so that msc is asymptotically equivalent to

$$\begin{aligned}
n^{-1}\sum_{k=1}^{2}\sum_{i=1}^{n_k} m_{ki}(\hat{p}_{ki}-p_k)^2 &= n^{-1}\sum_{i=1}^{n_1} m_{1i}\text{var}(\hat{p}_{1i}) + n^{-1}\sum_{i=1}^{n_2} m_{2i}\text{var}(\hat{p}_{2i}) + o_p(1)\\
&= n^{-1}\sigma_1^2\sum_{i=1}^{n_1}\{1+(m_{1i}-1)\rho_1\} + n^{-1}\sigma_2^2\sum_{i=1}^{n_2}\{1+(m_{2i}-1)\rho_2\} + o_p(1)\\
&= r_1\sigma_1^2\{1+(\bar{m}_1-1)\rho_1\} + r_2\sigma_2^2\{1+(\bar{m}_2-1)\rho_2\} + o_p(1).
\end{aligned}$$

Noting that

$$\begin{aligned}
E(\hat{p}_{ki}-\hat{p}_{ki}^2) &= p_k - p_k^2 - \text{var}(\hat{p}_{ki})\\
&= \sigma_k^2 - \sigma_k^2\{1+(m_{ki}-1)\rho_k\}/m_{ki}\\
&= \sigma_k^2(1-\rho_k)(1-1/m_{ki})
\end{aligned}$$

mse $= (M-n)^{-1}\sum_{k=1}^{2}\sum_{i=1}^{n_k} m_{ki}\hat{p}_{ki}(1-\hat{p}_{ki})$ is asymptotically identical to

$$\begin{aligned}
&\sigma_1^2(1-\rho_1)\frac{M_1-n_1}{M-n} + \sigma_2^2(1-\rho_2)\frac{M_2-n_2}{M-n}\\
&= r_1\sigma_1^2(1-\rho_1)\frac{\bar{m}_1-1}{\bar{m}-1} + r_2\sigma_2^2(1-\rho_2)\frac{\bar{m}_2-1}{\bar{m}-1}.
\end{aligned}$$

Hence, after some tedious calculations, the limit of $\hat{\rho}$ is expressed as

$$\rho^* = \frac{r_1\sigma_1^2\{r_2(\bar{m}_2-\bar{m}_1)+\bar{m}(\bar{m}_1-1)\rho_1\} + r_2\sigma_2^2\{r_1(\bar{m}_1-\bar{m}_2)+\bar{m}(\bar{m}_2-1)\rho_2\}}{(\bar{m}-1)(r_1\bar{m}_1\sigma_1^2 + r_2\bar{m}_2\sigma_2^2)}. \tag{3.2}$$

Under H_0, we have $\sigma_1^2 = \sigma_2^2$ and (3.2) is simplified to

$$\rho^* = \frac{r_1(\bar{m}_1-1)\rho_1 + r_2(\bar{m}_2-1)\rho_2}{\bar{m}-1}. \tag{3.3}$$

We simplify the expression of ρ^* in (3.2) and (3.3) in more specific cases.

Case 1 (When $\rho_1 = \rho_2 (= \rho_0)$): Under H_0, $\rho^* = \rho_0$ from (3.2). Under H_1, (2) is expressed as

$$\rho^* = \frac{r_1r_2(\bar{m}_2-\bar{m}_1)(\sigma_1^2-\sigma_2^2) + \bar{m}\rho_0\{r_1\sigma_1^2(\bar{m}_1-1)+r_2\sigma_2^2(\bar{m}_2-1)\}}{(\bar{m}-1)(r_1\bar{m}_1\sigma_1^2 + r_2\bar{m}_2\sigma_2^2)},$$

which is reduced to ρ_0 if $\bar{m}_1 = \bar{m}_2 = \bar{m}$.

Case 2 (When $\rho_1 \neq \rho_2$): In this case, the common ICC estimator $\hat{\rho}$ may be meaningless. Note that (3.2) is the expression of ρ^* under H_1. If $\bar{m}_1 = \bar{m}_2 = \bar{m}$, then ρ^* under H_1 is expressed as a weighted average of ρ_1 and ρ_2, i.e.,

$$\rho^* = \frac{r_1\sigma_1^2\rho_1 + r_2\sigma_2^2\rho_2}{r_1\sigma_1^2 + r_2\sigma_2^2}$$

Under H_0, if $\bar{m}_1 = \bar{m}_2 = \bar{m}$, then we have $\rho^* = r_1\rho_1 + r_2\rho_2$.
[End of proof]

When $\rho_1 = \rho_2$ (Case 1), $\hat{\rho}$ is always consistent under H_0. Under H_1, $\hat{\rho}$ is not a consistent estimator for the common ICC ρ_0 if $\bar{m}_1 \neq \bar{m}_2$. Note that, in this case, $\hat{\rho}$ is not consistent whether the allocation is balanced (i.e., $r_1 = r_2 = 1/2$) or not.

If X_D^2 in (3.1) has χ_1^2 distribution under H_0,

$$V_D = \frac{M^2\hat{\sigma}^2}{M_1^2 M_2^2}\left(\frac{1}{M_1 C_1^0} + \frac{1}{M_2 C_2^0}\right)^{-1}$$

should be the variance of $\hat{p}_1 - \hat{p}_2$.

On the other hand, since $\hat{p}_{ki}$ are independent random variables with mean p_k and variance $\sigma_k^2\{1 + (m_{ki} - 1)\rho_k\}/m_{ki}$, by the central limit theorem, $\hat{p}_k = M_k^{-1}\sum_{i=1}^{n_k} m_{ki}\hat{p}_{ki}$ is approximately normal with mean p_k and variance $\sigma_k^2 C_k/M_k$, where

$$C_k = 1 + \left(\sum_{i=1}^{n_k} m_{ki}^2/M_k - 1\right)\rho_k.$$

Hence, in order for X_D^2 to be valid, V_D should be asymptotically equivalent to the variance of $\hat{p}_1 - \hat{p}_2$ under H_0 (under which $\sigma_1^2 = \sigma_2^2 = \sigma^2$) that is given as

$$V = \hat{\sigma}^2\left(\frac{C_1}{M_1} + \frac{C_2}{M_2}\right).$$

As a measure of validity of the test statistic X_D^2, we use the ratio

$$\frac{V}{V_D} = \frac{(M_2C_1 + M_1C_2)(M_2/C_1^0 + M_1/C_2^0)}{M^2} \tag{3.4}$$

which should converge to 1 as $n \to \infty$ if X_D^2 is valid.

C_k^0 converges to $c_k^0 = 1 + (\bar{\bar{m}}_k/\bar{m}_k - 1)\rho^*$, where $\bar{\bar{m}}_k = \lim_{n\to\infty} n_k^{-1}\sum_{i=1}^{n_k} m_{ki}^2$ is the second moment of the cluster size distribution. Also, C_k converges to $c_k = 1 + (\bar{\bar{m}}_k/\bar{m}_k - 1)\rho_k$. Thus, from (4), we have

$$\frac{V}{V_D} = \frac{(r_2\bar{m}_2 c_1 + r_1\bar{m}_1 c_2)(r_2\bar{m}_2/c_1^0 + r_1\bar{m}_1/c_2^0)}{(r_1\bar{m}_1 + r_2\bar{m}_2)^2} + o_p(1). \tag{3.5}$$

The validity of X_D^2 is investigated when $\rho_1 = \rho_2$ and when $\rho_1 \neq \rho_2$.

Equal ICC case: $\rho_1 = \rho_2 (= \rho_0)$

In this case, from the Lemma, $\rho^* = \rho_0$ under H_0 so that we have $c_k = c_k^0 = 1 + (\bar{\bar{m}}_k/\bar{m}_k - 1)\rho_0$. Now, it is easy to show that the ratio (5) converges to 1 when

$$\bar{\bar{m}}_1/\bar{m}_1 = \bar{\bar{m}}_2/\bar{m}_2 \tag{3.6}$$

whether the two groups are balanced ($r_1 = r_2 = 1/2$) or not.

Hence, X_D^2 is valid in a randomized study, where two treatment groups have an equal ICC under H_0. When X_D^2 is applied to data from an observational study, however, it is necessary to verify the condition (3.6) as well as the equality of ICCs. We have just derived following theorem.

Theorem 1: X_D^2 is valid if $\rho_1 = \rho_2$ and $\bar{\bar{m}}_1/\bar{m}_1 = \bar{\bar{m}}_2/\bar{m}_2$.

When two groups have equal ICCs, the assumption of Theorem 1 is equivalent to Donner and Klar's (1994) equal design effect assumption. Note that X_D^2 is always valid in an experimental study since the randomization assures the assumptions of Theorem 1 under H_0. Rao and Scott (1992) note that X_D^2 is invalid when $\rho_1 \neq \rho_2$, and consequently possibly may be invalid in observational studies. In the following subsection, we show that X_D^2 is still valid for such studies provided that some additional assumptions are made.

Unequal ICC Case: $\rho_1 \neq \rho_2$

When $\rho_1 \neq \rho_2$, the validity of X_D^2 requires that

$$\bar{m}_1 = \bar{m}_2 (= \bar{m}_0, \text{ say}) \text{ and } \bar{\bar{m}}_1 = \bar{\bar{m}}_2 (= \bar{\bar{m}}_0, \text{ say}) \tag{3.7}$$

and

$$n_1 = n_2 \text{ (i.e., } r_1 = r_2 = 1/2). \tag{3.8}$$

Balanced cluster randomization studies satisfy the assumptions (3.7) and (3.8). Note that assumption (3.7) is stronger than assumption (3.6).

Under (3.7), we have $c_1^0 = c_2^0 = 1 + (\bar{\bar{m}}_0/\bar{m}_0 - 1)\rho^*$ and $c_k = 1 + (\bar{\bar{m}}_0/\bar{m}_0 - 1)\rho_k$, so that (3.5) becomes

$$\frac{V}{V_D} = \frac{1 + (\bar{\bar{m}}_0/\bar{m}_0 - 1)(r_2\rho_1 + r_1\rho_2)}{1 + (\bar{\bar{m}}_0/\bar{m}_0 - 1)\rho^*} + o_p(1). \tag{3.9}$$

Also, from the lemma, we have $\rho^* = (\rho_1 + \rho_2)/2$ under (3.7) and (3.8), which makes (3.9) converge to 1. This result is rephrased in the following theorem.

Theorem 2: X_D^2 is valid for balanced data with $\bar{m}_1 = \bar{m}_2$ and $\bar{\bar{m}}_1 = \bar{\bar{m}}_2$.

In an unbalanced observational study with $\rho_1 \neq \rho_2$, X_D^2 is invalid because of the discrepancy between ρ^* and $r_2\rho_1 + r_1\rho_2$ in (9). Recall that ρ^* is the limit of the ANOVA estimator $\hat{\rho}$. Without the common ICC assumption, by Donner and Donald (1987) and Donner and Klar (1993), a consistent ANOVA estimator for ρ_k is given as

$$\hat{\rho}_k = \frac{\text{msc}_k - \text{mse}_k}{\text{msc}_k + (\tilde{m}_k - 1)\text{mse}_k},$$

where

$$\text{msc}_k = \sum_{i=1}^{n_k} m_{ki}(\hat{p}_{ki} - \hat{p}_k)^2/(n_k - 1),$$
$$\text{mse}_k = \sum_{i=1}^{n_k} y_{ki}(1 - \hat{p}_{ki})/(M_k - n_k),$$

and $\tilde{m}_k = (M_k - M_k^{-1}\sum_{i=1}^{n_k} m_{ki}^2)/(n_k - 1)$.

If we use a consistent estimator of $r_2\rho_1 + r_1\rho_2$, such as $\tilde{\rho} = n^{-1}(n_2\hat{\rho}_1 + n_1\hat{\rho}_2)$, instead of $\hat{\rho}$, X_D^2 is valid whether the groups are balanced or not.

So far, we have investigated the limit of V/V_D under H_0. If the validity conditions are violated, X_D^2 converges to V/V_D times a χ_1^2 random variable. Using similar methods, we can show that V/V_D converges to 1 under H_1 in the cases where it converges to 1 under H_0, i.e., when (3.6) holds and $\rho_1 = \rho_2$ or when (3.7) and (3.8) hold. Hence, X_D^2 is asymptotically equivalent to

$$X^2 = (\hat{p}_1 - \hat{p}_2)^2/V$$

when X_D^2 is valid. $X^2 \sim \chi_1^2$ regardless of conditions (3.6)–(3.8) so that it can be a good alternative to the statistic X_D^2 if ρ_k in V is replaced by a consistent estimator, e.g., $\hat{\rho}_k$ given above.

A simple algorithm for checking the validity conditions of X_D^2 is provided in Figure 3.1.

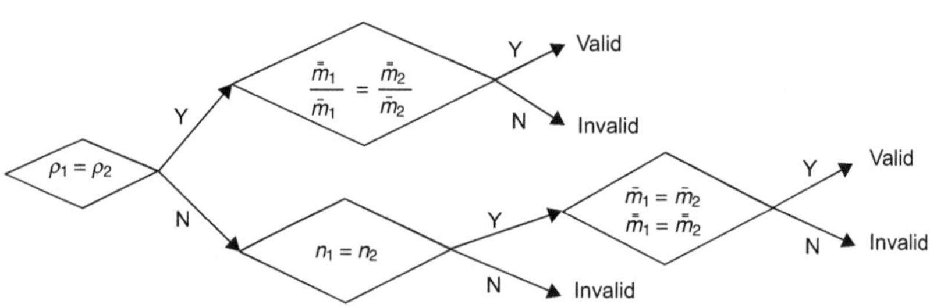

FIGURE 3.1
Procedure for checking the validity conditions of X_D^2. Here $\bar{m}_k = \lim_{n\to\infty} n_k^{-1}\sum_{i=1}^{n_k} m_{ki}$ and $\bar{\bar{m}}_k = \lim_{n\to\infty} n_k^{-1}\sum_{i=1}^{n_k} m_{ki}^2$.

Numerical Studies

Simulations are conducted to investigate the impact of violating validity conditions of X_D^2. Suppose that the cluster sizes in each group follow one of three discrete uniform distributions, $U(1,5)$, $U(3,7)$, and $U(1,9)$, for which $(\bar{m}_k, \bar{\bar{m}}_k) = (3, 11)$, $(5, 27.9)$, and $(5, 57)$ respectively. Different allocation proportions with $r_1 = 0.1, 0.3, 0.5, 0.7$, or 0.9 are considered. In a common ICC case, we consider $\rho_0 = 0.1, 0.4$, or 0.7. In an unequal ICC case, we consider $(\rho_1, \rho_2) = (0.1, 0.4)$, $(0.4, 0.7)$, or $(0.1, 0.7)$. The ratio V/V_D is calculated for each of these design settings.

To investigate the finite sample performance of X_D^2, we conduct simulations under these settings. For each setting, we generate 5,000 random data sets under $H_0 : p_1 = p_2 = 0.5$, each data set having $n_1 + n_2 = 100$ clusters. Using each data set, X_D^2 is calculated to test $H_0 : p_1 = p_2$ and compared with the critical value of chi-square distribution with 1 degree of freedom at two-sided $\alpha = 5\%$ level. An empirical type I error rate is estimated as the proportion of data sets rejecting the null hypothesis among the 5,000 data sets.

For comparisons, we also consider some chi-square test statistics using different variance estimators of $\hat{p}_1 - \hat{p}_2$. These include the use of V with the common ANOVA estimator $\hat{\rho}$, i.e.,

$$V_1 = \hat{\sigma}^2 \left(\frac{C_1^0}{M_1} + \frac{C_2^0}{M_2} \right)$$

and with separately estimated correlations, i.e.,

$$V_2 = \hat{\sigma}^2 \left(\frac{\hat{c}_1}{M_1} + \frac{\hat{c}_2}{M_2} \right),$$

where $\hat{c}_k = 1 + (\sum_{i=1}^{n_k} m_{ki}^2 / M_k - 1)\hat{\rho}_k$. Rao and Scott (1992) proposed χ_1^2 test statistic given by

$$X_R^2 = \frac{(\tilde{y}_1 - \tilde{M}_1 \tilde{p})^2}{\tilde{M}_1 \tilde{p}(1 - \tilde{p})} + \frac{(\tilde{y}_2 - \tilde{M}_2 \tilde{p})^2}{\tilde{M}_2 \tilde{p}(1 - \tilde{p})}$$

where $\tilde{y}_k = y_k/d_k$, $\tilde{M}_k = M_k/d_k$, $\tilde{p} = (\tilde{y}_1 + \tilde{y}_2)/(\tilde{M}_1 + \tilde{M}_2)$, $d_k = M_k v_k / \hat{\sigma}_k^2$, and

$$v_k = \frac{n_k}{M_k^2(n_k - 1)} \sum_{i=1}^{n_k} (y_{ki} - m_{ki}\hat{p}_k)^2.$$

It can be shown that X_R^2 is also expressed as

$$X_R^2 = \frac{(\hat{p}_1 - \hat{p}_2)^2}{V_R}$$

with $V_R = \tilde{p}(1 - \tilde{p})(1/\tilde{M}_1 + 1/\tilde{M}_2)$.

Note that calculation of V_R does not require the estimation of ICC. Moreover, V_2 and V_R are always valid, while V_1 is valid only when $\rho_1 = \rho_2$ or when the two groups are balanced. Under H_0, all three variance estimators are asymptotically equivalent to V_D when X_D^2 is valid. In this case, it can also be shown that V_1 and V_2 are asymptotically equivalent to V_D under H_1 as well. Hence, the test statistics using these variance estimators have exactly the same asymptotic power as the statistic X_D^2. The difference in power between the test statistics using V_D and V_R results from the discrepancy in limit between $\hat{p}$ and $\tilde{p}$ under H_1. We did not conduct small sample power comparisons among these test statistics due to their asymptotic equivalence.

The ratio V/V_D and simulation results under the various simulation settings reported in Table 3.1. When $\rho_1 = \rho_2$ (Table 3.1(a)), V/V_D is always larger than 1 for the simulation settings we are considering. The ratio increases as ρ_0 increases or as the ratio between $\bar{\bar{m}}_1/\bar{m}_1$ and $\bar{\bar{m}}_2/\bar{m}_2$ deviates from 1. Empirical type I error rates in Table 3.1 are marked with an asterisk if they are significantly different from the nominal $\alpha = 0.05$ at 1% of significance level, i.e., if they lie out of the 99% confidence interval $0.05 \pm 2.575\sqrt{0.05 \times 0.95/5{,}000} = (0.0421, 0.0579)$. When $\rho_1 = \rho_2$, X_D^2 has empirical type I error rates close to nominal level. At $\rho_1 = \rho_2$, its performance is only slightly influenced by the violation of condition (3.6). The performance of the test statistic using V_1 is very similar to that of X_D^2. We observe that the test statistic using V_1 is valid under all simulation settings of Table 3.1(a), while V_2 and V_R are anticonservative if $r_1 = 0.1$ or 0.9. Since V_2 uses separate estimates $\hat{\rho}_k$, it can be unstable if ICCs are estimated from small samples. Although V_R does not explicitly estimate ICCs, it does not require a common ICC and may also be unstable when one group has a small sample size.

When $\rho_1 \neq \rho_2$ (Table 3.1(b)), V/V_D can be very far from 1 and X_D^2 becomes very unreliable except when two groups are balanced (i.e., $r_1 = 1/2$). In general, when $r_1 = 1/2$, the statistic X_D^2 seems to be less influenced by unequal ICCs and/or cluster size distributions. The statistic using V_1, which is also based on a common ICC assumption, behaves very similarly to X_D^2. Test statistics using V_1 and V_D are conservative when fewer clusters are assigned to the group having the smaller ICC (i.e., $r_1 = 0.1$ or 0.3 and $\rho_1 < \rho_2$). Test statistics using V_1 and V_D are anticonservative when less clusters are assigned to the group with a larger ICC (i.e., $r_1 = 0.7$ or 0.9, and $\rho_1 < \rho_2$). When $\rho_1 \neq \rho_2$, the test statistic X_D^2 is unreliable if conditions (3.7) and (3.8) are violated. The test statistics using V_2 and V_R have empirical type I error rates close to the nominal level when $r_1 = 0.3$, 0.5, or 0.7. However, these statistics do not perform well when one group has a small number of clusters, i.e., $r_1 = 0.1$ or 0.9.

TABLE 3.1 (a)

The ratio V/V_D and empirical type I error rate of various chi-square test statistics using different variance formulas. The three rows corresponding to each ρ_0 or (ρ_1, ρ_2) value are for $m_{1i} \sim U(1,5)$ and $m_{2i} \sim U(3,7)$; $m_{1i} \sim U(3,7)$ and $m_{2i} \sim U(1,9)$; $m_{1i} \sim U(1,5)$ and $m_{2i} \sim U(1,9)$, respectively. Empirical type I error rates marked with an asterisk are significantly different from the nominal level 0.05 at 1% of significance level

(a) $\rho_1 = \rho_2 (= \rho_0)$

		Variance for Chi-Square Test			
ρ_0	V/V_D	V_D	V_1	V_2	V_R
$r_1 = 0.1$					
0.1	1.001	0.0474	0.0474	0.0500	0.0672*
	1.010	0.0548	0.0548	0.0572	0.0658*
	1.014	0.0514	0.0512	0.0532	0.0692*
0.4	1.006	0.0504	0.0498	0.0630*	0.0638*
	1.033	0.0508	0.0508	0.0694*	0.0674*
	1.053	0.0494	0.0488	0.0658*	0.0658*
0.7	1.009	0.0526	0.0514	0.0584*	0.0606*
	1.043	0.0514	0.0510	0.0586*	0.0522
	1.072	0.0540	0.0522	0.0588*	0.0588*
$r_1 = 0.3$					
0.1	1.003	0.0556	0.0550	0.0578	0.0586*
	1.024	0.0514	0.0514	0.0502	0.0510
	1.038	0.0508	0.0506	0.0522	0.0550
0.4	1.016	0.0500	0.0478	0.0484	0.0490
	1.078	0.0514	0.0512	0.0516	0.0508
	1.146	0.0554	0.0534	0.0532	0.0528
0.7	1.024	0.0548	0.0530	0.0530	0.0514
	1.100	0.0556	0.0548	0.0564	0.0538
	1.201	0.0574	0.0534	0.0514	0.0506
$r_1 = 0.5$					
0.1	1.005	0.0584*	0.0580*	0.0582*	0.0584*
	1.028	0.0548	0.0548	0.0532	0.0540
	1.054	0.0538	0.0526	0.0522	0.0530
0.4	1.023	0.0552	0.0526	0.0518	0.0512
	1.093	0.0466	0.0462	0.0458	0.0474
	1.210	0.0570	0.0536	0.0536	0.0546
0.7	1.035	0.0500	0.0472	0.0484	0.0466
	1.119	0.0498	0.0492	0.0494	0.0482
	1.289	0.0614*	0.0534	0.0540	0.0540

(Continued)

TABLE 3.1(a) (Continued)

The ratio V/V_D and empirical type I error rate of various chi-square test statistics using different variance formulas. The three rows corresponding to each ρ_0 or (ρ_1, ρ_2) value are for $m_{1i} \sim U(1,5)$ and $m_{2i} \sim U(3,7)$; $m_{1i} \sim U(3,7)$ and $m_{2i} \sim U(1,9)$; $m_{1i} \sim U(1,5)$ and $m_{2i} \sim U(1,9)$, respectively. Empirical type I error rates marked with an asterisk are significantly different from the nominal level 0.05 at 1% of significance level

(a) $\rho_1 = \rho_2 (= \rho_0)$

		Variance for Chi-Square Test			
ρ_0	V/V_D	V_D	V_1	V_2	V_R
$r_1 = 0.7$					
0.1	1.005	0.0594*	0.0590*	0.0598*	0.0598*
	1.024	0.0532	0.0532	0.0566	0.0570
	1.056	0.0536	0.0528	0.0524	0.0536
0.4	1.024	0.0586*	0.0552	0.0546	0.0544
	1.078	0.0538	0.0536	0.0564	0.0572
	1.218	0.0566	0.0520	0.0526	0.0536
0.7	1.036	0.0566	0.0538	0.0544	0.0532
	1.100	0.0520	0.0518	0.0506	0.0522
	1.300	0.0616*	0.0524	0.0532	0.0534
$r_1 = 0.9$					
0.1	1.003	0.0546	0.0544	0.0594*	0.0700*
	1.010	0.0500	0.0500	0.0596*	0.0748*
	1.031	0.0556	0.0554	0.0646*	0.0766*
0.4	1.013	0.0492	0.0482	0.0612*	0.0606*
	1.033	0.0516	0.0514	0.0662*	0.0746*
	1.118	0.0554	0.0526	0.0690*	0.0732*
0.7	1.020	0.0496	0.0476	0.0572	0.0512
	1.043	0.0502	0.0502	0.0554	0.0634*
	1.163	0.0526	0.0486	0.0568	0.0618*

Example

In a follow-up study of caries on the exposed roots of teeth, $n = 40$ chronically ill subjects ($n_1 = 11$ males and $n_2 = 29$ females) were followed for the development of root lesions (cavities localized to the root area of the tooth) over one year. Donner and Banting (1988) reported the data of the number of surfaces with lesions y_{ki} out of the number of surfaces examined m_{ki} for each subject as shown in Table 3.2. We want to test if the two gender groups have an equal incidence of surfaces with root lesions over the one year time period, a comparison which may have implications for preventive care. For these data, we have $\hat{\rho}_1 = 0.50$, $\hat{\rho}_2 = 0.35$, and $\hat{\rho} = 0.43$.

Whether conditions (3.6)–(3.8) hold or not depends on the design of the study. So, for observational or retrospective studies, the equal cluster size condition is particularly important.

TABLE 3.1(b)

$\rho_1 \neq \rho_2$

		Variance for Chi-Square Test			
ρ_0	V/V_D	V_D	V_1	V_2	V_R
$r_1 = 0.1$					
(0.1,0.4)	0.663	0.0138*	0.0136*	0.0496	0.0628*
	0.648	0.0104*	0.0104*	0.0612*	0.0674*
	0.718	0.0172*	0.0166*	0.0502	0.0660*
(0.4,0.7)	0.764	0.0254*	0.0246*	0.0672*	0.0658*
	0.789	0.0216*	0.0216*	0.0658*	0.0644*
	0.834	0.0222*	0.0212*	0.0648*	0.0660*
(0.1,0.7)	0.511	0.0056*	0.0054*	0.0566	0.0664*
	0.518	0.0022*	0.0022*	0.0546	0.0600*
	0.588	0.0088*	0.0084*	0.0532	0.0670*
$r_1 = 0.3$					
(0.1,0.4)	0.781	0.0288*	0.0282*	0.0542	0.0540
	0.925	0.0272*	0.0272*	0.0496	0.0500
	0.944	0.0266*	0.0248*	0.0518	0.0538
(0.4,0.7)	0.860	0.0348*	0.0320*	0.0504	0.0494
	1.007	0.0354*	0.0352*	0.0514	0.0506
	1.062	0.0360*	0.0326*	0.0504	0.0500
(0.1,0.7)	0.678	0.0196*	0.0184*	0.0544	0.0532
	0.890	0.0232*	0.0232*	0.0592*	0.0586*
	0.908	0.0216*	0.0186*	0.0570	0.0566
$r_1 = 0.5$					
(0.1,0.4)	0.936	0.0504	0.0484	0.0556	0.0554
	1.231	0.0552	0.0550	0.0508	0.0518
	1.195	0.0480	0.0466	0.0510	0.0514
(0.4,0.7)	0.977	0.0496	0.0472	0.0510	0.0498
	1.203	0.0512	0.0512	0.0502	0.0502
	1.285	0.0566	0.0524	0.0546	0.0544
(0.1,0.7)	0.905	0.0406*	0.0390*	0.0494	0.0478
	1.331	0.0544	0.0542	0.0496	0.0500
	1.279	0.0536	0.0484	0.0570	0.0566
$r_1 = 0.7$					
(0.1,0.4)	1.163	0.0824*	0.0806*	0.0606*	0.0594*
	1.602	0.0968*	0.0964*	0.0586*	0.0598*
	1.494	0.0802*	0.0786*	0.0572	0.0588*
(0.4,0.7)	1.125	0.0730*	0.0682*	0.0534	0.0514
	1.378	0.0752*	0.0750*	0.0534	0.0528
	1.476	0.0732*	0.0652*	0.0512	0.0514
(0.1,0.7)	1.257	0.0904*	0.0872*	0.0524	0.0498
	1.935	0.1188*	0.1186*	0.0490	0.0492
	1.749	0.1042*	0.0978*	0.0560	0.0564

(Continued)

TABLE 3.1(b) (Continued)

$\rho_1 \neq \rho_2$

		Variance for Chi-Square Test			
ρ_0	V/V_D	V_D	V_1	V_2	V_R
$r_1 = 0.9$					
(0.1,0.4)	1.565	0.1276*	0.1270*	0.0644*	0.0636*
	2.133	0.1448*	0.1448*	0.0688*	0.0716*
	1.977	0.1388*	0.1366*	0.0688*	0.0752*
(0.4,0.7)	1.333	0.0930*	0.0914*	0.0562	0.0522
	1.533	0.1074*	0.1074*	0.0628*	0.0722*
	1.593	0.0988*	0.0956*	0.0604*	0.0696*
(0.1,0.7)	1.991	0.1764*	0.1758*	0.0548	0.0498
	3.005	0.2170*	0.2170*	0.0576	0.0680*
	2.630	0.1942*	0.1914*	0.0604*	0.0660*

TABLE 3.2

Data of caries on the exposed roots of teeth: y = number of lesions, m = number of surfaces examined

Sex	y/m										
Male	0/4	1/1	2/2	0/2	2/4	0/3	0/3	0/3	0/1	1/2	0/2
Female	1/2	1/6	0/8	1/5	0/4	0/4	1/2	0/4	0/4	0/4	0/6
	0/2	0/4	0/4	0/2	0/3	0/2	0/2	0/4	2/2	0/2	0/2
	0/2	0/4	0/4	0/4	0/3	0/2	0/2				

From the root lesions example, we obtain $\bar{m}_1 = 2.5$, $\bar{m}_2 = 3.4$, $\bar{\bar{m}}_1 = 7.0$, and $\bar{\bar{m}}_2 = 13.9$. We calculate the ratio V/V_D using the observed values of the limiting parameters in (3.5). The calculated ratio V/V_D for the data set is 1.037. Since this value is quite close to 1, condition (3.6) should not be of an issue for the validity of X_D^2. Note that from Table 3.1(a), we also observe that X_D^2 performs very well at this level of V/V_D.

Since $\hat{p}_1 = 0.22$, $\hat{p}_2 = 0.06$, and $\hat{p} = 0.10$, and the value of X_D^2 for testing the hypothesis of equal incidence of surfaces with root lesions between the two gender groups is given by 3.401 ($p = 0.063$). The use of other variance formulas gives 3.364 ($p = 0.065$) for V_1, 3.291 ($p = 0.068$) for V_2 and 4.257 ($p = 0.038$) for the Rao-Scott statistic using V_R. Note that use of V_D, V_1, and V_2 results in similar p-values, while V_R gives slightly more significance.

To assess the validity of X_D^2 for the given data set, simulations are conducted under conditions reflecting the data set. With the number of clusters, cluster sizes, and ICCs fixed at the observed ones, 5,000 samples of clustered binary data are generated from a beta-binomial distribution. Under $H_0 : p_1 = p_2 = 0.22$ (and $H_0 : p_1 = p_2 = 0.06$), the empirical type I error rates are 0.056 (and 0.059) for X_D^2, 0.055 (and 0.057) using V_1, 0.057 (and 0.055) using V_2, and 0.074 (and 0.063) for Rao-Scott statistic. We observe that Rao-Scott test is slightly anticonservative, while the other tests perform well. From the simulation results of Table 3.1(a), we observe similar results when the two groups are heavily unbalanced. For our example data, we have $r_1 = 11/40 = 0.275$. On the other hand, under $H_1 : (p_1, p_2) = (0.22, 0.06)$, the empirical powers are 0.466 for X_D^2, 0.461 using V_1, 0.459 using V_2, and 0.463 for Rao-Scott test. All four test statistics have similar power. Since the incidence rates are small and the ICCs are large under the simulation settings, we observe many samples with no events in one or both groups. Note that, if a group has no events, we cannot calculate V_2 (because $\text{msc}_k = 0$) and V_R (because $v_k = d_k = 0$). If both groups have no events, V_D and V_1 cannot be calculated (because $\text{msc} = 0$) either. Therefore, the simulation results above are obtained excluding those samples with no events in a group. For example, under $H_1 : (p_1, p_2) = (0.22, 0.06)$, we have 95 and 116 such samples in the male and female groups, respectively, until 5,000 samples are generated with at least one event in both groups.

References

Brier S. Analysis of contingency tables under cluster sampling. Biometrika 1980; 67: 591–596.

Donner A. Statistical methods in ophthalmology: an adjusted chi-square approach. Biometrics 1989; 45: 605–611.

Donner A, Banting D. Analysis of site-specific data in dental studies. Journal of Dental Research 1988; 67: 1392–1395.

Donner A, Eliasziw M, Klar N. A comparison of methods for testing homogeneity of proportions in teratologic studies. Statistics in Medicine 1994; 13: 1253–1264.

Donner A, Klar N. Methods for comparing event rates in intervention studies when the unit of allocation is a cluster. American Journal of Epidemiology 1994; 140: 279–289.

Jung SH, Ahn C, Donner A. A study of an adjusted chi-square statistic as applied to observational studies involving clustered binary data. Statistics in Medicine 2001; 20: 2149–2161.

Rao JNK, Scott AJ. A simple method for the analysis of clustered binary data. Biometrics 1992; 48: 577–585.

4

Chi-Square Test for Two-Sample Clustered Binary Data (II)

GEE Adjustment

In Chapter 2, we have investigated GEE-type (Liang and Zeger 1986) adjustment of inference for one-sample clustered binary data based on weighted estimation of response rate. Kang et al. (2003) and Ahn et al. (2003) extend the GEE-type adjustment to two-sample testing problems. Kang et al. (2003) consider two-sample resting using estimators with equal weights to subunits and propose its sample size calculation method. Ahn et al. (2003) propose two-sample tests based on weighted estimators of response rates, called GEE-type adjustment. These methods are for cluster randomization trials. In this chapter, we will discuss these chi-square tests based on GEE-type adjustment, as an alternative to Donner's (1989) adjustment, and investigate a sample size method for two-sample testing based on general weighted estimators.

Modified Chi-Square Test with GEE-Type Adjustment

We assume that n_k clusters are assigned to treatment group $k(=1,2)$. Cluster $i(=1,...,n_k)$ in group k has m_{ki} subunits. For subunit j $(j=1,...,m_{ki})$ of cluster i in group k, we assume that x_{kij} is a binary variable taking value 1 with probability of success p_k. Usually subunits in each cluster share a common frailty so that they tend to have a positive intracluster correlation coefficient (ICC) $\rho_k = \text{corr}(x_{kij}, x_{kij'})$ for $j \neq j'$.

Let $y_{ki} = \sum_{j=1}^{m_{ki}} x_{kij}$, $\hat{p}_{ki} = y_{ki}/m_{ki}$, $y_k = \sum_{i=1}^{n_k} y_{ki} = \sum_{i=1}^{n_k}\sum_{j=1}^{m_{ki}} x_{kij}$, $M_k = \sum_{i=1}^{n_k} m_{ki}$, $M = M_1 + M_2$ and $n = n_1 + n_2$. Asymptotic theories are applied with respect to n, while $\max_{k=1}^{2} \max_{i=1}^{n_k} m_{ki} \leq \bar{M} < \infty$.

We want to test $H_0: p_1 = p_2$ against $H_1: p_1 \neq p_2$. From Chapter 2, a weighted estimator of p_k is given by

$$\hat{p}_k = \sum_{i=1}^{n_k} w_{ki}\hat{p}_{ki},$$

DOI: 10.1201/9781003221951-4

where $w_{ki} > 0$ and $\sum_{i=1}^{n_k} w_{ki} = 1$. As stated in Chapter 2, the estimator assigning equal weights to subunits uses $w_{ki} = m_{ki}/\sum_{i'=1}^{n_k} m_{ki'}$ and that assigning equal weights to clusters uses $w_{ki} = 1/n$. By the natural definition of weights, we have $w_{ki} = O_p(n^{-1})$.

Since $\hat{p}_{k1}, ..., \hat{p}_{k,n_k}$ are independent with mean p_k, $\epsilon_{ki} = \hat{p}_{ki} - p_k$ are independent random variables with mean 0. Hence, by the central limit theorem, $\hat{p}_k - p_k$ is asymptotically normal with mean 0 and variance σ_k^2 that can be consistently estimated by

$$\hat{\sigma}_k^2 = \sum_{i=1}^{n_k} w_{ki}^2 \hat{\epsilon}_{ki}^2,$$

where $\hat{\epsilon}_{ki}$ are obtained from ϵ_{ki} by replacing p_k with its consistent estimator $\hat{p}_k$, i.e., $\hat{\epsilon}_{ki} = \hat{p}_{ki} - \hat{p}_k$. This variance estimator is motivated by the GEE method (Liang and Zwgwr 1988). Hence, $Z = (\hat{p}_1 - \hat{p}_2)/\sqrt{\hat{\sigma}_1^2 + \hat{\sigma}_2^2}$ asymptotically $N(0,1)$ under H_0 so that we reject H_0 if $|Z| > z_{1-\alpha/2}$ or $Z^2 > \chi^2_{1,1-\alpha}$, the $100(1-\alpha)$ percentile of χ^2 distribution with 1 degree of freedom.

Test Statistic based on Optimal Estimators

If cluster size is constant, i.e., $m_{ki} = m$, equal weights to subunits and those to clusters result in the same estimators. From Chapter 2, when cluster sizes are random, the estimator with equal weights to clusters is more (less) efficient than that with equal weights to subunits if ICC is high (low). When cluster sizes are random, the optimal estimator uses optimal weights to $w_{ki} = \text{var}(\hat{p}_{ki})^{-1}/\sum_{i'=1}^{n_k} \text{var}(\hat{p}_{ki'})^{-1}$, i.e., weights

$$w_{ki} = \frac{m_{ki}\{1 + (m_{ki} - 1)\rho_k\}^{-1}}{\sum_{i'=1}^{n_k} m_{ki'}\{1 + (m_{ki'} - 1)\rho_k\}^{-1}}.$$

The optimal weights include an unknown parameter ρ_k so that we need a consistent estimator of ρ_k to use the optimal estimator for testing. One of most popular is the ANOVA estimator (Donner and Donald 1987, Donner and Klar 1993) that is given as

$$\hat{\rho}_k = \frac{\text{msc}_k - \text{mse}_k}{\text{msc}_k + (\tilde{m}_k - 1)\text{mse}_k},$$

where $\text{msc}_k = \sum_{i=1}^{n_k} m_{ki}(\hat{p}_{ki} - \tilde{p}_k)^2/(n_k - 1)$, $\text{mse}_k = \sum_{i=1}^{n_k} y_{ki}(1 - \hat{p}_{ki})/(M_k - n_k)$, $\tilde{m}_k = (M_k - \sum_{i=1}^{n_k} m_{ki}^2/M_k)/(n_k - 1)$, and $\tilde{p}_k = y_k/M_k$. Assuming common ICC model (Mak 1988), $\rho_1 = \rho_2 = \rho$, Donner (1989) and Donner and Banting (1988) propose to estimate it by

$$\hat{\rho} = \frac{\text{msc} - \text{mse}}{\text{msc} + (\tilde{m} - 1)\text{mse}},$$

where

$$\text{msc} =(n-2)^{-1}\sum_{k=1}^{2}\sum_{i=1}^{n_k} m_{ki}(\hat{p}_{ki}-\tilde{p}_k)^2$$
$$\text{mse} =(M-n)^{-1}\sum_{k=1}^{2}\sum_{i=1}^{n_k} y_{ki}(1-\hat{p}_{ki})$$

$\tilde{m} = (M - \sum_{k=1}^{2} M_k^{-1}\sum_{i=1}^{n_k} m_{ki}^2)/(n-2)$.

As an alternative to the ANOVA estimator, we may use a method of moments estimator. Note that $\rho_k = \text{cov}(x_{kij}, x_{kij'})/\text{var}(x_{kij}) = (c_k - p_k^2)/\{p_k(1-p_k)\}$, where $c_k = E(x_{kij}x_{kij'})$ for $j \neq j'$. Since

$$\sum\sum_{j\neq j'}^{n_{ki}} x_{kij}x_{kij'} = (\sum_{j=1}^{n_k} x_{kij})^2 - \sum_{j=1}^{n_k} x_{kij}^2 = y_{ki}(y_{ki}-1)$$

we can estimate c_k by

$$\hat{c}_k = \frac{\sum_{i=1}^{n_k} y_{ki}(y_{ki}-1)}{\sum_{i=1}^{n_k} m_{ki}(m_{ki}-1)}$$

Consequently, using the method of moments, we can consistently estimate by ρ_k by

$$\hat{\rho}_k = \frac{\hat{c}_k - \hat{p}_k}{\hat{p}_k(1-\hat{p}_k)},$$

where $\hat{p}_k$ is any consistent estimator of p_k, such as the one using equal weights to subunits.

Efficiency of Weighted Estimators

We assume common ICC (Mak 1988), i.e., $\rho_1 = \rho_2 = \rho$ and an alternative hypothesis of $H_1 : p_1 \neq p_2$. From Chapter 2, we have $\text{var}(\hat{p}_{ki}) = p_k(1-p_k)\{1+(m_{ki}-1)\rho\}/m_{ki}$ so that the variance of the weighted estimator $\hat{p}_k$ is given as

$$\sigma_k^2 = p_k(1-p_k)\sum_{i=1}^{n_k} w_{ki}^2 \frac{\{1+(m_{ki}-1)\rho\}}{m_{ki}}.$$

More specifically, we have

$$\sigma_k^2 = \frac{p_k(1-p_k)}{n_k^2}\sum_{i=1}^{n_k}\frac{1+(m_{ki}-1)\rho}{m_{ki}}$$

for the equal weights to clusters,

$$\sigma_k^2 = \frac{p_k(1-p_k)}{M_k^2}\sum_{i=1}^{n_k} m_{ki}\{1+(m_{ki}-1)\rho\}$$

for the equal weights to subunits, and

$$\sigma_k^2 = p_k(1-p_k)\left\{\sum_{i=1}^{n_k}\frac{m_{ki}}{1+(m_{ki}-1)\rho}\right\}^{-1}$$

for the optimal weights.

Suppose that the probability mass function (PMF) of a cluster size distribution is denoted as $f(l) = P(m_{ki} = l)$ for $l \in \mathcal{M}$, the support of the distribution. Then for a function $h(\cdot)$, $n_k^{-1}\sum_{i=1}^{n_k} h(m_{ki})$ converges to $E\{h(m)\} = \sum_{l\in\mathcal{M}} h(l)f(l)$. Hence, for large n, we have

$$\sigma_k^2 = n_k^{-1} p_k(1-p_k)d_w, \tag{4.1}$$

where $\bar{m}d_w$ is the variance inflation factor (VIF) due to the clustering effect that is expressed as

$$d_c = \nu + (1-\nu)\rho$$

for the equal weights to clusters,

$$d_u = \frac{\bar{m} + (\bar{\bar{m}} - \bar{m})\rho}{\bar{m}^2}$$

for the equal weights to subunits,

$$d_o = \left[E\left\{\frac{m}{1+(m-1)\rho}\right\}\right]^{-1}$$

for the optimal weights, and $\nu = E(m^{-1})$. Here, the expectations are applied to the distribution of cluster sizes which will be identical between two groups in a cluster randomization trial. We find that the VIF depends only on ICC and distribution of cluster size.

We have

$$d_c - d_u = \nu - 1/\bar{m} + (1 - \bar{\bar{m}}/\bar{m}^2 + 1/\bar{m} - \nu)\rho.$$

Here, by Jensen's inequality, $1 - \bar{\bar{m}}/\bar{m}^2 < 0$ and $1/\bar{m} - \nu < 0$ so that $d_c - d_u$ is linearly decreasing in ρ and crosses 0 at

$$\rho_0 = \frac{\nu - 1/\bar{m}}{(\bar{\bar{m}} - \bar{m})/\bar{m}^2 - 1 + \nu} = \frac{\nu - 1/\bar{m}}{\{\text{var}(m) - \bar{m}\}/\bar{m}^2 + \nu}$$

which depends on cluster size distribution through ν and var(m) even when $\bar{m}$ is fixed.

Hence, between the two weighted estimators, the estimator with equal weights to subunits is more efficient if $\rho < \rho_0$ and that with equal weights to clusters is more efficient if $\rho > \rho_0$.

The ratio between two VIFs is the relative efficiency of two corresponding weighted estimators. Figure 4.1 displays the efficiency of the estimator with equal weights to clusters $\text{RE}_c = d_o/d_c$ and that with equal weights to subunits $\text{RE}_u = d_o/d_u$ relative to the optimal estimator. We assume that the cluster size distribution is either discrete $U(4,8)$ or $U(2,10)$ with PMF

$$f_1(l) = 1/5 \qquad \text{for } l = 4, 5, 6, 7, 8$$

and

$$f_2(l) = 1/9 \qquad \text{for } l = 2, 3, 4, 5, 6, 7, 8, 9, 10$$

respectively. The two distributions have the same mean $\bar{m} = 6$, but f_1 has a smaller variance than f_2 (2.00 vs. 6.67).

From Figure 4.1, the two relative frequencies cannot be larger than 1 for any $\rho \in [0,1]$ so that the two weighted estimators (with equal weights to clusters or with equal weights to subunits) cannot be more efficient than the optimal estimator. For the both distributions, the estimator with equal weights to subunits has almost the same efficiency as the optimal estimator if ρ is close to 0, whereas the estimator with equal weights to clusters has almost the same efficiency as the optimal estimator if ρ is close to 1. For f_1, the estimator with equal weights to clusters is more efficient than that with equal weights to clusters if $\rho \le 0.155$, but the latter is more efficient than the former otherwise. On the other hand, for f_2, the estimator with equal weights to clusters is more efficient than that with equal weights to clusters if $\rho \le 0.204$, but the latter is more efficient than the former otherwise.

Sample Size Calculation

We derive a sample size formula for the test statistics based on weighted estimators.

The power for a given sample size n is

$$1 - \beta = P\left(\frac{|\hat{p}_1 - \hat{p}_2|}{\sqrt{\hat{\sigma}_1^2 + \hat{\sigma}_2^2}} > z_{1-\alpha/2} \,\Big|\, p_1, p_2 \right)$$

$$= P\left\{ \frac{\hat{p}_1 - \hat{p}_2 - (p_1 - p_2)}{\sqrt{\sigma_1^2 + \sigma_2^2}} > z_{1-\alpha/2} - \frac{p_1 - p_2}{\sqrt{\sigma_1^2 + \sigma_2^2}} \,\Big|\, p_1, p_2 \right\}$$

Since asymptotically $\{(\hat{p}_1 - \hat{p}_2) - (p_1 - p_2)\}/\sqrt{\sigma_1^2 + \sigma_2^2} \sim N(0,1)$ under H_1, we have

$$-z_{1-\beta} = z_{1-\alpha/2} - \frac{p_1 - p_2}{\sqrt{\sigma_1^2 + \sigma_2^2}} \tag{4.2}$$

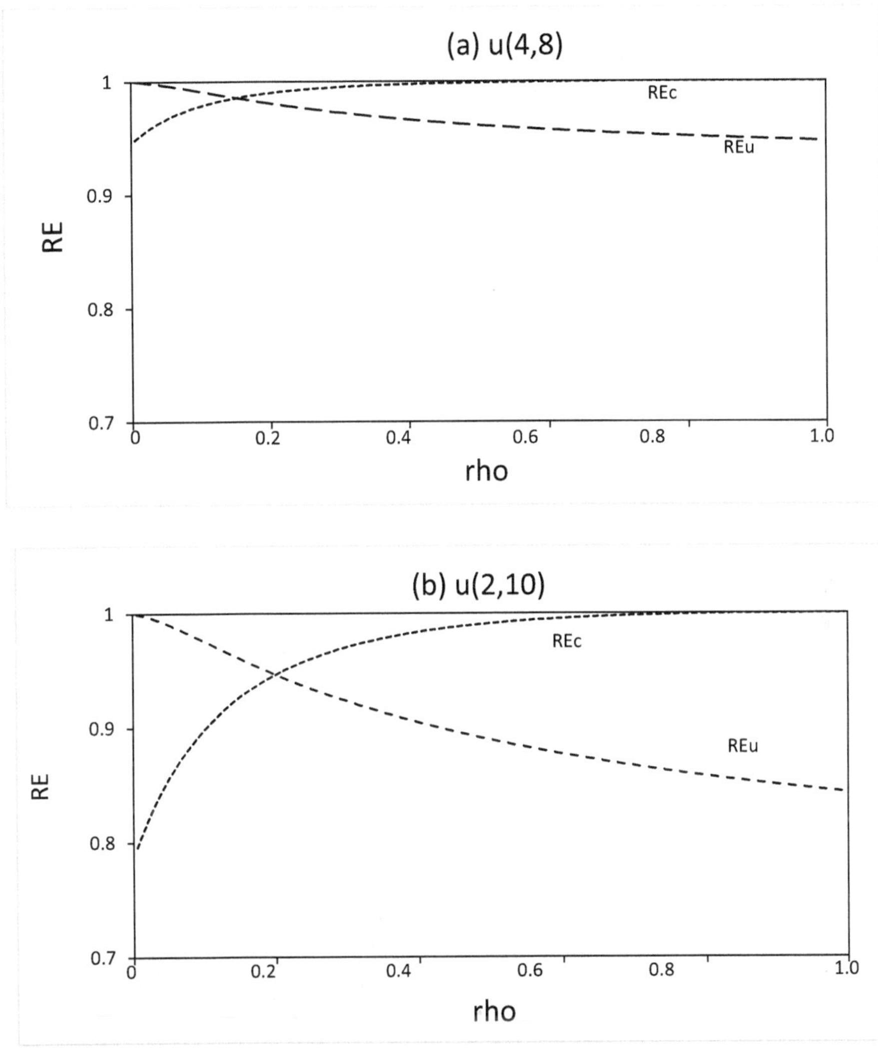

FIGURE 4.1
Relative efficiency of estimator with equal weights to clusters and that with equal weights to subunits relative to the optimal estimator when cluster sizes are U(4,8) or U(2,10).

Let $a_k = n_k/n$ denote the allocation proportion of group k ($a_1 + a_2 = 1$). From (4.1), we have

$$\begin{aligned}\sigma_1^2 + \sigma_2^2 =& \left\{\frac{p_1(1-p_1)}{n_1} + \frac{p_2(1-p_2)}{n_2}\right\} d_w \\ =& \frac{1}{n}\left\{\frac{p_1(1-p_1)}{a_1} + \frac{p_2(1-p_2)}{a_2}\right\} d_w \end{aligned} \tag{4.3}$$

By plugging (4.3) in (4.2) and solving equation (4.2) with respect to n, the required sample size is obtained as

$$n = d_w \left\{ \frac{p_1(1-p_1)}{a_1} + \frac{p_2(1-p_2)}{a_2} \right\} \frac{(z_{1-\alpha/2} + z_{1-\beta})^2}{(p_1 - p_2)^2} \tag{4.4}$$

Note that $n_0 = n/d_w$ is the required number of subunits by the sample size formula for independent dichotomous data. The required number of subunits is given as $M = n\bar{m}$.

The Donner (1989) test that is investigated in Chapter 3 assigns equal weights to subunits so that, if it is valid, it will have an equal power as our test statistic assigning equal weights to subunits.

Numerical Studies

Example

Donner and Banting (1988) introduce a study of caries on the exposed roots of teeth. Investigators followed $n = 40$ chronically ill subjects, including $n_1 = 11$ males and $n_2 = 29$ females, for the development of root lesions (cavities localized to the root area of the tooth) over one year and reported the data of the number of surfaces with lesions y_{ki} out of the number of surfaces examined m_{ki} for each subject as shown in Table 4.1. The objective of this study was to investigate if the two gender groups had an equal incidence of surfaces with root lesions over the one year time period, which might have implications for preventive care. To demonstrate the sample size methods, suppose that we want to design a new prospective study using this data set as pilot data. From the data set, we have $\hat{\rho} = 0.43$ by the ANOVA method (Donner 1989), cluster size distribution $(f(1), f(2), f(3), f(4), f(5), f(6), f(7), f(8)) = (0.05, 0.4, 0.125, 0.325, 0.025, 0.05, 0, 0.025)$, and $(\hat{p}_1, \hat{p}_2) = (0.273, 0.082)$ using equal weights to clusters, $(0.222, 0.061)$ using equal weights to subunits and using optimal weights. For a sample calculation, we use these estimates as the true parameter values with $(p_1, p_2) = (0.222, 0.061)$. Based on these

TABLE 4.1

Data of caries on the exposed roots of teeth: y = number of lesions, m = number of surfaces examined

Sex	y/m									
Male	0/4	1/1	2/2	0/2	2/4	0/3	0/3	0/3	0/1	1/2	0/2
Female	1/2	1/6	0/8	1/5	0/4	0/4	1/2	0/4	0/4	0/4	0/6
	0/2	0/4	0/4	0/2	0/3	0/2	0/2	0/4	2/2	0/2	0/2
	0/2	0/4	0/4	0/4	0/3	0/2	0/2				

design parameter values, we obtain $\nu = 0.389$, $\bar{m} = 3.150$, $\bar{\bar{m}} = 12.000$, $d_c = 652$, $d_u = 701$, and $d_u = 637$. Further, we assume balanced allocation $(a_1, a_2) = (1/2, 1/2)$, two-sided $\alpha = 0.05$ ($z_{1-\alpha/2} = 1.96$) and power of $1 - \beta = 0.8$ ($z_{1-\beta} = 0.842$). Hence, from our sample size formula (4.4), we obtain $n = 91, 97$, and 88 for estimators using equal weights to clusters, equal weights to subunits, and optimal weights, respectively. Due to the high ICC, the test statistic based on equal weights to subunits require a large sample size, while that based on optimal weights require the smallest sample size.

Simulations

We conduct simulations to evaluate the performance of the modified chi-square tests based on the three weighted estimators and their sample size formulas. We fix the type I error rate at two-sided $\alpha = 0.05$ and allocation proportions at $a_1 = a_2 = 1/2$ for balanced allocation. Other design parameters are set at $1 - \beta = 0.8, 0.85$, or 0.9, $\rho = 0.3, 0.6$, or $0{,}9$, cluster size distribution of discrete $U(4, 8)$ or $U(2, 10)$, and response rates of $(p_1, p_2) = (0.2, 0.3)$, $(0.2, 0.35)$, $(0.4, 0.5)$, or $(0.4, 0.55)$ under H_1. Under each combination of design parameter values, the sample size n for the test statistic based on each weighted estimator is calculated. And then, we generate 5,000 data sets of size n under the design setting and apply the modified chi-square test based on the weighted estimator to each data set and calculate an empirical power by the proportion of data sets rejecting the null hypothesis among the 5,000 sets. We also generate 5,000 data sets of size n under H_0, for which p_2 is the same as p_1, while other design parameters are the same as those used for the sample calculation. By applying the modified chi-square test based on the weighted estimator to each data set, we calculate an empirical type I error rate $\hat{\alpha}$ by the proportion of data sets rejecting the null hypothesis among the 5,000 sets. We conduct these numerical studies for the three weighted estimators.

We generate clustered binary data y_{ki} with cluster size m_{ki} from the beta-binomial distribution with the PMF

$$g(y_{ki}|m_{ki}, p_k, \rho) = \binom{m_{ki}}{y_{ki}} \frac{B(\alpha + y_{ki}, \beta + m_{ki} - y_{ki})}{B(\alpha, \beta)}$$

for $y_{ki} = 0, 1, ..., m_{ki}$, where $\alpha = p_k(1-\rho)/\rho$, $\beta = (1-p_k)(1-\rho)/\rho$, $B(a,b) = \Gamma(a)\Gamma(b)/\Gamma(a+b)$, and $\Gamma(a) = \int_0^\infty t^{a-1}\exp(-t)dt$. We assume common ICC between groups and estimate it by Donner (1989) method for the weights of optimal estimators.

Table 4.2 reports calculated the sample size n, and empirical type I error rate $\hat{\alpha}$ and power $1 - \hat{\beta}$ for each of design settings. Sample size increases in $1-\beta$, ρ, and variance of cluster sizes, or as p_1 and p_2 are closer to $1/2$, and decreases in $|p_1 - p_2|$. The test using equal weights to subunits requires smaller sample size than that using equal weights to clusters when ICC is low (i.e.,

TABLE 4.2

Sample size n (and empirical type I error rate $\hat{\alpha}$ and power $1-\hat{\beta}$ within parenthesis). Here, CSD stands for cluster size distribution and $\hat{p}_c$, $\hat{p}_u$, and $\hat{p}_o$ denote the test statistics based on estimators using equal weights to clusters, using equal weights to subunits, and optimal weights, respectively

ρ	CSD	(p_1, p_2)	$\hat{p}_c$	$\hat{p}_u$	$\hat{p}_o$
(I) $1-\beta=0.8$					
0.1	$U(4,8)$	(0.20, 0.30)	151(0.055, 0.808)	149(0.053, 0.804)	148(0.054, 0.810)
		(0.20, 0.35)	71(0.065, 0.802)	70(0.066, 0.801)	69(0.065, 0.798)
		(0.40, 0.50)	200(0.048, 0.795)	197(0.050, 0.796)	195(0.049, 0.793)
		(0.40, 0.55)	89(0.057, 0.807)	87(0.056, 0.808)	87(0.054, 0.810)
	$U(2,10)$	(0.20, 0.30)	171(0.055, 0.801)	156(0.056, 0.787)	153(0.056, 0.790)
		(0.20, 0.35)	80(0.057, 0.807)	73(0.058, 0.806)	71(0.055, 0.803)
		(0.40, 0.50)	226(0.056, 0.808)	207(0.056, 0.800)	202(0.056, 0.802)
		(0.40, 0.55)	100(0.060, 0.819)	92(0.057, 0.811)	90(0.057, 0.808)
0.3	$U(4,8)$	(0.20, 0.30)	247(0.046, 0.801)	252(0.047, 0.797)	245(0.047, 0.803)
		(0.20, 0.35)	115(0.057, 0.794)	118(0.055, 0.794)	114(0.057, 0.792)
		(0.40, 0.50)	327(0.054, 0.802)	334(0.056, 0.798)	325(0.056, 0.800)
		(0.40, 0.55)	145(0.054, 0.811)	148(0.055, 0.811)	144(0.055, 0.812)
	$U(2,10)$	(0.20, 0.30)	262(0.053, 0.797)	275(0.059, 0.808)	254(0.057, 0.799)
		(0.20, 0.35)	122(0.054, 0.801)	128(0.058, 0.805)	118(0.056, 0.805)
		(0.40, 0.50)	347(0.053, 0.813)	364(0.052, 0.816)	336(0.052, 0.810)
		(0.40, 0.55)	154(0.051, 0.787)	161(0.051, 0.791)	149(0.049, 0.786)
0.5	$U(4,8)$	(0.20, 0.30)	342(0.048, 0.810)	355(0.050, 0.805)	342(0.049, 0.814)
		(0.20, 0.35)	160(0.053, 0.809)	166(0.055, 0.806)	159(0.050, 0.808)
		(0.40, 0.50)	453(0.050, 0.804)	471(0.051, 0.808)	453(0.051, 0.805)
		(0.40, 0.55)	201(0.053, 0.791)	208(0.055, 0.792)	200(0.054, 0.791)
	$U(2,10)$	(0.20, 0.30)	353(0.050, 0.802)	393(0.052, 0.809)	350(0.049, 0.806)
		(0.20, 0.35)	165(0.053, 0.795)	183(0.057, 0.805)	163(0.056, 0.796)
		(0.40, 0.50)	468(0.046, 0.801)	520(0.047, 0.806)	463(0.045, 0.796)
		(0.40, 0.55)	207(0.046, 0.795)	230(0.047, 0.804)	205(0.049, 0.796)
(II) $1-\beta=0.9$					
0.1	$U(4,8)$	(0.20, 0.30)	202(0.054, 0.903)	199(0.056, 0.903)	198(0.054, 0.905)
		(0.20, 0.35)	94(0.054, 0.901)	93(0.056, 0.909)	92(0.059, 0.909)
		(0.40, 0.50)	267(0.047, 0.908)	264(0.050, 0.913)	261(0.049, 0.907)
		(0.40, 0.55)	119(0.055, 0.893)	117(0.057, 0.893)	116(0.054, 0.893)
	$U(2,10)$	(0.20, 0.30)	228(0.052, 0.900)	209(0.056, 0.897)	204(0.054, 0.900)
		(0.20, 0.35)	107(0.056, 0.901)	98(0.059, 0.904)	95(0.058, 0.903)
		(0.40, 0.50)	302(0.054, 0.908)	277(0.054, 0.902)	271(0.054, 0.905)
		(0.40, 0.55)	134(0.058, 0.898)	123(0.057, 0.896)	120(0.055, 0.896)
0.3	$U(4,8)$	(0.20, 0.30)	330(0.054, 0.898)	337(0.055, 0.898)	328(0.052, 0.901)
		(0.20, 0.35)	154(0.056, 0.899)	157(0.057, 0.901)	153(0.056, 0.902)
		(0.40, 0.50)	437(0.053, 0.899)	447(0.056, 0.903)	435(0.053, 0.902)
		(0.40, 0.55)	193(0.052, 0.896)	198(0.053, 0.901)	192(0.053, 0.898)
	$U(2,10)$	(0.20, 0.30)	350(0.053, 0.897)	368(0.050, 0.900)	340(0.054, 0.897)
		(0.20, 0.35)	163(0.058, 0.902)	171(0.054, 0.898)	158(0.057, 0.898)
		(0.40, 0.50)	464(0.048, 0.901)	487(0.055, 0.901)	450(0.049, 0.898)
		(0.40, 0.55)	205(0.063, 0.893)	216(0.057, 0.894)	199(0.060, 0.891)

(Continued)

TABLE 4.2 (Continued)

Sample size n (and empirical type I error rate $\hat{\alpha}$ and power $1-\hat{\beta}$ within parenthesis). Here, CSD stands for cluster size distribution and $\hat{p}_c$, $\hat{p}_u$, and $\hat{p}_o$ denote the test statistics based on estimators using equal weights to clusters, using equal weights to subunits, and optimal weights, respectively

ρ	CSD	(p_1, p_2)	$\hat{p}_c$	$\hat{p}_u$	$\hat{p}_o$
0.5	$U(4,8)$	(0.20, 0.30)	458(0.051, 0.906)	476(0.056, 0.901)	457(0.051, 0.904)
		(0.20, 0.35)	213(0.049, 0.903)	222(0.049, 0.901)	213(0.048, 0.904)
		(0.40, 0.50)	606(0.058, 0.905)	630(0.056, 0.900)	606(0.056, 0.905)
		(0.40, 0.55)	268(0.051, 0.889)	279(0.053, 0.890)	268(0.051, 0.891)
	$U(2,10)$	(0.20, 0.30)	473(0.051, 0.896)	526(0.052, 0.896)	468(0.051, 0.901)
		(0.20, 0.35)	220(0.050, 0.905)	245(0.051, 0.905)	218(0.051, 0.908)
		(0.40, 0.50)	626(0.048, 0.894)	697(0.050, 0.898)	620(0.047, 0.897)
		(0.40, 0.55)	277(0.053, 0.900)	308(0.052, 0.898)	274(0.054, 0.899)

$\rho = 0.1$), but the latter requires smaller sample size than the former otherwise. The test statistic based on the optimal weights always requires a smaller sample size than the other two. The calculated sample sizes maintain the power accurately because the empirical powers are close to the nominal level $1-\beta$. The tests based on weighted estimators can be slightly anti-conservative for a few cases, but controls the type I error rate accurately overall.

References

Ahn C, Jung SH, Kang SH. An evaluation of weighted chi-square statistics for site-specific binary data. Drug Information Journal 2003; 37: 91–99.

Donner A. Statistical methods in ophthalmology: an adjusted chi-square approach. Biometrics 1989; 45: 605–611.

Donner A, Banting D. Analysis of site-specific data in dental studies. Journal of Dental Research 1988; 67: 1392–1395.

Donner A, Donald A. Analysis of data from a stratified design with the cluster as unit of randomization. Statistics in Medicine 1987; 6: 43–52.

Donner A, Klar N. Methods for comparing event rates in intervention studies when the unit of allocation is a cluster. American Journal of Epidemiology 1994; 140: 279–289.

Kang SH, Ahn C, Jung SH. Sample size calculation for dichotomous outcomes in cluster randomization trials with varying cluster size. Drug Information Journal 2003; 37: 109–114.

Liang KY, Zeger SL. Longitudinal data analysis using generalized linear models. Biometrika 1986; 73: 13–22.

Mak TK. Analysing intraclass correlation for dichotomous variables. Applied Statistics 1988; 37: 344–352.

5

Subunit Randomization Trials

GEE-Type Test for Two-Sample Clustered Binary Data

In the previous chapters, we have assumed that clusters allocated to different treatments so that all subunits in each cluster receive the same treatment as in a cluster randomization trial. In such a trial, dependency is limited within each treatment group and the data between two groups are independent.

In this chapter, we consider randomizing subunits in each cluster between two treatment groups, resulting in clustered data with subunit randomization. In this case, dependency exists both within and between treatment groups. While the clustered data in each group have exchangeable dependency structure, those combining the two groups may not, especially if two groups have different response rates or different intracluster correlation coefficients (ICCs). We investigate two sample tests to compare response rates between treatment groups and their sample size calculation methods under subunit randomization.

Suppose that there are n clusters and cluster $i(=1,...,n)$ has m_i subunits, among which m_{1i} are randomized into treatment 1 and m_{2i} are randomized into treatment 2 ($m_i = m_{1i} + m_{2i}$). Let $M_k = \sum_{i=1}^{n} m_{ki}$ denote the total number subunits randomized into treatment k and $M = M_1 + M_2$. A binary outcome x_{kij} is observed from subunit $j(=1,...,m_{ki})$ that is randomized into treatment $k(=1,2)$ from cluster $i(=1,...,n)$. Let $E(x_{kij}) = p_k$, within-treatment ICC $\text{corr}(x_{kij}, x_{kij'}) = \rho_k$ for $j \neq j'$, and between-treatment ICC $\text{corr}(x_{1ij}, x_{2ij'}) = \rho_{12}$. Since x_{kij} are Bernoulli random variables, we have $\text{var}(x_{kij}) = p_k(1-p_k)$.

Usually, this kind of data structure arises from cluster randomization trials with matched clusters. For example, in Stanton and Clemens (1987), families are matched based on selected stratification factors and the matched families are randomized between two treatment arms. In this case, two matched families will be counted as a cluster because they share common frailties within each family and the two families share stratification factors used for matchings. The members (subunits) within each family share both the common frailties and stratification factors, while two individual in matched families

DOI: 10.1201/9781003221951-5

share only stratification factors. As a result, the ICC within each family, denoted as ρ_k, will be larger than that between matched families, denoted as ρ_{12}. The testing and sample size calculation methods discussed in this chapter do not require this assumption. But, the algorithm used to generate simulation data does.

Modified Chi-Square Test with GEE-Type Adjustment

We want to test $H_0 : p_1 = p_2$ using clustered binary data $\{(x_{1i1}, ..., x_{1i,m_{1i}}, x_{2i1}, ..., x_{1i,m_{1i}}), i = 1, ..., n\}$. Let $y_{ki} = \sum_{j=1}^{m_{ki}} x_{kij}$ and $\hat{p}_{ki} = y_{ki}/m_{ki}$. When cluster sizes are varying, we can consider a weighted estimator of p_k

$$\hat{p}_k = \sum_{i=1}^{n} w_{ki}\hat{p}_{ki}$$

using positive weights $w_{ki} = O_p(n^{-1})$ such that $\sum_{i=1}^{n} w_i = 1$. The estimator with equal weights to clusters uses $w_{ki} = 1/n$ and that with equal weights to subunits uses $w_{ki} = m_{ki}/\sum_{i'=1}^{n_k} m_{ki'}$. Since $E(\hat{p}_{ki}) = p_k$, $\hat{p}_k$ is an unbiased estimator of p_k.

Under H_0, we have

$$\sqrt{n}(\hat{p}_1 - \hat{p}_2) = \sqrt{n}\sum_{i=1}^{n} \epsilon_i,$$

where $\epsilon_i = \sqrt{n}\{w_{1i}(\hat{p}_{1i} - p_1) - w_{2i}(\hat{p}_{2i} - p_2)\}$. Since ϵ_i are independent random variables with mean 0, by the central limit theorem, $\sqrt{n}(\hat{p}_1 - \hat{p}_2)$ is approximately normal with mean 0 and variance that can be consistently estimated by

$$\hat{\sigma}^2 = n\sum_{i=1}^{n} \hat{\epsilon}_i^2,$$

where $\hat{\epsilon}_i$ is obtained from ϵ_i by replacing p_k with its consistent estimator $\hat{p}_k$.

Hence, we reject H_0 if $|Z| > z_{1-\alpha/2}$, where

$$Z = \frac{\sqrt{n}(\hat{p}_1 - \hat{p}_2)}{\hat{\sigma}}.$$

Test Statistic using Optimal Weights

If cluster sizes are constant, i.e., $m_i = m$ and the allocation proportion between two treatments is fixed across clusters, then equal weights to subunits and those to clusters result in the same estimators and identically optimal among all possible weighting methods.

Since $\hat{p}_{1i}$ and $\hat{p}_{2i}$ are paired, we consider a weighted test statistic

$$\sqrt{n}(\hat{p}_1 - \hat{p}_2) = \sqrt{n}\sum_{i=1}^{n} w_i(\hat{p}_{1i} - \hat{p}_{2i}).$$

From this expression, the optimal weights will be

$$w_i = \frac{1/\text{var}(\hat{p}_{1i} - \hat{p}_{2i})}{\sum_{i'=1}^{n} 1/\text{var}(\hat{p}_{1i'} - \hat{p}_{2i'})}.$$

Note that $\hat{p}_k = \sum_{i=1}^{n} w_i \hat{p}_{kij}$ is a consistent estimator of p_k, but is not an unbiased one as a point estimator.

We assume that the within-group ICC, $\rho_k = \text{corr}(x_{kij}, x_{kij'})$ for $j \neq j'$ is identical between two treatment groups, i.e., $\rho = \rho_1 = \rho_2$. We have another ICC, called between-group ICC, $\rho_{12} = \text{corr}(x_{1ij}, x_{2ij'})$. Due to different treatment effect or design effect, such as cluster matching as discussed above, it is likely that the between-group ICC cannot be stronger than that of within-treatment, i.e., $\rho_1 \geq \rho_2$. We have

$$\text{var}(\hat{p}_{1i} - \hat{p}_{2i}) = \text{var}(\hat{p}_{1i}) + \text{var}(\hat{p}_{2i}) - 2\text{cov}(\hat{p}_{1i}, \hat{p}_{2i}). \tag{5.1}$$

And from Chapter 4,

$$\text{var}(\hat{p}_{ki}) = p_k(1 - p_k)\{m_{ki}^{-1} + (1 - m_{ki}^{-1})\rho_1\}. \tag{5.2}$$

In (5.2) and in the calculation of the optimal weights, we replace p_k with a consistent estimator, such as that using equal weights to subunits. Also, using the ANOVA method that is proposed by Donner (1989) and Donner and Banting (1988), ρ_1 is estimated by

$$\hat{\rho}_1 = \frac{\text{msc} - \text{mse}}{\text{msc} + (\tilde{m} - 1)\text{mse}},$$

where

$$\begin{aligned}
\text{msc} =& (2n-2)^{-1}\sum_{k=1}^{2}\sum_{i=1}^{n} m_{ki}(\hat{p}_{ki} - \hat{p}_k)^2 \\
\text{mse} =& (M-2n)^{-1}\sum_{k=1}^{2}\sum_{i=1}^{n} y_{ki}(1 - \hat{p}_{ki}) \\
\tilde{m} =& (M - \sum_{k=1}^{2} M_k^{-1}\sum_{i=1}^{n} m_{ki}^2)/(2n-2).
\end{aligned}$$

Further,

$$\text{cov}(\hat{p}_{k1}, \hat{p}_{2i}) = \text{cov}(x_{1ij}, x_{2ij'}),$$

which can be consistently estimated by

$$\hat{c}_{12} = \frac{\sum_{i=1}^{n}\sum_{j=1}^{m_{1i}}\sum_{j'=1}^{m_{2i}}(x_{1ij}-\hat{p}_1)(x_{2ij'}-\hat{p}_2)}{\sum_{i=1}^{n} m_{1i}m_{2i}}.$$

Hence, the optimal weights are given as

$$w_i = \frac{[\hat{p}_1(1-\hat{p}_1)\{m_{1i}^{-1}+(1-m_{1i}^{-1})\hat{\rho}_1\}+\hat{p}_2(1-\hat{p}_2)\{m_{2i}^{-1}+(1-m_{2i}^{-1})\hat{\rho}_1\}-2\hat{c}_{12}]^{-1}}{\sum_{i'=1}^{n}[\hat{p}_1(1-\hat{p}_1)\{m_{1i'}^{-1}+(1-m_{1i'}^{-1})\hat{\rho}_1\}+\hat{p}_2(1-\hat{p}_2)\{m_{2i'}^{-1}+(1-m_{2i'}^{-1})\hat{\rho}_1\}-2\hat{c}_{12}]^{-1}}.$$

Note that the optimal test statistic requires the subunit level data, x_{kij}, for calculating $\hat{c}_{12}$, whereas those with equal weights to clusters or subunits require only cluster level data y_{ki} within each treatment group.

The variance of the test statistic with optimal weights $\sqrt{n}\sum_{i=1}^{n} w_i(\hat{p}_{1i}-\hat{p}_{2i})$ is

$$\begin{aligned}\hat{\sigma}^2 =& n\sum_{i=1}^{n} w_i^2\{(\hat{p}_{1i}-\hat{p}_1)-(\hat{p}_{2i}-\hat{p}_2)\}^2\\ =& n\left(\sum_{i=1}^{n}[\hat{p}_1(1-\hat{p}_1)\{m_{1i}^{-1}+(1-m_{1i}^{-1})\hat{\rho}_1\}+\hat{p}_2(1-\hat{p}_2)\right.\\ &\left.\{m_{2i}^{-1}+(1-m_{2i}^{-1})\hat{\rho}_1\}-2\hat{c}_{12}]^{-1}\right)^{-1}.\end{aligned}$$

We reject H_0 if $|Z| > z_{1-\alpha/2}$, where

$$Z = \frac{\sum_{i=1}^{n} w_i(\hat{p}_{1i}-\hat{p}_{2i})}{\hat{\sigma}}.$$

The modified McNemar's (1947) test that was discussed in Chapter 2 is a special example of the weighted test statistics. In the cases of McNemar test, we have $m_{1i} = m_{2i}$ since two diagnostic tests will be applied to each site (subunit). Our test statistic using equal weights to subunits is asymptotically identical to Obuchowski's (1998) as a modified McNemar's test.

Sample size Calculation

Let $a_k = m_{ki}/m_i$ denote the allocation proportion $(a_1 + a_2 = 1)$. We need the limit of $\text{var}(\hat{p}_k)$ and $\text{cov}(\hat{p}_1, \hat{p}_2)$ to derive the sample size formula for a weighted test statistic. Since $\sigma_{ki}^2 = \text{var}(\hat{p}_{ki}) = p_k(1-p_k)\{m_{ki}^{-1}+(1-m_{ki}^{-1})\rho_1\}$,

$$\text{var}(\hat{p}_k) = \sum_{i=1}^{n} w_{ki}^2\sigma_{ki}^2.$$

From (5.2), we have

$$\text{var}(\hat{p}_k) = \frac{p_k(1-p_k)}{n^2}\sum_{i=1}^{n}\{m_{ki}^{-1} + (1-m_{ki}^{-1})\rho_1\}$$

for equal weights to clusters with $w_{ki} = 1/n$ and

$$\text{var}(\hat{p}_k) = \frac{p_k(1-p_k)}{M_k^2}\sum_{i=1}^{n}\{m_{ki} + (m_{ki}^2 - m_{ki})\rho_1\}$$

for equal weights to subunits with $w_{ki} = m_{ki}/M_k$.

On the other hand, we have

$$\text{cov}(\hat{p}_1, \hat{p}_2) = \sum_{i=1}^{n} w_{1i}w_{2i}\text{cov}(\hat{p}_{1i}, \hat{p}_{2i}) = c_{12}\sum_{i=1}^{n} w_{1i}w_{2i},$$

which is expressed as

$$\text{cov}(\hat{p}_1, \hat{p}_2) = \frac{c_{12}}{n}$$

for equal weights to clusters and

$$\text{cov}(\hat{p}_1, \hat{p}_2) = c_{12}\frac{\sum_{i=1}^{n} m_{1i}m_{2i}}{M_1M_2}$$

for equal weights to subunits, where

$$c_{12} = \text{cov}(\hat{p}_{1i}, \hat{p}_{2i}) = \text{cov}(x_{1ij}, x_{2ij}) = \rho_{12}\sqrt{p_1p_2(1-p_1)(1-p_2)}.$$

Hence, from (5.1), $\sigma_n^2 = \text{var}\{\sqrt{n}(\hat{p}_1 - \hat{p}_2)\}$ is expressed as

$$\begin{aligned}\sigma_n^2 =& \frac{p_1(1-p_1)}{n}\sum_{i=1}^{n}\{m_{1i}^{-1} + (1-m_{1i}^{-1})\rho\} \\ &+ \frac{p_2(1-p_2)}{n}\sum_{i=1}^{n}\{m_{2i}^{-1} + (1-m_{2i}^{-1})\rho\} - 2c_{12}\end{aligned}$$

for equal weights to clusters, and

$$\begin{aligned}\sigma_n^2 =& \frac{p_1(1-p_1)n}{M_1^2}\sum_{i=1}^{n}\{m_{1i} + (m_{1i}^2 - m_{1i})\rho\} \\ &+ \frac{p_2(1-p_2)n}{M_2^2}\sum_{i=1}^{n}\{m_{2i} + (m_{2i}^2 - m_{2i})\rho_1)\rho\} \\ &- 2c_{12}\frac{n\sum_{i=1}^{n} m_{1i}m_{2i}}{M_1M_2}\end{aligned}$$

for equal weights to subunits.

Let $\bar{m} = E(m_i)$ and $\bar{\bar{m}} = E(m_i^2)$, and $\nu = E(1/m_i)$. If cluster size is constant $m_i = m$, then we have $\bar{m} = m$ and $\bar{\bar{m}} = m^2$, and $\nu = 1/m$, and the weighted estimators all identical. By replacing m_{ki} with $a_k m_i$, $n^{-1}\sum_{i=1}^n m_{ki} \to a_k \bar{m}$, we have $n^{-1}\sum_{i=1}^n m_{ki}^2 \to a_k^2 \bar{\bar{m}}$, $n^{-1}\sum_{i=1}^n m_{1i}m_{2i} \to a_1 b_1 \bar{\bar{m}}$, and $n^{-1}\sum_{i=1}^n m_{ki}^{-1} \to a_k^{-1}\nu$ as $n \to \infty$.

Hence, as $n \to \infty$, σ_n^2 converges to

$$\begin{aligned}\sigma^2 =& p_1(1-p_1)\{\nu/a_1 + (1-\nu/a_1)\rho\} + p_2(1-p_2)\{\nu/a_2 + (1-\nu/a_2)\rho\} \\ &- 2\rho_{12}\sqrt{p_1 p_2 (1-p_1)(1-p_2)}\}\end{aligned}$$

for equal weights to clusters, and

$$\begin{aligned}\sigma^2 =& \frac{1}{\bar{m}}\Big[p_1(1-p_1)\{1/a_1 + (\bar{\bar{m}}/\bar{m} - 1/a_1)\rho\} \\ &+ p_2(1-p_2)\{1/a_2 + (\bar{\bar{m}}/\bar{m} - 1/a_2)\rho\} \\ &-2\bar{\bar{m}}/\bar{m}\rho_{12}\sqrt{p_1 p_2(1-p_1)(1-p_2)}\Big]\end{aligned}$$

for equal weights to subunits by replacing c_{12} with $\rho_2\sqrt{p_1 p_2 (1-p_1)(1-p_2)}$.

Note that

$$\begin{aligned}\text{var}(\hat{p}_{1i} - \hat{p}_{2i}) =& p_1(1-p_1)\{m_{1i}^{-1} + (1-m_{1i}^{-1})\rho_1\} \\ &+ p_2(1-p_2)\{m_{2i}^{-1} + (1-m_{2i}^{-1})\rho_1\} \\ &- 2c_{12}.\end{aligned}$$

So, using the optimal weights $w_i = \text{var}(\hat{p}_{1i} - \hat{p}_{2i})^{-1}/\sum_{i'=1}^n \text{var}(\hat{p}_{1i'} - \hat{p}_{2i'})^{-1}$, the variance of $\sum_{i=1}^n w_i(\hat{p}_{1i} - \hat{p}_{2i})$ is

$$\begin{aligned}\sigma_n^2 =& n\left[\sum_{i=1}^n \{\text{var}(\hat{p}_{1i} - \hat{p}_{2i})\}^{-1}\right]^{-1} \\ =& n\left(\sum_{i=1}^n \Big[p_1(1-p_1)\{m_{1i}^{-1} + (1-m_{1i}^{-1})\rho_1\}\right. \\ &\left.+p_2(1-p_2)\left\{m_{2i}^{-1} + (1-m_{2i}^{-1})\rho_1 - 2c_{12}\right\}\Big]^{-1}\right)^{-1},\end{aligned}$$

which converges to

$$\begin{aligned}\sigma^2 =& \left(E\left[p_1(1-p_1)\left\{\frac{1}{a_1 m_i} + \left(1 - \frac{1}{a_1 m_i}\right)\rho\right\} + p_2(1-p_2)\right.\right. \\ &\left.\left.\left\{\frac{1}{a_2 m_i} + \left(1 - \frac{1}{a_2 m_i}\right)\rho\right\} - 2\rho_{12}\sqrt{p_1 p_2 (1-p_1)(1-p_2)}\right]^{-1}\right)^{-1},\end{aligned}$$

where the expectation is applied to the distribution of cluster sizes m_i.

For a given number of clusters n, the power under $H_1: p_1 \neq p_2$ is

$$\begin{aligned}1-\beta =& P\left(\frac{\sqrt{n}|\hat{p}_1-\hat{p}_2|}{\hat{\sigma}} > z_{1-\alpha/2} \,\middle|\, H_1\right)\\ =& P\left(\frac{\sqrt{n}\{(\hat{p}_1-\hat{p}_2)-(p_1-p_2)\}}{\sigma} > z_{1-\alpha/2} - \frac{\sqrt{n}(p_1-p_2)}{\sigma} \,\middle|\, H_1\right).\end{aligned}$$

Since $\sqrt{n}\{(\hat{p}_1-\hat{p}_2)-(p_1-p_2)\}/\sigma$ is asymptotically $N(0,1)$ under H_1, we have

$$z_{1-\alpha/2} - \frac{\sqrt{n}(p_1-p_2)}{\sigma} = -z_{1-\beta}.$$

By solving this equation with respect to n, we obtain the number of clusters n required for a power of $1-\beta$ under $H_1: p_1 \neq p_2$

$$n = \frac{\sigma^2(z_{1-\alpha/2}+z_{1-\beta})^2}{(p_1-p_2)^2}.$$

Numerical Studies

Simulations

In this section, we use (ρ_1, ρ_2) in place of (ρ, ρ_{12}). We conduct simulations to evaluate the finite sample performance of the modified chi-square tests under subunit randomization based on the three weighting methods. We fix the type I error rate at two-sided $\alpha = 0.05$ and assume balanced allocation, i.e., $a_1 = a_2 = 1/2$. Other design parameters are specified as $n = 80$ or 120, $(p_1, p_2) = (0.2, 0.3)$ or $(0.4, 0.5)$ under H_1 and p_2 is set at p_1 under H_0, $(\rho_1, \rho_2) = (0.3, 0.1)$, (0.3,0.2), (0.4,0.2), or (0.4,0.3), cluster size distribution with PMF

$$(f_1(8), f_1(10), f_1(12), f_1(14), f_1(16)) = (0.2, 0.2, 0.2, 0.2, 0.2)$$

or

$$(f_2(4), f_2(8), f_2(12), f_2(16), f_2(10)) = (0.2, 0.2, 0.2, 0.2, 0.2).$$

Half of subunits are randomized into each treatment from each cluster so that $a_1 = 1/2$. Note that the two distributions have the same mean of $E(m) = 12$, but a variance of $\text{var}(m) = 8$ for f_1 and 32 for f_2.

For each combination of the design parameter values, clustered binary data under subunit randomization are generated by dichotomizing multivariate normal random variables as introduced in Chapter 6. $B = 5,000$ simulation data sets of size n are generated, and test statistics using the three weighting methods are applied to each data set and empirical type I error rate $\hat{\alpha}$ and

TABLE 5.1

Empirical type I error rate $\hat{\alpha}$ and power $1-\hat{\beta}$ within each parenthesis. CSD stands for cluster size distribution, f_1 or f_2, and Cluster, Unit, and Optimal denote the test statistics based on equal weights to clusters, using equal weights to subunits, and optimal weights, respectively

(ρ_1, ρ_2)	(p_1, p_2)	CSD	Cluster	Unit	Optimal
(I) $n = 80$					
(0.3,0.1)	(0.2,0.3)	f_1	(0.055, 0.903)	(0.057, 0.909)	(0.056, 0.910)
		f_2	(0.055, 0.859)	(0.055, 0.878)	(0.057, 0.882)
	(0.4,0.5)	f_1	(0.052, 0.810)	(0.056, 0.814)	(0.055, 0.817)
		f_2	(0.052, 0.744)	(0.059, 0.773)	(0.054, 0.779)
(0.3,0.2)	(0.2,0.3)	f_1	(0.062, 0.907)	(0.059, 0.909)	(0.061, 0.911)
		f_2	(0.050, 0.863)	(0.052, 0.887)	(0.051, 0.890)
	(0.4,0.5)	f_1	(0.055, 0.800)	(0.060, 0.797)	(0.058, 0.802)
		f_2	(0.058, 0.749)	(0.060, 0.775)	(0.058, 0.780)
(0.4,0.2)	(0.2,0.3)	f_1	(0.057, 0.764)	(0.057, 0.754)	(0.058, 0.767)
		f_2	(0.054, 0.718)	(0.057, 0.712)	(0.055, 0.737)
	(0.4,0.5)	f_1	(0.054, 0.643)	(0.053, 0.637)	(0.053, 0.645)
		f_2	(0.057, 0.597)	(0.055, 0.589)	(0.057, 0.617)
(0.4,0.3)	(0.2,0.3)	f_1	(0.052, 0.907)	(0.053, 0.909)	(0.052, 0.912)
		f_2	(0.057, 0.855)	(0.057, 0.888)	(0.057, 0.885)
	(0.4,0.5)	f_1	(0.055, 0.810)	(0.055, 0.811)	(0.056, 0.816)
		f_2	(0.060, 0.744)	(0.056, 0.778)	(0.058, 0.782)
(II) $n = 120$					
(0.3, 0.1)	(0.2, 0.3)	f_1	(0.054, 0.980)	(0.052, 0.979)	(0.054, 0.981)
		f_2	(0.054, 0.960)	(0.056, 0.972)	(0.055, 0.972)
	(0.4, 0.5)	f_1	(0.055, 0.934)	(0.054, 0.934)	(0.053, 0.937)
		f_2	(0.051, 0.912)	(0.052, 0.924)	(0.050, 0.933)
(0.3, 0.2)	(0.2, 0.3)	f_1	(0.054, 0.979)	(0.055, 0.980)	(0.053, 0.980)
		f_2	(0.055, 0.960)	(0.056, 0.972)	(0.057, 0.972)
	(0.4, 0.5)	f_1	(0.055, 0.934)	(0.055, 0.937)	(0.054, 0.936)
		f_2	(0.053, 0.892)	(0.055, 0.914)	(0.053, 0.916)
(0.4, 0.2)	(0.2, 0.3)	f_1	(0.053, 0.896)	(0.052, 0.890)	(0.052, 0.899)
		f_2	(0.056, 0.873)	(0.055, 0.872)	(0.055, 0.890)
	(0.4, 0.5)	f_1	(0.052, 0.815)	(0.055, 0.804)	(0.051, 0.816)
		f_2	(0.059, 0.778)	(0.052, 0.761)	(0.054, 0.798)
(0.4, 0.3)	(0.2, 0.3)	f_1	(0.045, 0.982)	(0.047, 0.980)	(0.046, 0.983)
		f_2	(0.056, 0.962)	(0.051, 0.972)	(0.053, 0.974)
	(0.4, 0.5)	f_1	(0.056, 0.934)	(0.058, 0.934)	(0.056, 0.937)
		f_2	(0.059, 0.895)	(0.059, 0.913)	(0.059, 0.917)

power $1-\hat{\beta}$ are estimated by the proportion of data sets, generated under H_0 and under H_1 respectively, rejecting H_0 out of 5,000 data sets.

Table 5.1 reports the simulation results. We find that the test statistics using the three weighting methods control the type I error accurately overall. Naturally, the power increases in n. In general, the test statistic using optimal weights has the highest power although it is similarly powerful as that using equal weights to subunits if ICCs are low, like $\rho_1 = 0.3$ and as that

TABLE 5.2

Sample size n (empirical type I error rate $\hat{\alpha}$ and power $1-\hat{\beta}$ within each parenthesis. CSD stands for cluster size distribution, f_1 or f_2, and Cluster, Unit, and Optimal denote the test statistics based on equal weights to clusters, using equal weights to subunits, and optimal weights, respectively

(ρ_1,ρ_2)	(p_1,p_2)	CSD	Cluster	Unit	Optimal
(I) $1-\beta=0.8$					
(0.3, 0.1)	(0.3, 0.4)	f_1	115(0.053, 0.804)	116(0.054, 0.800)	114(0.054, 0.801)
		f_2	128(0.054, 0.801)	128(0.055, 0.811)	120(0.054, 0.772)
	(0.4, 0.5)	f_1	125(0.055, 0.812)	127(0.059, 0.812)	124(0.056, 0.808)
		f_2	139(0.055, 0.799)	139(0.056, 0.805)	130(0.055, 0.781)
(0.3, 0.2)	(0.3, 0.4)	f_1	80(0.047, 0.812)	79(0.048, 0.809)	78(0.050, 0.802)
		f_2	92(0.052, 0.802)	85(0.059, 0.801)	82(0.054, 0.753)
	(0.4, 0.5)	f_1	87(0.056, 0.809)	86(0.059, 0.802)	85(0.055, 0.795)
		f_2	100(0.055, 0.805)	92(0.056, 0.806)	89(0.053, 0.759)
(0.4, 0.2)	(0.3, 0.4)	f_1	109(0.049, 0.796)	111(0.050, 0.795)	108(0.050, 0.796)
		f_2	120(0.057, 0.807)	122(0.056, 0.802)	113(0.054, 0.779)
	(0.4, 0.5)	f_1	118(0.050, 0.800)	120(0.049, 0.801)	117(0.051, 0.797)
		f_2	130(0.053, 0.799)	133(0.055, 0.796)	123(0.052, 0.775)
(0.4, 0.3)	(0.3, 0.4)	f_1	74(0.051, 0.811)	73(0.051, 0.801)	72(0.050, 0.800)
		f_2	84(0.049, 0.811)	79(0.051, 0.816)	76(0.050, 0.768)
	(0.4, 0.5)	f_1	80(0.057, 0.817)	80(0.054, 0.815)	79(0.056, 0.815)
		f_2	92(0.051, 0.803)	86(0.062, 0.799)	82(0.053, 0.758)
(II) $1-\beta=0.85$					
(0.3, 0.1)	(0.3, 0.4)	f_1	131(0.050, 0.847)	133(0.052, 0.850)	130(0.051, 0.846)
		f_2	146(0.048, 0.849)	147(0.051, 0.851)	137(0.052, 0.823)
	(0.4, 0.5)	f_1	143(0.051, 0.847)	145(0.052, 0.843)	142(0.049, 0.844)
		f_2	159(0.047, 0.849)	159(0.052, 0.845)	149(0.046, 0.827)
(0.3, 0.2)	(0.3, 0.4)	f_1	91(0.052, 0.856)	90(0.056, 0.855)	89(0.054, 0.850)
		f_2	106(0.060, 0.856)	97(0.057, 0.851)	94(0.057, 0.813)
	(0.4, 0.5)	f_1	99(0.055, 0.851)	98(0.057, 0.852)	97(0.057, 0.846)
		f_2	115(0.049, 0.851)	106(0.047, 0.854)	102(0.053, 0.813)
(0.4, 0.2)	(0.3, 0.4)	f_1	124(0.051, 0.853)	126(0.050, 0.850)	123(0.053, 0.851)
		f_2	137(0.050, 0.841)	140(0.050, 0.851)	130(0.054, 0.823)
	(0.4, 0.5)	f_1	135(0.053, 0.856)	137(0.049, 0.857)	134(0.054, 0.852)
		f_2	149(0.056, 0.848)	152(0.054, 0.854)	141(0.057, 0.831)
(0.4, 0.3)	(0.3, 0.4)	f_1	84(0.053, 0.861)	84(0.048, 0.862)	83(0.051, 0.857)
		f_2	97(0.052, 0.867)	91(0.050, 0.862)	87(0.053, 0.820)
	(0.4, 0.5)	f_1	91(0.059, 0.864)	91(0.059, 0.862)	90(0.058, 0.859)
		f_2	105(0.052, 0.858)	98(0.060, 0.857)	94(0.050, 0.823)
(III) $1-\beta=0.9$					
(0.3, 0.1)	(0.3, 0.4)	f_1	154(0.052, 0.897)	156(0.049, 0.894)	152(0.052, 0.894)
		f_2	171(0.050, 0.904)	171(0.053, 0.903)	160(0.050, 0.881)
	(0.4, 0.5)	f_1	167(0.051, 0.900)	169(0.049, 0.897)	166(0.050, 0.896)
		f_2	186(0.047, 0.895)	186(0.049, 0.893)	174(0.049, 0.872)
(0.3, 0.2)	(0.3, 0.4)	f_1	107(0.051, 0.897)	106(0.054, 0.898)	105(0.052, 0.889)
		f_2	124(0.052, 0.906)	114(0.053, 0.902)	110(0.054, 0.872)
	(0.4, 0.5)	f_1	116(0.048, 0.902)	115(0.048, 0.904)	114(0.047, 0.894)
		f_2	134(0.052, 0.899)	124(0.055, 0.902)	119(0.053, 0.866)

(Continued)

TABLE 5.2 (Continued)

Sample size n (empirical type I error rate $\hat{\alpha}$ and power $1-\hat{\beta}$ within each parenthesis. CSD stands for cluster size distribution, f_1 or f_2, and Cluster, Unit, and Optimal denote the test statistics based on equal weights to clusters, using equal weights to subunits, and optimal weights, respectively

(ρ_1, ρ_2)	(p_1, p_2)	CSD	Cluster	Unit	Optimal
(0.4, 0.2)	(0.3, 0.4)	f_1	145(0.051, 0.899)	148(0.052, 0.902)	144(0.050, 0.896)
		f_2	160(0.056, 0.886)	164(0.060, 0.888)	152(0.055, 0.868)
	(0.4, 0.5)	f_1	158(0.055, 0.896)	161(0.053, 0.889)	157(0.056, 0.892)
		f_2	174(0.049, 0.901)	178(0.049, 0.897)	165(0.050, 0.886)
(0.4, 0.3)	(0.3, 0.4)	f_1	98(0.058, 0.907)	98(0.058, 0.907)	97(0.058, 0.902)
		f_2	113(0.048, 0.899)	106(0.052, 0.901)	102(0.049, 0.871)
	(0.4, 0.5)	f_1	107(0.052, 0.910)	106(0.052, 0.907)	105(0.051, 0.901)
		f_2	123(0.048, 0.902)	115(0.051, 0.904)	110(0.047, 0.869)

TABLE 5.3

Specificity data of PET ($k = 1$) and SPECT ($k = 2$): m_i = number of glands, and, for patient i and test k, y_{ki} = number of negative glands and $x_{kij} = 1$ if gland $j(= 1, ..., m_i)$ is negative

		PET	SPECT			PET	SPECT
i	m_i	$y_{1i}[x_{1ij}]$	$y_{2i}[x_{2ij}]$	i	m_i	$y_{1i}[x_{1ij}]$	$y_{2i}[x_{2ij}]$
1	3	0[0, 0, 0]	2[0, 1, 1]	12	2	2[1, 1]	2[1, 1]
2	3	2[1, 1, 0]	3[1, 1, 1]	13	3	3[1, 1, 1]	3[1, 1, 1]
3	3	3[1, 1, 1]	3[1, 1, 1]	14	2	2[1, 1]	2[1, 1]
4	1	1[1]	1[1]	15	2	0[0, 0]	2[1, 1]
5	3	2[1, 1, 0]	3[1, 1, 1]	16	3	2[1, 1, 0]	2[1, 1, 0]
6	4	4[1, 1, 1, 1]	4[1, 1, 1, 1]	17	3	2[1, 1, 0]	2[1, 1, 0]
7	3	3[1, 1, 1]	3[1, 1, 1]	18	3	2[1, 1, 0]	3[1, 1, 1]
8	2	2[1, 1]	2[1, 1]	19	2	2[1, 1]	2[1, 1]
9	2	2[1, 1]	1[1, 0]	20	1	1[1]	1[1]
10	1	1[1]	1[1]	21	2	2[1, 1]	2[1, 1]
11	3	2[1, 1, 0]	2[1, 1, 0]				

using equal weights to clusters if ICCs are high, like $\rho_1 = 0.4$, Because f_2 has a higher variance than f_1, the test statistics are less powerful with f_2. It is less clear with $\rho_1 = 0.3$, but when $\rho_1 = 0.4$, the power increases in ρ_2. This is very much like the power of paired tests increases in the correlation coefficient between powered data. The test statistics are less powerful if p_1 and p_2 are closer to 50%, i.e., $(p_1, p_2) = (0.4, 0.5)$ compared to $(0.2, 0.3)$.

We perform more simulations to investigate the performance of our sample size formulas that are derived using large sample approximation. Under each of above design settings and for two-sided $\alpha = 0.05$ and a power of $1-\beta = 0.8, 0.85,$ or 0.9, we calculate the sample size n for each test statistic using equal weights to clusters, equal weights to subunits, or optimal weights. After then, we generate 5,000 simulation data sets of size n under the design setting, apply the weighted test statistic to each data set, and calculate empirical power $1 - \hat{\beta}$ by the proportion of data sets rejecting H_0. We also generate simulation data sets under $H_0 : p_2 = p_1$ and calculate empirical type I error rate $\hat{\alpha}$ similarly.

Table 5.2 reports the simulation results. We find that the sample size increases in $1 - \beta$, variance of cluster size distribution (i.e., f_2 has a larger variance than f_1), and ρ_1, and decreases as ρ_2 increases and as p_1 and p_2 are far from $1/2$. For ICCs ρ_1 and ρ_2 considered here, the test statistic using equal weights to clusters has slightly smaller sample size than that using equal weights to subunits. The test statistic with optimal weights always has a sample size smaller than the other two weighted test statistics, but can be slightly underpowered, especially with cluster size distribution f_2. Otherwise, these sample sizes maintain the nominal power quite closely over all. Also these weighted test statistics control the type I error rate quite accurately for the calculated sample sizes.

Real Data Example

As a real data example, we apply the weighted tests to we use the data from Neumann et al. (1996) that are used for adjusted McNemar's test in Chapter 2. In this study, two diagnostic tests in radiology, positron emission tomography (PET, $k = 1$) and single photon emission tomography (SPECT, $k = 2$), are compared for the detection of hyperparathyroidism using matched data from multiple glands. Table 5.3 presents, the specificity data taken from Obuchowski (1989), consisting of 51 glands with no hyperparathyroidism (as confirmed by surgery) from $\tilde{n} = 21$ patients. Since both PET and SPECT are applied to each gland, we have $m_{1i} = m_{2i}$ for each cluster. We have specificity estimates $(\hat{p}_1, \hat{p}_2) = (0.810, 0, 913)$ and p-value = 0.053 using equal weights to clusters, $(\hat{p}_1, \hat{p}_2) = (0.784, 0, 902)$ and p-value = 0.028 using equal weights to clusters, and $(\hat{p}_1, \hat{p}_2) = (0.809, 0, 912)$ and p-value = 0.053 using optimal weights. These tests give smaller p-values than those using discordant cases only as given in Chapter 2.

References

Donner A, Donald A. Analysis of data from a stratified design with the cluster as unit of randomization. Statistics in Medicine 1987; 6: 43–52.

Donner A, Klar N. Methods for comparing event rates in intervention studies when the unit of allocation is a cluster. American Journal of Epidemiology 1994; 140: 279–289.

Jung SH, Ahn C. Estimation of response probability in correlated binary data: a new approach. Drug Information Journal 2000; 34: 599–604.

McNemar Q. Note on the sampling error of the difference between correlated proportions or percentages. Psychometrika 1947; 12: 153–157.

Obuchowski NA. On the comparison of correlated proportions for clustered data. Statistics in Medicine 1998; 17: 1495–1507.

Stanton BF, Clemens JD. An educational intervention for altering water-sanitation behaviors to reduce childhood diarrhea in urban Bangladesh. American Journal of Epidemiology 1987; 125, 292–301.

6

Random Number Generation of Clustered Binary Data

As seen in the previous chapters, the standard analysis methods are based on large sample theories so that we evaluate their finite sample performance through simulations. In the simulations, we need to generate clustered binary data. In this chapter, we investigate some methods of generating clustered binary data for such simulations. Note that the asymptotic distribution of the test statistics depends only on the first and second moments of the correlated Bernoulli random variables. Hence, we can evaluate the finite sample property of the asymptotic tests as we generate dependent Bernoulli random variables with mean and correlation coefficient specified for simulations.

Lunn-Davies Method

Lunn and Davies (1998) propose a simple method to generate exchangeable correlation structure. Clustered binary data that have been considered in the previous chapters have exchangeable structure so that their method is suitable to generate such data.

Suppose that we want to generate clustered binary random variables $(x_1, ..., x_m)$ with $E(x_j) = p$ and $\text{corr}(x_j, x_{j'}) = \rho$ for $j \neq j'$. Let $e_0, e_1, ..., e_m$ are independent and identically distributed Bernoulli random variable with mean p, denoted as IID $B(1, p)$, and $u_1, ..., u_m \sim$ IID $B(1, \sqrt{\rho})$ that are independent of $e_0, e_1, ..., e_m$. Then, $x_j = (1 - u_j)e_j + u_j e_0$ are Bernoulli random variables with $E(x_j) = p$ and $\text{var}(x_j) = p(1 - p)$. Further, for $j \neq j'$,

$$\begin{aligned}\text{cov}(x_j, x_{j'}) =& \text{cov}\{(1 - u_j)e_j + u_j e_0, (1 - u_{j'})e_{j'} + u_{j'} e_0\} \\ =& \text{cov}(u_j e_0, u_{j'} e_0) = E(u_j u_{j'} e_0) - E(u_j e_0)E(u_{j'} e_0) \\ =& p\rho - p^2\rho = p(1 - p)\rho\end{aligned}$$

so that $\text{corr}(x_j, x_{j'}) = p(1 - p)\rho/p/(1 - p) = \rho$. This proves that $(x_1, ..., x_m)$ are Bernoulli random variables with mean $E(x_j) = p$ and $\text{corr}(x_j) = \rho$.

This algorithm is very suitable to generate Bernoulli random for cluster randomization trials. Lunn and Davies (1998) also propose algorithms to generate Bernoulli random variables with autoregressive correlation structure

DOI: 10.1201/9781003221951-6

and M-dependent correlation structure, but it seems difficult to expand their method to other correlation structures, such as the one for trials with subunit randomization that is discussed in Chapter 4.

Kang-Jung Method

Kang and Jung (2001) propose a simple method for generating correlated binary variables from any given m-variate joint distribution. The key idea is to assign probabilities to all possible 2^m outcomes and to partition the $(0,1)$ interval into the same number of subintervals whose lengths equal the probabilities. Then, an m-variate binary random vector is generated from a uniform (0,1), denoted as $U(0,1)$, depending on which subinterval it belongs to.

Basic Algorithm

Let $(X_1, \ldots, X_m)$ be m dependent binary random variables and an integer h be the binary sequence of length m that is the binary representation of the integer h satisfying $0 \le h \le 2^m - 1$. Thus if $m = 3$, we express the integer 0 as the binary sequence 000, 1 as 001, 2 as 010, and so forth. For $0 \le h \le 2^m - 1$, let λ_h be the probability

$$\lambda_h = P(X_1 = h_1, \ldots, X_m = h_m),$$

where the binary sequence $(h_1, \ldots, h_m)$ is the binary representation of the integer h.

For a given m-variate joint distribution of binary random variables, $(\lambda_h, 0 \le h \le 2^m - 1)$, the algorithm generates binary sequence h if $z_{h-1} \le U < z_h$, where U is a random number from $U(0,1)$, and $z_0 = 0$ and $z_h = z_{h-1} + \lambda_h$ for $h = 0, 1, \ldots, 2^m - 1$. For example, when $m = 2$,

$$(X_1, X_2) = \begin{cases} (0,0) & \text{if } 0 < U < \lambda_{00} \\ (0,1) & \text{if } \lambda_{00} \le U < \lambda_{00} + \lambda_{01} \\ (1,0) & \text{if } \lambda_{00} + \lambda_{01} \le U < \lambda_{00} + \lambda_{01} + \lambda_{10} \\ (1,1) & \text{if } \lambda_{00} + \lambda_{01} + \lambda_{10} \le U < 1. \end{cases}$$

Kang and Jung (2001) use this algorithm to generate correlated binary data with various dependence structures, including clustered binary data that has an exchangeable structure.

Exchangeable Binary Variables

$X_1, \ldots, X_m$ is said to be exchangeable if for any $k(\leq m)$ and any vector $(x_1, x_2, \ldots, x_k)$, with $x_i = 0, 1, i = 1, 2, \ldots, k$,

$$P(X_{\pi(1)} = x_1, \ldots, X_{\pi(k)} = x_m) = P(X_1 = x_1, \ldots, X_k = x_k)$$

for any permutation $\pi(1), \ldots, \pi(k)$ of $1, \ldots, k$. In most studies under exchangeability assumption, one generates only the number of successes $\sum_{i=1}^{k} X_i$. Denote the probability of y successes ($y = 0, 1, \ldots, m$), $P(\sum_{i=1}^{m} X_i = y) = \sum_{\{(x_1,\ldots,x_m):\sum_{i=1}^{m} x_i = y\}} P(X_1 = x_1, \ldots, X_m = x_m)$, by τ_y. Then we divide the interval $(0, 1)$ into $m + 1$ subintervals and apply the algorithm described above. In other words,

1. Define $z_0, \ldots, z_m$ by $z_j = z_{j-1} + \tau_j, z_{-1} = 0$ for $j = 0, 1, \ldots, m$.
2. Generate a random number U from $U(0, 1)$.
3. Let $\sum_{i=1}^{m} X_i = j$ if $z_{j-1} \leq U \leq z_j$ for $j = 0, 1, \ldots, m$.

Note that Kang and Jung (2001) method is very simple to generate m-variate correlated binary data if we know the joint distribution (e.g., Beta-Binomial distribution for dependent binary data under cluster randomization as discussed in the next section) or all the moments of up to the mth moment. Since the large sample property of inferences depend on the first and second moments of clustered binary data, it will be better if we can generate them without specifying the higher moments or with a known full joint PDF, which is tough, especially with high dimensions and complicated marginal and second moment structures (e.g., clustered binary data under subunit randomization).

Beta-Binomial Distribution

Suppose that p follows beta distribution Beta(α, β) and, given p, Y follows $B(m, p)$. Then, Y follows Beta-Binomial distribution with

$$E(Y) = m\frac{\alpha}{\alpha + \beta}$$
$$E(Y^2) = m\frac{\alpha}{\{m(1 + \alpha) + \beta\}}$$

and probability mass function (PMF)

$$f(y|m, \alpha, \beta) = \binom{m}{y}\frac{B(\alpha + y, \beta + m - y)}{B(\alpha, \beta)} \tag{6.1}$$

for $y = 0, 1, ..., m$, where $\alpha = p(1-\rho)/\rho$, $\beta = (1-p)(1-\rho)/\rho$, $B(a,b) = \Gamma(a)\Gamma(b)/\Gamma(a+b)$, and $\Gamma(a) = \int_0^\infty t^{a-1}\exp(-t)dt$. It is easy to show that $E(y) = mp$ and $\text{var}(y) = mp(1-p)\{1+(m-1)\rho\}$ like the sum of clustered Bernoulli random variables y that was investigated in the previous chapters.

We generate Y from the PMF (6.1) for specified p and ρ by generating a random number u from $U(0,1)$. If $u \in [\tau_y, \tau_{y+1})$, then we have $Y = y$, where $\tau_y = \sum_{j=0}^{y} f(j|m,\alpha,\beta)$ denotes the cumulative mass function of the beta-binomial distribution. This can be counted as a specific application of Kang and Jung (2001).

Beta-binomial distribution is very convenient to generate clustered binary random variables with exchangeable correlation structure, such as clustered binary data from cluster randomization trials. But, the binary random variables from a subunit randomization trial are not exchangeable so that beta-binomial distribution is not appropriate to generate such clustered Bernoulli random variables.

Method based on Multivariate Normal Random Variables

We discuss an algorithm to generate clustered standard normal random variables and dichotomize them to generate clustered binary random variables. This method provides more flexible algorithms to generate clustered binary data than the previous methods.

Under Cluster Randomization

We want to generate clustered Bernoulli random variables $(x_1, ..., x_m)$ with $E(x_j) = p$ and $\text{corr}(x_j, x_{j'}) = \rho$ for $j \neq j'$. To this end, we generate $Z_1, ..., Z_m$ with marginally $N(0,1)$ and $\text{corr}(Z_j, Z_{j'}) = r$. and dichotomize them as follows. Let z_p denote the $100p$ percentile of $N(0,1)$ distribution. Then, for the indication function $I(\cdot)$,

$$x_j = I(Z_j \leq z_p)$$

for $j = 1, ..., m$ are clustered Bernoulli random variable with mean p and ICC ρ that can be obtained as a function of r using a numerical method as follows.

Given p and ρ, we want to find r satisfying

$$\rho = \frac{\text{cov}(x_1, x_2)}{\text{var}(x_1)} = \frac{P(Z_1 \leq z_p, Z_2 \leq z_p) - p^2}{p(1-p)}$$

or

$$P(Z_1 \leq z_p, Z_2 \leq z_p) = \rho p(1-p) + p^2. \quad (6.2)$$

Since (Z_1, Z_2) is bivariate $N(0,1)$ with $\text{corr}(Z_1, Z_2) = r$ with joint probability density function (PDF) $f(z_1, z_2)$ and $Z_1|Z_2 = z_2 \sim N(rz_2, 1-r^2)$, the left-hand side of (6.2) is

$$\begin{aligned}
P(Z_1 \leq z_p, Z_2 \leq z_p) &= \int_{-\infty}^{z_p}\int_{-\infty}^{z_p} f(z_1, z_2)dz_1dz_2 \\
&= \int_{-\infty}^{z_p}\int_{-\infty}^{z_p} f(z_2)f(z_1|z_2)dz_1dz_2 \\
&= \int_{-\infty}^{z_p} \phi(z_2)P(Z_1 \leq z_p|z_2)dz_2 \\
&= \int_{-\infty}^{z_p} \phi(z_2)P\left(\frac{Z_1 - rz_2}{\sqrt{1-r^2}} \leq \frac{z_p - rz_2}{\sqrt{1-r^2}} \;\middle|\; z_2\right)dz_2 \\
&= \int_{-\infty}^{z_p} \phi(z_2)\Phi\left(\frac{z_p - rz_2}{\sqrt{1-r^2}}\right)dz_2
\end{aligned}$$

where $\phi(\cdot)$ and $\Phi(\cdot)$ are the PDF and cumulative density function (CDF), respectively, of $N(0,1)$ distribution. Here, the last equality holds because we have $(Z_1 - rz_2)/\sqrt{1-r^2} \sim N(0,1)$ conditioning on $Z_2 = z_2$.

By plugging this result in (6.2), we obtain an equation on r

$$\int_{-\infty}^{z_p} \phi(z)\Phi\left(\frac{z_p - rz}{\sqrt{1-r^2}}\right)dz = \rho p(1-p) + p^2. \tag{6.3}$$

If we find the r value corresponding to ρ, $(x_1, ..., x_m)$ are clustered Bernoulli random variables with mean p and ICC ρ.

Given (p, ρ), we solve (6.3) with respect to r using numerical integration and bisection methods. Table 6.1 reports r value for given p, ρ. Note that, given ρ, r value slightly depends on p and is identical for p and $1-p$. And, r increases in ρ.

TABLE 6.1

r value for given p and ρ ('−' means not available)

	ρ								
p	**0.1**	**0.2**	**0.3**	**0.4**	**0.5**	**0.6**	**0.7**	**0.8**	**0.9**
0.1	0.243	0.424	0.572	0.690	0.788	0.867	0.926	0.966	–
0.2	0.191	0.359	0.507	0.637	0.746	0.838	0.909	0.958	0.989
0.3	0.170	0.329	0.476	0.608	0.723	0.821	0.899	0.955	0.989
0.4	0.160	0.313	0.459	0.593	0.712	0.811	0.893	0.953	0.987
0.5	0.156	0.310	0.453	0.587	0.708	0.809	0.891	0.951	0.987
0.6	0.160	0.313	0.459	0.593	0.712	0.811	0.893	0.953	0.987
0.7	0.170	0.329	0.476	0.608	0.723	0.821	0.899	0.955	0.989
0.8	0.191	0.359	0.507	0.637	0.746	0.838	0.909	0.958	0.989
0.9	0.243	0.424	0.572	0.690	0.788	0.867	0.926	0.966	–

Once we find r for given (p, ρ), we generate z_j as follows. Let $u_0, u_1, ..., u_m \sim$ IID $N(0, 1)$ random variables. For $j = 1, ..., m$, we generate $N(0, 1)$ random variables, $Z_1, ..., Z_m$, with ICC r by

$$Z_j = u_j\sqrt{1-r} + u_0\sqrt{r}.$$

It is easy to show that $z_1, ..., z_m$ are $N(0, 1)$ random variables with intracluster correlation coefficient (ICC) r.

Under Subunit Randomization

Suppose that we randomize subunits of each cluster between two treatment arms. For example, we may randomize siblings of each litter to different treatments. From each cluster, we observe $x_{11}, ..., x_{1m_1}, x_{21}, ..., x_{2m_2}$ that are Bernoulli random variables with $E(x_{1j}) = p_1$, $E(x_{2j}) = p_2$, $\text{corr}(x_{1j}, x_{1j'}) = \text{corr}(x_{2j}, x_{2j'}) = \rho_1$ for $j \neq j'$ and $\text{corr}(x_{1j}, x_{2j'}) = \rho_2 (\leq \rho_1)$. Note that, in a statistical testing, $p_1 = p_2$ under H_0 and $p_1 \neq p_2$ under H_1. We want to generate these correlated binary random variables from multivariate normal random variables.

Suppose that $(Z_{11}, ..., Z_{1m_1}, Z_{21}, ..., Z_{2m_2})$ are marginally $N(0, 1)$ with $\text{corr}(Z_{1j}, Z_{1j'}) = r_1$, $\text{corr}(Z_{2j}, Z_{2j'}) = r_2$, and $\text{corr}(Z_{1j}, Z_{2j'}) = r_0$. From $(Z_{11}, .., Z_{1m_1}, Z_{21}, ..., Z_{2m_2})$, we generate $(x_{1m_1}, ..., x_{1m_1}, x_{21}, ..., x_{2m_2})$ by

$$x_{kj} = I(Z_{kj} \leq z_{p_k})$$

for $k = 1, 2$.

These binary random variables should have a correlation structure, $\text{corr}(x_{kj}, x_{kj'}) = \rho_1$ for $k = 1, 2$ and $\text{corr}(x_{1j}, x_{2j'}) = \rho_2$. So, we want to find (r_1, r_2, r_0) corresponding to given $(p_1, p_2, \rho_1, \rho_2)$. Given (p_1, p_2), (r_0, r_1, r_2) corresponding to (ρ_1, ρ_2) are identified using a numerical method as follows. Since $(x_{k1}, ..., x_{km_k})$ has an exchangeable structure, we can find r_k for given (p_k, ρ_1) from Table 6.1 as in the cluster randomization case.

Now, given (p_1, p_2, ρ_2), we want to find r_0 satisfying

$$\rho_2 = \frac{\text{cov}(x_{1j}, x_{2j'})}{\sqrt{\text{var}(x_{1j})\text{var}(x_{2j'})}} = \frac{P(Z_{1j} \leq z_{p_1}, Z_{2j'} \leq z_{p_2}) - p_1 p_2}{\sqrt{p_1(1-p_1)p_2(1-p_2)}}$$

or

$$P(Z_{1j} \leq z_{p_1}, Z_{2j'} \leq z_{p_2}) = \rho_2\sqrt{p_1(1-p_1)p_2(1-p_2)} + p_1 p_2. \tag{6.4}$$

For $Z_1 = Z_{1j}$ and $Z_2 = Z_{2j'}$, (Z_1, Z_2) is bivariate $N(0, 1)$ with $\text{corr}(Z_1, Z_2) = r_0$ with joint PDF $f(z_1, z_2)$ and $Z_2|Z_1 = z_1 \sim N(r_0 z_1, 1 - r_0^2)$, the left-hand side of (6.4) is

$$
\begin{aligned}
P(Z_1 \leq z_{p_1}, Z_2 \leq z_{p_2}) &= \int_{-\infty}^{z_{p_1}} \int_{-\infty}^{z_{p_2}} f(z_1, z_2) dz_2 dz_1 \\
&= \int_{-\infty}^{z_{p_1}} \int_{-\infty}^{z_{p_2}} f(z_1) f(z_2 | z_1) dz_2 dz_1 \\
&= \int_{-\infty}^{z_{p_1}} \phi(z_1) P(Z_2 \leq z_{p_2} | z_1) dz_1 \\
&= \int_{-\infty}^{z_{p_1}} \phi(z_1) P\left(\frac{Z_2 - r_0 z_1}{\sqrt{1 - r_0^2}} \leq \frac{z_{p_2} - r_0 z_1}{\sqrt{1 - r_0^2}} \,\Big|\, w \right) dz_1 \\
&= \int_{-\infty}^{z_{p_1}} \phi(z_1) \Phi\left(\frac{z_{p_2} - r_0 z_1}{\sqrt{1 - r_0^2}} \right) dz_1.
\end{aligned}
$$

Here, the last equality holds because we have $(Z_2 - r_0 z_1)/\sqrt{1 - r_0^2} \sim N(0, 1)$ conditioning on $Z_1 = z_1$.

By plugging this result in (6.4), we obtain an equation on r_0

$$
\int_{-\infty}^{z_{p_1}} \phi(z) \Phi\left(\frac{z_{p_2} - r_0 z}{\sqrt{1 - r_0^2}} \right) dz = \rho_2 \sqrt{p_1(1 - p_1) p_2 (1 - p_2)} + p_1 p_2. \tag{6.5}
$$

If we find the r_0 value corresponding to ρ_2, we have $E(x_{kj}) = p_k$ and $\text{corr}(x_{1j}, x_{2j'}) = \rho_2$.

Given (p_1, p_2, ρ_2), we solve (6.5) with respect to r_0 using numerical integration and bisection methods. Table 6.2 reports r_0 value for given (p_1, p_2, ρ_2).

Note that, given ρ_2, r_0 value slightly depends on (p_1, p_2), and is identical for (p_1, p_2) and $(1 - p_2, 1 - p_1)$. There exist no r_0 values for large ρ_2 values, such as 0.9, for most (p_1, p_2) combinations. We have r_0 values for a wider range of ρ_2 values if p_1 and p_2 are close to $1/2$.

Once we find (r_0, r_1, r_2) corresponding to given $(p_1, p_2, \rho_1, \rho_2)$, we generate multivariate normal random vector with marginal $N(0, 1)$ distribution $(Z_{11}, ..., Z_{1m_1}, Z_{21}, ..., Z_{2m_2})$ with $\text{corr}(Z_{kj}, Z_{kj'}) = r_k$ and $\text{corr}(Z_{1j}, Z_{2j'}) = r_0$ as follows.

Assuming that the impact of shared frailty within each cluster is lowered by different treatments, we assume that $\rho_2 \leq \rho_1$ and $r_0 \leq \min(r_1, r_2)$. Suppose that e_0, e_1, e_2 and $\epsilon_{11}, ..., \epsilon_{1m_1}, ..., \epsilon_{21}, ..., \epsilon_{2m_2}$ IID $N(0, 1)$ random variables. Then, for $k = 1, 2$,

$$
Z_{kj} = \epsilon_{kj} \sqrt{1 - r_k} + e_k \sqrt{r_k - r_0} + e_0 \sqrt{r_0}.
$$

It is easy to show that $(Z_{11}, ..., Z_{1m_1}, Z_{21}, ..., Z_{2m_2})$ has the required correlation structure.

While the previous methods are useful to generate clustered binary data only under cluster randomization, this method is very convenient to generate

TABLE 6.2

r_0 value for given (p_1, p_2, ρ_2) ('−' means not available)

		ρ_2							
p_1	p_2	0.1	0.2	0.3	0.4	0.5	0.6	0.7	0.8
0.1	0.1	0.242	0.425	0.571	0.690	0.788	0.865	0.926	0.967
	0.2	0.218	0.400	0.556	0.690	0.805	0.905	–	–
	0.25	0.214	0.398	0.560	0.708	0.842	–	–	–
	0.3	0.210	0.400	0.572	0.734	0.918	–	–	–
0.2	0.2	0.191	0.359	0.507	0.637	0.747	0.836	0.908	0.959
	0.3	0.181	0.346	0.497	0.633	0.752	0.853	0.935	–
	0.35	0.179	0.346	0.501	0.641	0.767	0.880	–	–
	0.4	0.177	0.346	0.507	0.656	0.794	0.937	–	–
0.3	0.3	0.170	0.327	0.476	0.608	0.723	0.821	0.899	0.955
	0.4	0.164	0.323	0.472	0.608	0.729	0.832	0.918	–
	0.45	0.164	0.323	0.474	0.614	0.742	0.853	0.953	–
	0.5	0.164	0.327	0.482	0.627	0.761	0.888	–	–
0.4	0.4	0.160	0.314	0.458	0.593	0.711	0.811	0.893	0.951
	0.5	0.158	0.313	0.461	0.597	0.719	0.824	0.911	0.979
	0.55	0.158	0.315	0.465	0.604	0.733	0.844	0.941	–
	0.6	0.160	0.321	0.474	0.620	0.754	0.878	–	–
0.5	0.5	0.156	0.310	0.454	0.589	0.708	0.809	0.891	0.951
	0.6	0.158	0.313	0.461	0.597	0.719	0.824	0.911	0.979
	0.65	0.160	0.317	0.468	0.602	0.734	0.847	0.945	–
	0.7	0.164	0.327	0.482	0.627	0.761	0.888	–	–
0.6	0.6	0.160	0.314	0.458	0.593	0.711	0.811	0.893	0.951
	0.7	0.164	0.323	0.472	0.608	0.729	0.832	0.918	–
	0.75	0.170	0.333	0.486	0.625	0.752	0.863	0.970	–
	0.8	0.177	0.346	0.507	0.656	0.794	0.937	–	–
0.7	0.7	0.170	0.327	0.476	0.608	0.723	0.821	0.899	0.955
	0.8	0.181	0.346	0.497	0.633	0.752	0.853	0.935	–
	0.85	0.193	0.365	0.524	0.666	0.794	0.911	–	–
	0.9	0.212	0.400	0.574	0.734	0.918	–	–	–

clustered binary data either under cluster randomization or under subunit randomization even when cluster sizes are big.

Example: Suppose that we want to find (r_0, r_1, r_2) for given $(p_1, p_2, \rho_1, \rho_2) = (0.1, 0.3, 0.2, 0.1)$. From Table 6.1, we have $r_1 = 0.424$ for $(p_1, \rho_1) = (0.1, 0.2)$ and $r_2 = 0.329$ for $(p_2, \rho_1) = (0.3, 0.2)$. For $(p_1, p_2, \rho_2) = (0.1, 0.3, 0.1)$, we have $r_0 = 0.210$ from Table 6.2.

References

Kang SH, Jung SH. Generating correlated binary variables with complete specification of joint distribution. Biometrical Journal 2001; 43: 263–269.

Lunn AD, Davies SJ. A note on generating correlated binary variables. Biometrika 1998; 85: 487–490.

7

Tests for $R \times C$ Contingency Tables with Clustered Categorical Data

In Chapters 3–5, we have considered two-sample tests with clustered binary data. Ignoring intracluster correlation coefficient (ICC), the resulting data can be summarized by a 2×2 table. Sometimes, the number of groups may be larger than 2 or the outcome variable may have more than two categories. This kind of data are summarized using $R \times C$ tables with $R, C \geq 2$. In this chapter, we investigate chi-square tests for $R \times C$ contingency tables with clustered categorical data. We consider both cluster and subunit randomization cases under various study designs.

Tests for $2 \times K$ Contingency Tables with Clustered Ordered Categorical Data

Ordered categorical data summarized in a $2 \times K$ contingency table may arise from a two-sample comparison of an ordered categorical outcome, called a two-sample multinomial test, or K-sample comparison of a binary outcome with ordered groups, called a K-sample binomial test. The Wilcoxon rank sum test (Wilcoxon 1945; Mann and Whitney 1947) and the linear trend test (Cochran 1954; Armitage 1958) are the standard methods for the former case, whereas the linear trend test may be one of the most popular choices in the latter case.

Although the two types of studies, appear to be quite different, the test statistics used can be formulated in a unified way. The linear trend test and the Wilcoxon rank sum test belong to a family of score tests for ordered categorical data. When subjects are independent, methodologies for score tests have been well developed. Basically, a score test for a $2 \times K$ table assigns scores to the ordered columns and compares the average scores of two groups defined by rows. Chapter 2 of Agresti (1996) provides a good review on this topic.

In this section, we consider clustered ordered categorical data that can be summarized by $2 \times K$ tables. We consider both cluster randomization and subunit randomization cases. There are multiple examples of real studies.

DOI: 10.1201/9781003221951-7

In a lung transplant study (Song et al. 1997), the investigators were interested in assessing whether one surgery method had better healing after transplant than the other. Twenty-six rabbits were randomized into two surgery methods. Healing was measured by the degree of inflammation (no, some, much, or very much), and observations were made from two sites of surgery area on each animal. In this case, clusters (animals) are randomized into two treatment groups so that subunits (sites) in different groups are independent.

On the other hand, in a dentistry study with split-mouth protocol (Barnett et al. 1989), some teeth (subunits) within a mouth (cluster) are randomly assigned to an experiment treatment, while the other teeth serving as controls. If the response is measured by an ordered discrete variable in this study, then the resulting data will have two multinomial samples with subunit randomization.

K-sample binomial data with cluster randomization often arise from developmental toxicity experiments. George and Kodell (1996) refer to a study where pregnant animals (clusters) are assigned to one of four doses of a compound during the period of organogenesis and then they are sacrificed just prior to the end of gestation to observe occurrence or no occurrence of malformation from each fetus (subunit).

In a dentistry study, we may consider assigning teeth (units) within each patient (cluster) to K ordered treatment groups and make binary observations from the teeth to result in K-sample binomial data with subunit randomization.

In this section, we investigate the unified method that was proposed by Jung and Kang (2001) to derive score tests suitable for these types of studies.

Score Tests for Independent Data

We briefly review the score tests for ordered categorical data with independent observations.

Suppose that two sample multinomial data or K sample binomial data are summarized by a $2 \times K$ contingency table. As displayed in Table 7.1, let n_{lk} denote (l, k)-cell frequencies and n_l and $n_{\cdot k}$ denote row and column totals, respectively, for $l = 1, 2$ and $k = 1, \ldots, K$, and let $n = n_1 + n_2 = \sum_{k=1}^{K} n_{\cdot k} = \sum_{l=1}^{2} \sum_{k=1}^{K} n_{lk}$ denote the total frequency. In a K sample binomial case, let p_k and q_k denote the success and the failure (or, row 1 and 2) probabilities, respectively, with $p_k + q_k = 1$ for $k = 1, ..., K$. On the other hand, in a two-sample multinomial case, let $(P_1, ..., P_K)$ and $(Q_1, ..., Q_K)$, satisfying $\sum_{k=1}^{K} P_k = 1$ and $\sum_{k=1}^{K} Q_k = 1$, denote the multinomial probabilities for groups 1 and 2, respectively. For unified notations to be used in both cases, we redefine the multinomial parameters as $p_k = P_k/(P_k + Q_k)$ and $q_k = Q_k/(P_k + Q_k)$ so that $p_k + q_k = 1$ as in the K sample binomial case.

TABLE 7.1
$2 \times K$ contingency table

	1	2	...	K	Total
1	n_{11}	n_{12}	...	n_{1K}	n_1
2	n_{21}	n_{22}	...	n_{2K}	n_2
Total	$n_{\cdot 1}$	$n_{\cdot 2}$	...	$n_{\cdot K}$	n

Then a score test tests the equality of $p_1, ..., p_K$ against a specific form of discrepancy. For example, the linear trend test considers the model $p_k = \beta_0 + \beta_1 k$ and tests $H_0 : \beta_1 = 0$ against $H_1 : \beta_1 \neq 0$.

A score test assigns scores s_k to the subjects belonging to column k and compares the average scores between two rows. A set of scores $(s_1, ..., s_K)$ is chosen depending on the testing used. For example, the linear trend test uses scores $s_k = k$, and the test statistic is given as

$$Z = \frac{\sum_{k=1}^{K} n_{\cdot k}(\hat{p}_k - \bar{p})(s_k - \bar{s})}{\sqrt{\bar{p}\bar{q}(\sum_{k=1}^{K} n_{\cdot k} s_k^2 - n\bar{s}^2)}},$$

where $\hat{p}_k = n_{1k}/n_{\cdot k}$ the proportion of row 1 for column k, $\bar{p} = n_1/n$ the proportion of row 1 for all K columns combined, $\bar{q} = 1 - \bar{p} = n_2/n$, and $\bar{s} = n^{-1} \sum_{k=1}^{K} n_{\cdot k} s_k$ the grand mean score.

This test statistic is asymptotically equivalent to the t-test statistic for the slope of a simple linear regression model using the binary variable representing whether a subject belongs to row 1 or not as the y-variable and the score assigned to the subject as the x-variable. Under H_0, Z is asymptotically $N(0, 1)$.

In the Wilcoxon rank sum test, also called the Mann-Whitney-Wilcoxon test or the Wilcoxon U-test, the score for a column corresponds to the rank of a subject belonging to the column among n subjects. Without loss of generality, suppose that K columns are in ascending order. Subjects in a column will be assigned by the same score, i.e., the average of possible ranks. For a subject belonging to column k, a possible rank would be $\sum_{j=1}^{k-1} n_{\cdot j} + 1$, $\sum_{j=1}^{k-1} n_{\cdot j} + 2$,..., or $\sum_{j=1}^{k} n_{\cdot j}$. Hence, we assign the average rank

$$\frac{(\sum_{j=1}^{k-1} n_{\cdot j} + 1) + (\sum_{j=1}^{k} n_{\cdot j})}{2} = \sum_{j=1}^{k-1} n_{\cdot j} + \frac{n_{\cdot k} + 1}{2}$$

to the subjects in column k. Using these scores, the Wilcoxon rank sum test is expressed as

$$Z = \frac{R_1 - n_1(n+1)/2}{\sqrt{\text{var}(R_1)}},$$

where R_1 is the total ranks for subjects in row 1 and

$$\text{var}(R_1) = \frac{n_1 n_2}{12}\left\{n+1-\frac{\sum_{k=1}^{K} n_{\cdot k}(n_{\cdot k}^2-1)}{n(n-1)}\right\}$$

see, for example, p. 20 of Lehmann (1975). Under H_0, Z is asymptotically $N(0,1)$.

While the Wilcoxon rank sum test is usually used for comparing two multinomial distributions with ordered categories, the linear trend test is used for comparing binomial proportions among K ordered groups as well as comparing two multinomial distributions with ordered categories (Yates 1948).

Score Tests for Clustered Data

Suppose that there are n clusters and cluster $i(=1,...,n)$ has m_i subunits. In a clustered ordered categorical data case, we assign the scores $s_1,...,s_K$ to K columns as in the independent data case. For subunit $j(=1,...,m_i)$ in cluster $i(=1,...,n)$, let x_{ij} be the score value, i.e., $x_{ij}=s_k$ if this subunit belongs to column k and δ_{ij} be the binary variable taking 1 if the subunit belongs to row 1 and 0 otherwise. Note that δ_{ij} and x_{ij} are variables identifying the row and column of the cell to which subunit j of cluster i belongs.

Ignoring the possible dependence among subunits, the difference of the total scores between row 1 and row 2 is expressed as

$$\bar{x}_1-\bar{x}_2=\frac{1}{M_1}\sum_{i=1}^{n}\sum_{j=1}^{m_i}\delta_{ij}x_{ij}-\frac{1}{M_2}\sum_{i=1}^{n}\sum_{j=1}^{m_i}(1-\delta_{ij})x_{ij},$$

where $M_1=\sum_{i=1}^{n}\sum_{j=1}^{m_i}\delta_{ij}$ and $M_2=\sum_{i=1}^{n}\sum_{j=1}^{m_i}(1-\delta_{ij})$ are the total number of subunits in rows 1 and 2, respectively. We prove in Appendix A that $\sqrt{n}(\bar{x}_1-\bar{x}_2)/\hat{\sigma}$ converges to the standard normal distribution under the null hypothesis of no treatment effect. Here,

$$\hat{\sigma}^2=n\sum_{i=1}^{n}\{\sum_{j=1}^{m_i}(\frac{\delta_{ij}}{M_1}-\frac{1-\delta_{ij}}{M_2})(x_{ij}-\bar{x})\}^2,$$

where $\bar{x}=(M_1\bar{x}_1+M_2\bar{x}_2)/(M_1+M_2)$ is the grand mean score for all M_1+M_2 subunits.

We reject H_0 with two-sided type I error rate α if the absolute value of test statistic

$$Z=\frac{\sqrt{n}(\bar{X}_1-\bar{X}_2)}{\hat{\sigma}} \tag{7.1}$$

is larger than $z_{1-\alpha/2}$, the $100(1-\alpha/2)$ percentile of $N(0,1)$.

This test statistic can be used for any type of clustered ordered categorical data discussed above. If $m_i = 1$ or subunits are independent, $\hat{\sigma}^2$ is asymptotically equivalent to the variance estimator for uncorrelated observations and hence (7.1) is reduced to the standard test statistics that was reviewed above.

Under different study designs, test statistic (7.1) can be expressed as follows.

Example 1 (Two-sample multinomial test with cluster randomization)
Suppose that n_r clusters are randomized into group $r(=1,2)$. For cluster i in group r, let m_{li} be the cluster size and x_{li} the sum of scores assigned to the m_{li} subunits. Then, we have $\bar{x}_r = M_r^{-1}\sum_{i=1}^{n_r} x_{ri}$ and

$$\hat{\sigma}^2 = \frac{n}{M_1^2}\sum_{i=1}^{n_1}(x_{1i} - m_{1i}\bar{x})^2 + \frac{n}{M_2^2}\sum_{i=1}^{n_2}(x_{2i} - m_{2i}\bar{x})^2,$$

where $M_r = \sum_{i=1}^{n_r} m_{ri}$ and $\bar{x} = (M_1\bar{x}_1 + M_2\bar{x}_2)/(M_1 + M_2)$.

Example 2 (Two-sample multinomial with subunit randomization)
Suppose that cluster $i(=1,...,n)$ has m_i subunits of which m_{ri} ($m_{1i} + m_{2i} = m_i$) are randomized into treatment $r(=1,2)$ and x_{ri} be the sum of scores assigned to the m_{ri} subunits. Then, we have $\bar{x}_r = M_l^{-1}\sum_{i=1}^{n} x_{ir}$ and

$$\hat{\sigma}^2 = n\sum_{i=1}^{n}(\frac{x_{1i} - m_{1i}\bar{x}}{M_1} - \frac{x_{2i} - m_{2i}\bar{x}}{M_2})^2,$$

where $M_r = \sum_{i=1}^{n} m_{ri}$ and $\bar{x} = (M_1\bar{x}_1 + M_2\bar{x}_2)/(M_1 + M_2)$.

Example 3 (K-sample binomial with cluster randomization)
Suppose that $n_{\cdot k}$ clusters are randomized into group k ($k = 1,...,K$). For cluster i ($i = 1,...,n_{\cdot k}$) in group k, let m_{ki} and y_{ki} denote the cluster size and the number of successes (or row 1 frequency) among the m_{ki} subunits, respectively. Also let $M_{\cdot k} = \sum_{i=1}^{n_{\cdot k}} m_{ki}$ be the total number of subunits in group k. Then, (7.1) is expressed as

$$Z = \frac{\sum_{k=1}^{K}(s_k - \bar{s})y_k}{\sqrt{\sum_{k=1}^{K}\{(s_k - \bar{s})^2\sum_{i=1}^{n_{\cdot k}}(y_{ki} - m_{ki}\bar{p})^2\}}},$$

where $y_k = \sum_{i=1}^{n_{\cdot k}} y_{ki}$, $\bar{p} = M_1/(M_1 + M_2)$, and $\bar{s} = (M_1 + M_2)^{-1}\sum_{k=1}^{K} M_{\cdot k}s_k$.

Example 4 (K-sample binomial with subunit randomization)
Suppose that cluster $i(=1,...,n)$ has m_i subunits of which m_{ik} ($m_{1i} + m_{2i} = m_i$), and y_{ki} denotes the number of successes (or row 1 frequency) among the m_{ki} subunits. Also let $M_{\cdot k} = \sum_{i=1}^{n} m_{ki}$ denote the total number of subunits assigned to group k. Then, test statistic (7.1) is expressed as

$$Z = \frac{\sum_{k=1}^{K}(s_k - \bar{s})y_k}{\sqrt{\sum_{i=1}^{n}\{\sum_{k=1}^{K}(s_k - \bar{s})(y_{ki} - m_{ki}\bar{p})\}^2}},$$

where $y_k = \sum_{i=1}^{n} y_{ki}$, $\bar{p} = M_1/(M_1 + M_2)$ and $\bar{s} = (M_1 + M_2)^{-1}\sum_{k=1}^{K} M_{\cdot k}s_k$.

TABLE 7.2

Empirical power for two independent multinomial case. (a) The Wilcoxon rank sum test: $(P_1, P_2, P_3, P_4) = (0.25, 0.25, 0.25, 0.25)$ for Case 1, (0.4, 0.3, 0.2, 0.1) for Case 2, and $(0.1, 0.4, 0.4, 0.1)$ for Case 3. Under H_1, (Q_1, Q_2, Q_3, Q_4) is obtained by shifting the multivariate normal distribution by 0.4 from that of group 1

		H_0			H_1		
ρ	n	Case 1	Case 2	Case 3	Case 1	Case 2	Case 3
0	40	0.052	0.053	0.053	0.725	0.723	0.718
	80	0.054	0.049	0.052	0.952	0.953	0.950
	160	0.050	0.051	0.050	0.999	0.999	0.999
0.3	40	0.053	0.051	0.053	0.404	0.404	0.402
	80	0.050	0.053	0.050	0.675	0.667	0.675
	160	0.050	0.048	0.051	0.931	0.932	0.932
0.6	40	0.052	0.054	0.051	0.280	0.279	0.284
	80	0.054	0.051	0.053	0.479	0.486	0.488
	160	0.050	0.051	0.050	0.779	0.777	0.782

Simulation Studies

In order to investigate the finite sample properties of the method, simulation studies were conducted. Reported here are the results in cluster randomization case only.

Correlated discrete data are generated by discretizing exchangeable multivariate normal random variables with marginally $N(0, 1)$ and ICC $\rho = 0$, 0.3, or 0.6 using appropriate cutoff values. In the first part of simulations, we consider the Wilcoxon's rank sum test for two-sample multinomial data with $K = 4$ ordered outcomes. With a balanced allocation, $n_1 = n_2 = 20, 40$, or 80 clusters are randomized into each of two treatment groups. The cluster size distribution has PMF

$$f(2) = f(4) = f(6) = f(8) = 1/4.$$

Under H_0, the two groups have a common multinomial distribution with probabilities $(P_1, P_2, P_3, P_4) = (0.25, 0.25, 0.25, 0.25)$ in Case 1, (0.4, 0.3, 0.2, 0.1) in Case 2, and (0.1, 0.4, 0.4, 0.1) in Case 3. Under H_1, the distributions in group 2 are generated by shifting the multivariate normal distribution of group 1 by 0.4 and using the same cutoff values. For each parameter value setting, $B = 5{,}000$ samples are generated and the Wilcoxon rank sum test with two-sided $\alpha = 0.05$ is applied to each sample. Empirical power is calculated as the proportion of simulation samples rejecting H_0 among the 5,000 samples.

The simulation results are reported in Table 7.2(a). We find that the Wilcoxon rank sum test has empirical power very close to the nominal type I

TABLE 7.2 (Continued)

(b) The linear trend test: Under H_0 the distributions are the same as those of Cases 1, 2, and 3 in (a). Under H_1, $(Q_1, Q_2, Q_3, Q_4) = (0.418, 0.276, 0.186, 0.120)$ for Case 1, (0.557, 0.279, 0.124, 0.040) for Case 2, and (0.175, 0.464, 0.310, 0.051) for Case 3. For the three cases, $(\beta_0, \beta_1) = (0.275, 0.1)$, (0.318, 0.1), and (0.265, 0.1), respectively

		H_0			H_1		
ρ	n	**Case 1**	**Case 2**	**Case 3**	**Case 1**	**Case 2**	**Case 3**
0	40	0.053	0.050	0.052	0.881	0.753	0.617
	80	0.055	0.051	0.056	0.992	0.962	0.905
	160	0.051	0.050	0.048	1.00	0.999	0.995
0.3	40	0.059	0.054	0.059	0.552	0.432	0.333
	80	0.051	0.055	0.054	0.845	0.718	0.582
	160	0.050	0.051	0.051	0.989	0.946	0.859
0.6	40	0.059	0.055	0.055	0.389	0.302	0.232
	80	0.054	0.054	0.058	0.662	0.522	0.409
	160	0.050	0.050	0.047	0.916	0.802	0.680

error probability $\alpha = 0.05$ under H_0. When n is large ($n = 160$) or ρ is small, it has a reasonable power. But, as ρ increases, the power decreases. This result is natural in cluster randomization case, since a high ICC diminishes the total information contained in data.

Now, we conduct simulations for the linear trend test. Null distributions are the same as those of the Wilcoxon test. Under H_1, group 2 has quadrinomial probabilities $(Q_1, Q_2, Q_3, Q_4) = (0.418, 0.276, 0.186, 0.120)$ in case 1, $(0.557, 0.279, 0.124, 0.040)$ in case 2, and $= (0.175, 0.464, 0.310, 0.051)$ in case 3 by shifting the multivariate normal random variables. Note that, for the three cases, the regression coefficients for a linear trend are $(\beta_0, \beta_1) = (0.275, 0.1)$, (0.318, 0.1), and (0.265, 0.1), respectively. Empirical power is calculated from 5,000 simulation samples as in the Wilcoxon rank sum test.

Table 7.2(b) reports the results of the linear trend test. Under H_0, our trend test has empirical type I error probabilities close to the nominal $\alpha = .05$. It also has a good power when sample size is large or ρ is small.

In the second part of simulation, we apply the trend test to four sample ($K = 4$) binomial data with cluster randomization. Le (1988) proposes a test for trend of K independent binomial trials with correlated binary data based on a reparameterization of Rosner's (1982) correlated binary data model. In order to obtain a modified chi-square statistic he applies a correction factor for intracluster correlation to the variance. This method is applicable only when the cluster size is two. Donner and Banting (1989) propose an adjustment of the chi-square test for linear trend. To account for the dependency of binary observations, they assume that the number of successes within

TABLE 7.3

Empirical power of the linear trend test for four independent binomial groups: under H_0, $p_1 = p_2 = p_3 = p_4 = 0.5$ and, under H_1, $(p_1, p_2, p_3, p_4) = (0.34, 0.42, 0.50, 0.58)$. Le = Le (1988) and DB = Donner and Banting (1988)

		Cluster size = 2				Cluster size = 2, 4, 6, or 8			
		H_0		H_1		H_0		H_1	
ρ	n	New	Le	New	Le	New	DB	New	DB
0	40	0.054	0.052	0.340	0.347	0.055	0.043	0.712	0.716
	80	0.056	0.054	0.627	0.632	0.048	0.042	0.941	0.944
	160	0.052	0.052	0.899	0.898	0.055	0.050	0.999	0.999
0.3	40	0.054	0.053	0.309	0.310	0.047	0.054	0.433	0.465
	80	0.050	0.050	0.551	0.555	0.046	0.048	0.714	0.727
	160	0.049	0.049	0.843	0.844	0.053	0.054	0.953	0.958
0.6	40	0.052	0.051	0.270	0.274	0.054	0.059	0.308	0.324
	80	0.049	0.048	0.489	0.491	0.049	0.048	0.539	0.545
	160	0.045	0.045	0.778	0.779	0.048	0.050	0.835	0.840

each cluster follows a beta-binomial distribution with ICC ρ. In our simulations, a balanced allocation of clusters ($n_k = 10$, 20, or 40) to each of four groups is considered. In comparison with Le's method, all clusters have two subunits, while in that with Donner and Banting's method, clusters have $m_i = 2$, 4, 6, or 8 subunits with equal probabilities, i.e., $f(2) = f(4) = f(6) = f(8) = 1/4$. Each subunit in clusters takes on a binary outcome. The marginal success probabilities are $p_k = 0.5$ under H_0 and $(p_1, p_2, p_3, p_4) = (0.34, 0.42, 0.50, 0.58)$ under H_1. $B = 5{,}000$ simulation samples are generated under each design setting to calculate an empirical power.

Table 7.3 summarizes the simulation results of the linear trend test to compare 4 groups of clustered binary data. Note that the score test, Le's test, and Donner and Banting's test all have empirical type I error rates close to the nominal 0.05. Under H_1, the three tests have similar empirical power.

Le's method assumes that all clusters have two subunits so that clusters with a missing subunit should be deleted in analysis. Note also that Donner and Banting's method assumes equal ICC among clustered binary observations in all treatment groups. However, the score test can be used under any cluster size distribution and with different ICCs among treatment groups. Furthermore, Le's method and Donner and Banting's method can be used only for K sample binomial data with cluster randomization, whereas our methods can be used for two-sample multinomial data as well as K ordered binomial data with subunit or cluster randomization.

Real Data Examples

A lung transplant study (Song et al. 1997)[6] was conducted to investigate whether one surgery method has better healing after transplant than the other. Twenty-six rabbits ($n = 26$) were randomized into two surgery methods, $n_1 = 12$ to one surgery and $n_2 = 14$ to the other. Degree of healing was measured by the degree of inflammation in $m_i = 2$ sites (subunits) of surgery area on each animal (cluster). The inflammation degree was graded as no, some, much, or very much inflammation so that the response variable is ordered quadrinomial ($K = 4$). Table 7.4 displays the resulting data of two sample multinomial with cluster randomization. For the Wilcoxon's rank sum test, statistic (and p-value) is $Z = -1.16$ (0.246) by our method and -1.53 (0.126) by the standard method ignoring dependency. For the linear trend test, we have $Z = -1.15$ (0.250) by our proposed method and -1.67 (0.095) by the standard method ignoring dependency.

In an otolaryngologic trial (Mandel et al. 1982), children (clusters) suffering from otitis media with effusion in both ears (subunits) were randomized into either cefaclor or amoxicillin group. After 14-day course of treatment, the children's ears were examined to determine if cured or not. Table 7.5 reports the data of cefaclor group taken from Mandel et al. (1982). Children's age was partitioned into three groups ($K = 3$) so that the data have three groups with clustered binary outcomes. The estimated cure rates are $\hat{p}_1 = 0.50$ for the children younger than 2 years of age, $\hat{p}_2 = 0.59$ for the children between 2 to 5 years of age, and $\hat{p}_3 = 0.88$ for the children of 6 years of age or older. The

TABLE 7.4

Lung Transplant Data: Inflammation grade of 12 animals in surgery A and 14 animals in surgery B. Two digits are for two sites, and for each digit 0 = no, 1 = some, 2 = much, and 3 = very much inflammation

Surgery A	00 00 00 11 11 11 21 21 22 22 32 32
B	11 11 11 11 12 12 12 12 22 22 22 22 22 32

TABLE 7.5

Status of otitis media with effusion after 14-day course of cefaclor

	Age (years)		
# of ears cured	**< 2**	**$2 - 5$**	**≥ 6**
2	8	10	3
1	2	6	1
0	8	6	0

p-values for the linear trend test are 0.206, 0.205, and 0.147 by Le's, Donner and Banting's, and the score tests, respectively.

Chi-Square Test for $R \times C$ Contingency Tables with Clustered Categorical Data

In the previous section, we assume that there are two rows and K columns are ordered. In this section, we extend this setting to the cases where both rows and columns can be either ordered or nominal categorical.

Let A and B be two categorical variables with R and C categories, respectively. Typically, variable A is an outcome variable with R different categories and variable B is C different treatment groups. We can classify subjects based on the two variables using an $R \times C$ contingency table. With the data summarized by a contingency table, we usually test the independence of the two variables using a χ^2-test that was proposed by Pearson (1922) and corrected later by Fisher (1922). If one variable is to distinguish different treatment groups and the other is to represent categorical outcomes, then independence of the two variables is identical to no treatment effect in the outcome variable.

In this section, the clustered categorical data can be from either cluster randomization or subunit randomization trials. We first discuss a simple test statistic for 2×2 tables and extend it to $R \times C$ tables.

Analysis of 2×2 Tables

We first discuss the χ^2 test for 2×2 tables. Extension to $R \times C$ tables will be discussed in the following section. At first, we briefly review the standard χ-squared test for 2×2 tables with independent binary data.

Independent Observation Case

Observations of two binary variables A and B are collected from n independent subjects, and the resulting frequencies are summarized in a 2×2 contingency table with rows and columns to classify two outcomes of A and B, respectively. To be more specific, suppose that the columns stand for two treatment groups and the rows stand for binary outcomes such as response and non-response. Let n_{rc} denote the observed frequency for (r, c)-cell ($r = 1, 2$, $c = 1, 2$) and $n_{r\cdot} = n_{r1} + n_{r2}$ and $n_{\cdot c} = n_{1c} + n_{2c}$. Let p_{rc} ($0 < p_{rc} < 1$) be the probability for (r, c)-cell, $p_{r\cdot} = p_{r1}+p_{r2}$ and $p_{\cdot c} = p_{1c}+p_{2c}$. We have $p_{11} + p_{12} + p_{21} + p_{22} = p_{1\cdot} + p_{2\cdot} = p_{\cdot 1} + p_{\cdot 2} = 1$. These probabilities are estimated by $\tilde{p}_{rc} = n_{rc}/n$, $\tilde{p}_{r\cdot} = n_{r\cdot}/n$, and $\tilde{p}_{\cdot c} = n_{\cdot c}/n$, respectively.

The null hypothesis for testing independence of the two variables is expressed as

$$H_0 : p_{rc} = p_{r\cdot}p_{\cdot c} \text{ for } r = 1, 2, c = 1, 2,$$

and that for homogeneity of two groups, i.e., equal response rate for two groups (columns), is expressed as

$$H_0 : P_1 = P_2,$$

where $P_c = p_{1c}/p_{\cdot c}$. In the former case no margin totals are fixed, whereas in the latter case the column totals are fixed at 1. However, it is easy to show that both hypotheses are identical and the standard large sample statistics for testing these hypotheses are exactly the same.

If n subjects are independent, it is known that $\sqrt{n}(\tilde{p}_{11} - \tilde{p}_{1\cdot}\tilde{p}_{\cdot 1})$ has an asymptotically normal distribution with mean 0 under H_0. Its variance can be consistently estimated by $\tilde{s}^2 = n_{1\cdot}n_{\cdot 1}n_{2\cdot}n_{\cdot 2}/n^4$. Therefore, under $H_0 : p_{rc} = p_{r\cdot}p_{\cdot c}$, the test statistic

$$X^2 = \frac{n(\tilde{p}_{11} - \tilde{p}_{1\cdot}\tilde{p}_{\cdot 1})^2}{\tilde{s}^2}$$

has asymptotically χ^2 distribution with 1 degree of freedom. We reject the null hypothesis when X^2 is larger than $\chi^2_{1,1-\alpha}$, where $\chi^2_{k,1-\alpha}$ is the $100(1-\alpha)$ percentile of χ^2 distribution with k degrees of freedom.

Clustered Data Case

Now, we consider cases where binary data are clustered either from cluster randomization trials or subunit randomization trials. Let n denote the number of clusters, m_i the number of subunits in cluster $i(= 1, ..., n)$, and $M = \sum_{i=1}^{n} m_i$ the total number of subunits. Also, let $x_{rc,ij}$ be a binary random variable taking 1 if observation $j(= 1, ..., m_i)$ in cluster i belongs to (r, c)-cell and 0 otherwise. Note that $\sum_{r=1}^{2}\sum_{j=1}^{2} x_{rc,ij} = 1$.

In clustered data, $x_{rc,ij}$ and $x_{r'c',i'j'}$ may be correlated if $i = i'$, although are independent if $i \neq i'$. We assume that subunits within each cluster are exchangeable in each treatment group. Denote $\mathrm{P}(x_{rc,ij} = 1) = p_{rc}$. In order to test the null hypothesis $H_0 : p_{rc} = p_{r\cdot}p_{\cdot c}, r = 1, 2, c = 1, 2$, we propose to use the test statistic

$$W = \sqrt{n}(\hat{p}_{11} - \hat{p}_{1\cdot}\hat{p}_{\cdot 1}), \tag{7.2}$$

where $\hat{p}_{rc} = M^{-1}\sum_{i=1}^{n}\sum_{j=1}^{m_i} x_{rc,ij}$, $\hat{p}_{r\cdot} = \hat{p}_{r1} + \hat{p}_{r2}$, and $\hat{p}_{\cdot c} = \hat{p}_{1c} + \hat{p}_{2c}$. As in the independent data case, these sample proportions are consistent estimators of the corresponding proportion parameters as $n \to \infty$.

Under H_0, by Appendix B, W is asymptotically normal with mean 0. A consistent estimator of its variance is given as

$$s^2 = n^{-1}\sum_{i=1}^{n}\hat{\epsilon}_i^2,$$

where

$$\hat{\epsilon}_i = nM^{-1}\sum_{j=1}^{m_i}(x_{11,ij} - \hat{p}_{1\cdot}x_{\cdot 1,ij} - \hat{p}_{\cdot 1}x_{1\cdot,ij} + \hat{p}_{1\cdot}\hat{p}_{\cdot 1}),$$

$x_{r\cdot,ij} = x_{r1,ij} + x_{r2,ij}$ and $x_{\cdot c,ij} = x_{1c,ij} + x_{2c,ij}$. Hence, we can reject H_0 when the absolute value of W/s is larger than $z_{1-\alpha/2}$ or equivalently when its squared value is larger than $\chi^2_{1,1-\alpha}$.

In a cluster randomization study with n_k clusters assigned to group $k(=1,2)$, let m_{ki} and y_{ki} denote the size and the number of successes of cluster $i(=1,...,n_k)$, respectively. Then, the χ^2 test statistic $(W/s)^2$ for testing $H_0 : P_1 = P_2$ is expressed as

$$\frac{(\hat{P}_1 - \hat{P}_2)^2}{\sum_{k=1}^{2} M_k^{-2} \sum_{i=1}^{n_k} (y_{ki} - m_{ki}\hat{P})^2},$$

where $M_k = \sum_{i=1}^{n_k} m_{ki}$ and $\hat{P}_k = M_k^{-1} \sum_{i=1}^{n_k} y_{ki}$ are the total number of units and estimated success probability in group k, respectively, and $\hat{P} = M^{-1} \sum_{k=1}^{2} \sum_{i=1}^{n_k} y_{ki}$ is the pooled estimator of success probability. In an ophthalmologic study, it can be shown that this test statistic is exactly the same as Rosner's (1982) test statistic if equal number of patients are randomized into two treatment groups and all patients contribute both eyes. Furthermore, this test statistic is identical to the test statistics Z in Chapter 4 under cluster randomization and that in Chapter 5 under subunit randomization with equal weights to subunits.

Extension to $R \times C$ Tables

Now, we extend the methods to $R \times C$ contingency tables with clustered categorical data. For $R \times C$ contingency tables, Jung et al. (2003) propose a unified testing method that can be used for various design settings resulting in different types of clustered categorical data. The variables defining columns and rows of contingency tables can be either ordinal or nominal in this section.

For $r = 1,...,R$ and $c = 1,...,C$, let $x_{rc,ij}$ be a binary random variable taking 1 if unit $j(=1,...,m_i)$ in cluster $i(=1,...,n)$ belongs to (r,c)-cell and 0 otherwise. Let $\mathrm{P}(x_{rc,ij} = 1) = p_{rc}$, $x_{r\cdot,ij} = \sum_{c=1}^{C} x_{rc,ij}$, and $x_{\cdot c,ij} = \sum_{r=1}^{R} x_{rc,ij}$. As in 2×2 tables, $x_{rc,ij}$ and $x_{r'c',i'j'}$ may be correlated if $i = i'$, although are independent if $i \neq i'$.

To test $H_0 : p_{rc} = p_{r\cdot}p_{\cdot c}$, $r = 1,...,R$, $c = 1,...,C$ against a general alternative, we use the statistic $\sqrt{n}(\hat{p}_{rc} - \hat{p}_{r\cdot}\hat{p}_{\cdot c})$, where $\hat{p}_{rc} = M^{-1} \sum_{i=1}^{n} \sum_{j=1}^{m_i} x_{rc,ij}$, $\hat{p}_{r\cdot} = \sum_{c=1}^{C} \hat{p}_{rc}$, and $\hat{p}_{\cdot c} = \sum_{r=1}^{R} \hat{p}_{rc}$. Noting that the *RC* statistics have only $(R-1)(C-1)$ degrees of freedom, let $W = (W_1, ..., W_{(R-1)(C-1)})^T$ be the vector of statistics with the full degrees of freedom of $(R-1)(C-1)$. For example, for $\{(r,c), 1 \leq r \leq R-1, 1 \leq c \leq C-1\}$ and $l = r + (c-1)(R-1)$, let $W_l = \sqrt{n}(\hat{p}_{rc} - \hat{p}_{r\cdot}\hat{p}_{\cdot c})$.

Then, we have

$$W_l = n^{-1/2} \sum_{i=1}^{n} \epsilon_{li} + o_p(1)$$

under H_0, where

$$\epsilon_{li} = nM^{-1} \sum_{j=1}^{m_i} (x_{rc,ij} - p_{r\cdot} x_{\cdot c,ij} - p_{\cdot c} x_{r\cdot,ij} + p_{r\cdot} p_{\cdot c})$$

as in Appendix B. Let $\epsilon_i = (\epsilon_{1i}, ..., \epsilon_{(R-1)(C-1),i})^T$ be a random vector of dimension $(R-1)(C-1)$, then $W = n^{-1/2} \sum_{i=1}^{n} \epsilon_i + o_p(1)$. Since $\epsilon_1, ..., \epsilon_n$ are independent 0-mean random vectors under H_0, by the multivariate central limit theorem, W is asymptotically normal with mean 0. Its variance-covariance matrix can be consistently estimated by $\hat{\Sigma} = n^{-1} \sum_{i=1}^{n} \hat{\epsilon}_i \hat{\epsilon}_i^T$, where $\hat{\epsilon}_i$ are obtained from ϵ_i by replacing p_{rc} with $\hat{p}_{rc}$. Hence, for large n, we can reject H_0 if $W^T \hat{\Sigma}^{-1} W$ is larger than $\chi^2_{(R-1)(C-1),1-\alpha}$.

Simulation Studies

The testing methods reviewed in this section are based on asymptotic results for large number of clusters. In order to investigate the finite sample property of these methods, simulation studies are conducted.

Total n = 20, 40, 60, or 80 clusters are equally randomized into two treatment groups. That is, each group has the number of clusters equal to $n_k = 10$, 20, 30, or 40. Within each group, cluster sizes of 2, 4, 6, and 8 are equally distributed with PMF $f(2) = f(4) = f(6) = f(8) = 1/4$. Beta-binomial distributions were used to generate the number of successes in clustered subunits. We assume common intracluster correlation coefficient ρ = 0, 0.3, 0.6, or 0.9 in two groups. For each setting, 5,000 simulation samples are generated.

Our test statistic, Donner and Banting's (1988) method (DB), Rao and Scott's (1992) method (RS), and Pearson's chi-square statistic are applied to each sample. Empirical power of a test is estimated as the proportion of samples out of 5,000 rejecting the null hypothesis of no difference with nominal level $\alpha = 0.05$.

The simulation results are summarized in Table 7.6. Under the null hypothesis $H_0 : P_1 = P_2 = 0.5$, our new test statistic is always within the 95% confidence limit of the nominal level 0.05 ± 0.006. However, Donner and Banting's test tends to be anticonservative when $\rho = 0$. Rao and Scott's test is anticonservative when sample size is small or when $\rho = 0$. As expected, the Pearson's chi-square test yields too high values of empirical type I errors when $\rho > 0$.

Under the alternative hypothesis $H_1 : P_1 = 0.2, P_2 = 0.5$, there are negligible differences in empirical powers among the proposed test, Donner and Banting's test, and Rao and Scott's test. As pointed out by Rao and Scott (1992), Donner and Banting's method assumes equal intracluster correlation between treatment groups. As shown in Chapter 3, Donner and Banting's test works well even under unequal intracluster correlations when two groups have an equal number of clusters. Different cluster size distribution does not seriously affect the validity of Donner and Banting's test.

TABLE 7.6

Empirical power in cluster randomization case: under $H_0 : P_1 = P_2 = 0.5$ and $H_1 : P_1 = 0.2, P_2 = 0.5$

		H_0				H_1			
ρ	n^*	New	DB	RS	X^2	New	DB	RS	X^2
0	10	0.053	0.061	0.057	0.040	0.878	0.884	0.885	0.903
	20	0.054	0.062	0.060	0.055	0.994	0.995	0.994	0.995
	30	0.054	0.055	0.055	0.045	10.000	10.000	10.000	10.000
	40	0.055	0.057	0.057	0.051	10.000	10.000	10.000	10.000
0.3	10	0.052	0.051	0.055	0.193	0.522	0.510	0.525	0.794
	20	0.052	0.056	0.059	0.225	0.821	0.826	0.819	0.952
	30	0.053	0.053	0.053	0.211	0.940	0.939	0.936	0.990
	40	0.051	0.054	0.053	0.218	0.983	0.983	0.982	0.999
0.6	10	0.058	0.053	0.061	0.334	0.372	0.350	0.383	0.750
	20	0.054	0.054	0.058	0.347	0.625	0.630	0.623	0.902
	30	0.053	0.050	0.052	0.323	0.797	0.793	0.784	0.966
	40	0.054	0.054	0.054	0.339	0.889	0.891	0.887	0.989
0.9	10	0.054	0.044	0.053	0.415	0.294	0.266	0.312	0.731
	20	0.056	0.057	0.057	0.426	0.497	0.495	0.484	0.870
	30	0.054	0.051	0.050	0.402	0.661	0.650	0.639	0.938
	40	0.056	0.056	0.056	0.408	0.786	0.785	0.777	0.972

DB = Donner and Banting (1989)
RS = Rao and Scott (1922)
X^2 = Pearson's chi-square test for independence
n^* = number of clusters per group
ρ = intracluster correlation coefficient

Real Data Analysis

Our testing method can be used to analyze diverse types of clustered categorical data. Four data sets from real experiments were taken to demonstrate the application of our method and to compare its analysis result with those by existing methods if applicable.

For the lung transplant study by Song et al. (1997) with data presented in Table 7.4, let $W = (W_1, W_2, W_3)^T$ be the test statistics of $\sqrt{n}(\hat{p}_{rc} - \hat{p}_{r\cdot}\hat{p}_{\cdot c})$ for $(r, c) = (1, 1)$, (2, 1), and (3, 1). Then, we have $W = (0.317, -0.121, -0.256)^T$,

$$\hat{\Sigma} = \begin{pmatrix} 0.0290 & -0.0127 & -0.0144 \\ -0.0127 & 0.0446 & -0.0262 \\ -0.0144 & -0.0262 & 0.0395 \end{pmatrix}$$

and the resulting χ^2 statistic with 3 degrees of freedom is $W^T \hat{\Sigma}^{-1} W = 4.812$ (p-value = 0.19). Ignoring dependency, we have the regular χ^2 statistic value 9.009 (p-value = 0.03), leading to a wrong conclusion.

In an ophthalmologic study (Berson et al. 1980), patients with retinitis pigmentosa from different families were classified into the genetic types of autosomal dominant RP (DOM), autosomal recessive RP (AR), sex-linked

TABLE 7.7

Eye infection data from Rosner (1982): Distribution of the number of affected eyes for persons in each genetic type. For each genetic type, n_l denotes the number of persons with l (=0, 1, 2) affected eyes

	n_0	n_1	n_2	Total
DOM	15	6	7	28
AR	7	5	9	21
SL	3	2	14	19
ISO	67	24	57	148

TABLE 7.8

Teratology study (Weil 1970, Williams 1975); Number, m, of pups alive at 4 days and the number, y, of pups that survived the 21-day lactation period for each litter

Group	(y, m)							
Control	(13,13)	(12,12)	(9,9)	(9,9)	(8,8)	(8,8)	(12,13)	(11,12)
	(9,10)	(9,10)	(8,9)	(11,13)	(4,5)	(5,7)	(7,10)	(7,10)
Treated	(12,12)	(11,11)	(10,10)	(9,9)	(10,11)	(9,10)	(9,10)	(8,9)
	(8,9)	(4,5)	(7,9)	(4,7)	(5,10)	(3,6)	(3,10)	(0,7)

RP (SL), and isolate RP (ISO). One of study objectives was to compare the proportion of affected eyes among the four groups of genetic types. In this case, patients are clusters and eyes of each patient are subunits. Rosner (1982) proposed a χ^2-test for homogeneity adjusting for ICC between the two eyes of each patient. Rosner's method assumes that all subjects contribute two eyes to study, so that subjects who have missing information from one eye should be excluded from analysis. Table 7.7 displays the data reported in Rosner (1982). We want to test if the prevalence of affected eyes varies among four different genetic type groups. The χ^2 test statistic (and p-value) with 3 degrees of freedom is 10.69 (0.01) by our method discussed in the section 'Extension to $R \times C$ Tables', 11.36 (0.01) by Rosner (1982), and 11.43 (0.01) by Donner (1989). Hence, we obtain the same conclusions from all testing methods.

In an experiment (Weil 1970; Williams 1975), a group of $n_1 = 16$ pregnant female rats were fed a control diet during pregnancy and lactation, while another of $n_2 = 16$ pregnant female rats were fed a diet treated with a chemical. For each litter, the number of pups alive at day 4 and the number of pups that survived the 21-day lactation period are shown in Table 7.8. Rao and Scott's (1992) χ^2 test statistic (and p-value) with 1 degree of freedom for testing equal survival probability between two dietary groups was 4.04 (0.044), showing significant result. In contrast, those were 2.89 (0.089) by our method and 2.76 (0.097) by Donner (1989), both methods giving not so significant results.

In order to investigate which method gives most reliable testing result for the data, a bootstrap study was conducted. A bootstrap data set was generated by randomly sampling $n_k = 16$ litters (clusters) for each group with replacement from the pooled original data. Test statistics by the three methods were calculated from each of 5,000 bootstrapped data sets. Bootstrap p-value of a testing method was obtained as the proportion of bootstrap samples whose test statistic values exceed the observed one from the original data. The bootstrap p-values were 0.072 by Rao and Scott's method, 0.090 by our method and 0.086 by Donner's method. All three test statistics by bootstrap method give insignificant results. Further, note that Rao and Scott's results based on the asymptotic distribution and bootstrap samples show much discrepancy, whereas ours based on the two approaches match well.

References

Agresti A. An introduction to categorical data analysis. Wiley, New York, 1996.

Armitage P. Tests for linear trends in proportions and frequencies. Biometrics 1955; 11: 375–386.

Barnett JD, Melloneg JT, Gray JL, Towie HJ. Comparison of freeze-dried bone allograft and porous hydroxylapatite in human periodontal defects. Journal of Periodontology 1989; 60: 231–237.

Berson EL, Rosner B, Simonoff E. An outpatient population of retinitis pigmentosa and their normal relatives: Risk factors for genetic typing and detection derived from their ocular examinations. American Journal of ophthalmology 1980; 89: 763–765.

Cochran WG. Some methods of strengthening the common χ^2 tests. Biometrics 1954; 10: 417–451.

Donner A. Statistical methods in ophthalmology: an adjusted chi-square approach. Biometrics 1989; 45: 605–611.

Donner A, Banting D. Adjustment of frequently used chi-square procedures for the effect of site-to-site dependencies in the analysis of dental data. Journal of Dental Research 1989; 68(9): 1350–1354.

Fisher, R. A. (1922). On the interpretation of X^2 from contingency tables, and the calculation of P. Journal of the Royal Statistical Society 85 (1): 87–94.

George EO, Kodell RL. Tests of independence, treatment heterogeneity, and dose-related trend with exchangeable binary data. Journal of the American Statistical Association 1996; 91: 602–1611.

Jung SH, Kang SH. Tests for 2xK contingency tables with clustered ordered categorical data. Statistics in Medicine 2001; 20: 785–794.

Jung SH, Kang SH, Ahn C. Chi-square test for RxC contingency tables with clustered data. Journal of Biopharmaceutical Statistics 2003; 13: 241–251.

Le CT. Testing for linear trends in proportions using correlated otolaryngology or ophthalmology data. Biometrics 1988; 44: 299–303.

Lehmann EL. Nonparametrics. Holden-Day, San Francisco, 1975.

Liang KY, Zeger SL. Longitudinal data analysis using generalized linear models. Biometrika 1986; 73: 13–22.

Mandel E, Bluestone CD, Rockette HE, Blatter MM, Reisinger KS, Wucher FP, Harper J. Duration of effusion after antibiotic treatment for acute Otitis Media: comparison of Cefaclor and Amoxicillin. Pediatric Infectious Diseases 1982; 1: 310–316.

Mann HB, Whitney DR. On a test of whether one of two random variables is stochastically larger than the other. Annals of Mathematical Statistics 1947; 18: 50–60.

Pearson K. On the χ^2 test of goodness of fit. Biometrika 1922; 14: 186–191.

Rao JNK, Scott AJ. A simple method for the analysis of clustered binary data. Biometrics 1922; 48: 577–585.

Rosner B. Statistical methods in ophthalmology: An adjustment for the intraclass correlation between eyes. Biometrics 1982; 38: 105–114.

Song WY, Lee YJ, Hwang SW, Kim HY, Yoo BH, Kwon OJ. Comparative study of tracheal anastomotic techniques. Korean Journal of Thoracic and Cardiovascular Surgery 1997; 30: 1–7.

Weil CS. Selection of the valid number of sampling units and a consideration of their combination in toxicological studies involving reproduction, teratogenesis or carcinogenesis. Food and Cosmetics Toxicology 1970; 8: 177–182.

Wilcoxon F. Individual comparisons by ranking methods. Biometrics 1945; 1: 80–83.

Williams DA. The analysis of binary responses from toxicological experiments involving reproduction and teratogenicity. Biometrics 1975; 31: 949–952.

Yates F. The analysis of contingency tables with groups based on quantitative characters. Biometrika 1948; 35: 176–181.

Appendix A. Asymptotic normality of test statistic (7.1)

At first, we prove the asymptotic normality of (7.1) for the two-sample test with K ordered categorical outcome, where δ_{ij} are fixed and x_{ij} are random. Let $E(x_{ij}|\delta_{ij}) = \mu_{2-\delta_{ij}}$. The hypotheses for a score test can be represented as $H_0 : \mu_1 = \mu_2 (= \mu)$ and $H_1 : \mu_1 \neq \mu_2$. Under H_0,

$$\bar{x}_1 - \bar{x}_2 = \frac{1}{n} \sum_{i=1}^{n} \epsilon_i,$$

where

$$\epsilon_i = n \sum_{j=1}^{m_i} (\frac{\delta_{ij}}{M_1} - \frac{1-\delta_{ij}}{M_2})(x_{ij} - \mu).$$

Without loss of generality, we assume that the scores are standardized so that they have variances of order $O_p(1)$. For example, in the Wilcoxon rank sum test, we use the ranks divided by n as scores. Under H_0, $\epsilon_1, ..., \epsilon_n$ are independent random variables with mean 0 so that, by the central limit theorem, $\sqrt{n}(\bar{x}_1 - \bar{x}_2)$ converges to the normal distribution with mean 0 and variance σ^2 that can be consistently estimated by

$$\hat{\sigma}^2 = \frac{1}{n} \sum_{i=1}^{n} \hat{\epsilon}_i^2,$$

where $\hat{\epsilon}_i$ are obtained from ϵ_i by replacing μ with $\bar{x}$. The standardization of scores is needed only to derive the asymptotic normality. The divided constants of a proper order of n will be canceled out from the numerator and the denominator of the standardized test statistic so that this step is unnecessary in data analysis.

Now let's consider the trend test for K ordered groups with clustered binary outcome. Given scores $s_1, ..., s_K$ for K groups, the trend test considers model

$$E(\delta_{ij}) = \beta_0 + \beta_1 x_{ij}$$

to test $H_0 : \beta_1 = 0$ against $H_1 : \beta_1 \neq 0$. Recall that x_{ij} is the score of subunit j in cluster i, i.e., $x_{ij} = s_k$ if subunit j in cluster i belongs to group k. Note that the role of dependent and independent variables is switched here from that of two sample multinomial cases discussed above. Generalized estimating equation estimator (Liang and Zeger 1986) of β_1 based on independent working correlation structure is given as

$$\hat{\beta}_1 = \frac{\sum_{i=1}^{n}\sum_{j=1}^{m_i}(x_{ij}-\bar{x})\delta_{ij}}{\sum_{i=1}^{n}\sum_{j=1}^{m_i}(x_{ij}-\bar{x})^2}.$$

Let $\varepsilon_i = \sum_{j=1}^{m_i}(x_{ij}-\bar{x})(\delta_{ij}-\beta_0)$. Since the numerator of $\hat{\beta}_1$ is expressed as $\sum_{i=1}^{n}\varepsilon_i$ and $\varepsilon_1, ..., \varepsilon_n$ are independent random variables with mean 0, by the central limit theorem, $\hat{\beta}_1$ is approximately normal with mean 0 and variance

$$\hat{\sigma}^2(\hat{\beta}_1) = \frac{\sum_{i=1}^{n}\hat{\varepsilon}_i^2}{\{\sum_{i=1}^{n}\sum_{j=1}^{m_i}(x_{ij}-\bar{x})^2\}^2}$$

under H_0, where $\hat{\varepsilon}_i = \sum_{j=1}^{m_i}(x_{ij}-\bar{x})(\delta_{ij}-\hat{\beta}_0)$ and $\hat{\beta}_0 = M_1/M$, which is a consistent estimator of β_0 under H_0. Now, it is easy to show that $\hat{\beta}_1/\hat{\sigma}(\hat{\beta}_1)$ equals $Z = \sqrt{n}(\bar{x}_1 - \bar{x}_2)/\hat{\sigma}$ in (7.1).

Appendix B. Asymptotic normality of test statistic (7.2)

Under $H_0 : p_{rc} = p_{r\cdot}p_{\cdot c}$, we have

$$\sqrt{n}(\hat{p}_{11} - \hat{p}_{1\cdot}\hat{p}_{\cdot 1}) = \sqrt{n}(\hat{p}_{11} - p_{11}) - \sqrt{n}\hat{p}_{1\cdot}(\hat{p}_{\cdot 1} - p_{\cdot 1}) - \sqrt{n}p_{\cdot 1}(\hat{p}_{1\cdot} - p_{1\cdot}).$$

Since $\hat{p}_{1\cdot}$ is a consistent estimator of $p_{1\cdot}$, we have

$$\sqrt{n}(\hat{p}_{11} - \hat{p}_{1\cdot}\hat{p}_{\cdot 1}) = \sqrt{n}(\hat{p}_{11} - p_{11}) - p_{1\cdot}\sqrt{n}(\hat{p}_{\cdot 1} - p_{\cdot 1}) - p_{\cdot 1}\sqrt{n}(\hat{p}_{1\cdot} - p_{1\cdot}) + o_p(1),$$

which becomes

$$\sqrt{n}M^{-1}\sum_{i=1}^{n}\sum_{j=1}^{m_i}\{x_{11,ij} - p_{11} - p_{1\cdot}(x_{\cdot 1,ij} - p_{\cdot 1}) - p_{\cdot 1}(x_{1\cdot,ij} - p_{1\cdot})\}.$$

Hence we have

$$\sqrt{n}(\hat{p}_{11} - \hat{p}_{1\cdot}\hat{p}_{\cdot 1}) = n^{-1/2}\sum_{i=1}^{n} \epsilon_i + o_p(1),$$

where

$$\epsilon_i = nM^{-1}\sum_{j=1}^{m_i}\{x_{11,ij} - p_{11} - p_{1\cdot}(x_{\cdot 1,ij} - p_{\cdot 1}) - p_{\cdot 1}(x_{1\cdot,ij} - p_{1\cdot})\},$$

which is equal to

$$\epsilon_i = nM^{-1}\sum_{j=1}^{m_i}(x_{11,ij} - p_{1\cdot}x_{\cdot 1,ij} - p_{\cdot 1}x_{1\cdot,ij} + p_{1\cdot}p_{\cdot 1})$$

under H_0.

Since ϵ_i $(i = 1, ..., n)$ are independent 0-mean random variables, by the central limit theorem, $\sqrt{n}(\hat{p}_{11} - \hat{p}_{1\cdot}\hat{p}_{\cdot 1})$ has an asymptotically normal distribution with mean 0. Its variance can be consistently estimated by $s^2 = n^{-1}\sum_{i=1}^{n}\hat{\epsilon}_i^2$, where $\hat{\epsilon}_i$ are obtained from ϵ_i by replacing p_{rc} with $\hat{p}_{rc}$.

8

Clustered Continuous Data

In the previous chapters, we investigated analysis methods for clustered binary data. In this chapter, we consider clustered continuous data for cluster randomization trials (CRTs) and subunit randomization trials (SRTs). We investigate modified two-sample t-test and its sample size formula for each type of trials. We also investigate a trial with clustered pairs.

Cluster Randomization Trials

Modified t-Test for CRTs

We investigate two-sample test on population mean between two arms for CRTs. Suppose that n_k clusters are randomized into treatment arm $k(=1,2)$. Cluster $i(=1,...,n_k)$ in arm k has m_{ki} subunits. A continuous observation x_{kij} is collected from subunit $j(=1,...,m_{ki})$ of cluster i in arm k. Usually subunits in each cluster share a common frailty, so that they tend to have a positive intracluster correlation coefficient (ICC) $\rho_k = \text{corr}(x_{kij}, x_{kij'})$ for $j \neq j'$.

Let $x_{ki} = \sum_{j=1}^{m_{ki}} x_{kij}$, $M_k = \sum_{i=1}^{n_k} m_{ki}$, $M = M_1 + M_2$ and $n = n_1 + n_2$. Asymptotic theories are applied with respect to large n, while $\max_{k=1}^{2} \max_{i=1}^{n_k} m_{ki} \leq c < \infty$.

For $\mu_k = E(x_{kij})$, we want to test $H_0: \mu_1 = \mu_2$ against $H_1: \mu_1 \neq \mu_2$. An unbiased and consistent estimator of θ_k is given as

$$\bar{x}_k = M_k^{-1} \sum_{i=1}^{n_k} \sum_{j=1}^{m_{ki}} x_{kij} = M_k^{-1} \sum_{i=1}^{n_k} x_{ki}.$$

We could consider weighted estimators as discussed in Chapter 2 for binary data, but we limit our discussion to this estimator assigning equal weights to subunits in this chapter.

Under H_0, we have

$$\sqrt{M}(\bar{x}_1 - \bar{x}_2) = \sqrt{M} \left\{ M_1^{-1} \sum_{i=1}^{n_1} \epsilon_{1i} - M_2^{-1} \sum_{i=1}^{n_2} \epsilon_{2i} \right\} \tag{8.1}$$

DOI: 10.1201/9781003221951-8

where $\epsilon_{ki} = x_{ki} - m_{ki}\mu_k$. Since $(\epsilon_{ki}, i = 1, ..., n_k, k = 1, 2)$ are independent 0-mean random variables, by the central limit theorem, $\sqrt{M}(\bar{x}_1 - \bar{x}_2)$ converges to a normal distribution with mean 0 and variance σ^2 that can be consistently estimated by

$$\hat{\sigma}^2 = M\left(M_1^{-2}\sum_{i=1}^{n_1}\hat{\epsilon}_{1i}^2 + M_2^{-2}\sum_{i=1}^{n_2}\hat{\epsilon}_{2i}^2\right),$$

where $\hat{\epsilon}_{ki} = x_{ki} - m_{ki}\bar{x}$ and $\bar{x} = M^{-1}\sum_{k=1}^{2}\sum_{i=1}^{n_k} x_{ki}$.

We reject H_0 if

$$\frac{\sqrt{M}|\bar{x}_1 - \bar{x}_2|}{\hat{\sigma}} > z_{1-\alpha/2}.$$

Sample Size Calculation for CRTs

Let $n_k/n = p_k$ denote the allocation proportion, and $\bar{m}$ and $\bar{\bar{m}}$ denote the first and second moments, respectively, of the cluster size distribution. If the cluster size is constant $m_{ki} = m$, then we have $\bar{m} = m$ and $\bar{\bar{m}} = m^2$.

Assuming that two arms have the same variance v and the same ICC $\rho = \text{corr}(x_{kij}, x_{kij'})$ for $j \neq j'$, we have

$$\text{var}(\epsilon_{ki}) = v\{m_{ki} + m_{ki}(m_{ki} - 1)\rho\}$$

so that the variance of $\bar{x}_k$ is given as

$$\sigma_k^2 = v\{1 + (\bar{\bar{m}}/\bar{m} - 1)\rho\}$$

and, from (8.1),

$$\sigma^2 = \frac{\bar{m}v}{p_1p_2}\{1 + (\bar{\bar{m}}/\bar{m} - 1)\rho\}$$

Assuming that two arms have the same variances and under nearby alternative hypothesis $\mu_1 - \mu_2 = o_p(1/\sqrt{n})$, $\hat{\sigma}^2$ converges to the common variance σ^2. So, under $H_1 : \mu_1 - \mu_2 = \delta(> 0)$, the power is given as

$$\begin{aligned} 1 - \beta =& P\left(\frac{\sqrt{M}|\bar{x}_1 - \bar{x}_2|}{\hat{\sigma}} > z_{1-\alpha/2}\middle|\delta\right) \\ \approx& P\left(\frac{\sqrt{M}(\bar{x}_1 - \bar{x}_2 - \delta)}{\sigma} > z_{1-\alpha/2} - \frac{\delta\sqrt{M}}{\sigma}\middle|\delta\right) \\ =& \bar{\Phi}\left(z_{1-\alpha/2} - \frac{\delta\sqrt{M}}{\sigma}\right) \end{aligned} \quad (8.2)$$

since $\sqrt{M}(\bar{x}_1 - \bar{x}_2 - \delta)/\sigma \sim N(0, 1)$ under H_1, where $\bar{\Phi}(\cdot)$ is the survival function of $N(0, 1)$ distribution.

From (8.2), we have

$$z_{1-\alpha/2} - \frac{\delta_0\sqrt{M}}{\sigma} = -z_{1-\beta}.$$

By solving this equation with respect to the required number of subunits M, we obtain

$$M = \frac{\sigma^2(z_{1-\alpha/2}+z_{1-\beta})^2}{\delta^2} = \frac{v(z_{1-\alpha/2}+z_{1-\beta})^2}{p_1p_2\delta^2}\text{IF},$$

where IF $= 1 + (\bar{\bar{m}}/\bar{m} - 1)\rho$ denote the inflation factor due to intracluster dependency.

Since $M = n\bar{m}$, the required number of patients is given as

$$n = \frac{v(z_{1-\alpha/2}+z_{1-\beta})^2}{\bar{m}p_1p_2\delta^2}\text{IF}.$$

The sample size increases in $1-\beta$, $|p_1 - 1/2|$, and variance of cluster size distribution $\bar{\bar{m}} - \bar{m}^2$ when the mean $\bar{m}$ is fixed, and decreases in α and δ.

Subunit Randomization Trials

Modified t-Test for SRTs

We investigate two-sample test on population mean between two arms for SRTs. Suppose that there are n clusters, and cluster $i(=1,...,n)$ has m_i subunits of which m_{ki} are randomized into treatment arm k $(m_{1i}+m_{2i}=m_i)$. A continuous observation x_{kij} is collected from subunit $j(=1,...,m_{ki})$ of cluster i randomized into arm $k(=1,2)$. Usually subunits in each cluster share a common frailty, so that they tend to have a positive ICC $\rho_k = \text{corr}(x_{kij}, x_{kij'})$ for $j \neq j'$ and $\rho_{12} = \text{corr}(x_{1ij}, x_{2ij'})$. We assume that $\rho_1 = \rho_2 = \rho$.

Let $x_{ki} = \sum_{j=1}^{m_{ki}} x_{kij}$, $M_k = \sum_{i=1}^{n} m_{ki}$, and $M = M_1 + M_2$. Asymptotic theories are applied with respect to large n, while $\max_{k=1}^{2}\max_{i=1}^{n} m_i \le c < \infty$.

For $\mu_k = E(x_{kij})$, we want to test $H_0: \mu_1 = \mu_2$ against $H_1: \mu_1 \neq \mu_2$. An unbiased and consistent estimator of θ_k is given as

$$\bar{x}_k = M_k^{-1}\sum_{i=1}^{n}\sum_{j=1}^{m_{ki}} x_{kij} = M_k^{-1}\sum_{i=1}^{n} x_{ki}.$$

We could consider weighted estimators as discussed in Chapter 4 for binary data, but we limit our discussion to this estimator assigning equal weights to subunits in this chapter.

Under H_0, we have

$$\sqrt{M}(\bar{x}_1 - \bar{x}_2) = \sqrt{M}\sum_{i=1}^{n} \epsilon_i, \tag{8.3}$$

where $\epsilon_i = \epsilon_{1i} - \epsilon_{2i}$ and $\epsilon_{ki} = (x_{ki} - m_{ki}\mu_k)/M_k$. Since $\epsilon_1, ..., \epsilon_n$ are independent 0-mean random variables, by the central limit theorem, $\sqrt{M}(\bar{x}_1 - \bar{x}_2)$ converges to a normal distribution with mean 0 and variance σ^2 that can be consistently estimated by

$$\hat{\sigma}^2 = M\sum_{i=1}^{n} \hat{\epsilon}_i^2,$$

where $\hat{\epsilon}_i = \hat{\epsilon}_{1i} - \hat{\epsilon}_{2i}$, $\hat{\epsilon}_{ki} = (x_{ki} - m_{ki}\bar{x})/M_k$, and $\bar{x} = M^{-1}\sum_{i=1}^{n}\sum_{k=1}^{2} x_{ki}$.

We reject H_0 if

$$\frac{\sqrt{M}|\bar{x}_1 - \bar{x}_2|}{\hat{\sigma}} > z_{1-\alpha/2}.$$

Sample Size Calculation for SRTs

Let $m_{ki}/m_i = p_k$ denote the allocation proportion, and $\bar{m}$ and $\bar{\bar{m}}$ denote the first and second moments, respectively, of the distribution of cluster sizes m_i. If the cluster size is constant $m_i = m$, then we have $\bar{m} = m$ and $\bar{\bar{m}} = m^2$.

By the definition of ϵ_i, we have

$$\text{var}(\epsilon_i) = \text{var}(\epsilon_{1i}) + \text{var}(\epsilon_{2i}) - 2\text{cov}(\epsilon_{1i}, \epsilon_{2i}).$$

Assuming that two arms have the same variance $v = v_k = \text{var}(x_{kij})$ and the same ICC $\rho = \rho_k = \text{corr}(x_{kij}, x_{kij'})$, we have

$$\text{var}(\epsilon_{ki}) = M_k^{-2}\{\sum_{j=1}^{m_{ki}} \text{var}(x_{kij}) + \sum_{j \neq j'}^{m_{ki}} \text{cov}(x_{kij}, x_{kij'})\} = M_k^{-2} v\{m_{ki} + m_{ki}(m_{ki}-1)\rho\}$$

and

$$\text{cov}(\epsilon_{1i}, \epsilon_{2i}) = (M_1M_2)^{-1}\sum_{j=1}^{m_{1i}}\sum_{j'=1}^{m_{2i}} \text{cov}(\epsilon_{1ij}, \epsilon_{2ij'}) = (M_1M_2)^{-1} m_{1i}m_{2i}v\rho_{12}.$$

Since $m_{ki} = p_k m_i$, $n^{-1}\sum_{i=1}^{n} m_i \to \bar{m}$, and $n^{-1}\sum_{i=1}^{n} m_i^2 \to \bar{\bar{m}}$, from (8.3), we have

$$\begin{aligned}\sigma^2 &= \bar{m}\left[\frac{v\{p_1\bar{m} + (p_1^2\bar{\bar{m}} - p_1\bar{m})\rho\}}{p_1^2\bar{m}^2} + \frac{v\{p_2\bar{m} + (p_2^2\bar{\bar{m}} - p_2\bar{m})\rho\}}{p_2^2\bar{m}^2} - \frac{2vp_1p_2\bar{\bar{m}}\rho_{12}}{p_1p_2\bar{m}^2}\right] \\ &= v\left\{(1-\rho)/(p_1p_2) + 2(\rho - \rho_{12})\bar{\bar{m}}/\bar{m}\right\}.\end{aligned}$$

Under nearby alternative hypothesis $p_1 - p_2 = o_p(1/\sqrt{n})$, $\hat{\sigma}^2$ converges to σ^2. So, under $H_1 : \mu_1 - \mu_2 = \delta(> 0)$, the power is given as

$$\begin{aligned} 1-\beta =& P\left(\frac{\sqrt{M}|\bar{x}_1 - \bar{x}_2|}{\hat{\sigma}} > z_{1-\alpha/2}\Big|\delta\right) \\ \approx& P\left(\frac{\sqrt{M}(\bar{x}_1 - \bar{x}_2 - \delta)}{\sigma} > z_{1-\alpha/2} - \frac{\delta\sqrt{M}}{\sigma}\Big|\delta\right) \\ =& \bar{\Phi}\left(z_{1-\alpha/2} - \frac{\delta\sqrt{M}}{\sigma}\right) \end{aligned} \tag{8.4}$$

since $\sqrt{M}(\bar{x}_1 - \bar{x}_2 - \delta)/\sigma \sim N(0,1)$ under H_1.

From (8.4), we have

$$z_{1-\alpha/2} - \frac{\delta_0\sqrt{M}}{\sigma} = -z_{1-\beta}.$$

By solving this equation with respect to the required number of subunits M, we obtain

$$M = \frac{\sigma^2(z_{1-\alpha/2} + z_{1-\beta})^2}{\delta^2}.$$

Since $M = n\bar{m}$, the required number of patients is given as

$$n = \frac{\sigma^2(z_{1-\alpha/2} + z_{1-\beta})^2}{\bar{m}\delta^2}.$$

An Equivalence Test for Clustered Pair Data

We discuss an equivalence test for clustered pair data using a real study. An objective of this study is to show that body temperature measured by a wearable is equivalent to that by a conventional thermometer for patients with hematologic malignancies undergoing an immunotherapy. Toward this end, body temperature of each patient will be measured regularly each day for 14 days while wearing the wearable device, and a measurement by the conventional thermometer is paired with that by the wearable collected at the measurement time. The wearable collects data passively and its measurements will be double-blinded.

Equivalence Test

Suppose that there are n patients. For patient $i(= 1, ..., n)$, body temperature is measured m_i times by a conventional thermometer ($k = 1$) or the wearable ($k = 2$). Let x_{kij} denote the body temperature measured by device $k(= 1, 2)$

at time $j(= 1, ..., m_i)$ from patient i and let $d_{ij} = x_{1ij} - x_{2ij}$. For $E(d_{ij}) = \delta$ and an equivalence limit $\delta_0(> 0)$, we want to drive an equivalence test $H_0 : |\delta| \geq \delta_0$ against $H_1 : |\delta| < \delta_0$ using

$$\hat{\delta} = \frac{1}{M}\sum_{i=1}^{n}\sum_{j=1}^{m_i} d_{ij},$$

where $M = \sum_{i=1}^{n} m_i$. We will reject H_0 if a $100(1-\alpha)\%$ two-sided CI of δ is within $[-\delta_0, \delta_0]$.

Note that

$$\sqrt{M}(\hat{\delta} - \delta) = \frac{1}{\sqrt{M}}\sum_{i=1}^{n} \epsilon_i,$$

where $\epsilon_i = \sum_{j=1}^{m_i}(d_{ij} - \delta)$. Since $\epsilon_1, ..., \epsilon_n$ are independent 0-mean random variables, by the central limit theorem, $\sqrt{M}(\hat{\delta} - \delta)$ converges to normal with mean 0 and variance σ^2 that can be consistently estimated by

$$\hat{\sigma}^2 = \frac{1}{M}\sum_{i=1}^{n} \hat{\epsilon}_i^2,$$

where $\hat{\epsilon}_i = \sum_{j=1}^{m_i}(d_{ij} - \hat{\delta})$.

Hence, a $100(1-\alpha)\%$ two-sided CI of δ is given as

$$\hat{\delta} \pm z_{1-\alpha/2}\frac{\hat{\sigma}}{\sqrt{M}}.$$

We reject H_0 if $\hat{\delta} - z_{1-\alpha/2}\hat{\sigma}/\sqrt{M} > -\delta_0$ and $\hat{\delta} + z_{1-\alpha/2}\hat{\sigma}/\sqrt{M} < \delta_0$, or equivalently if $-\delta_0 + z_{1-\alpha/2}\hat{\sigma}/\sqrt{M} < \hat{\delta} < \delta_0 - z_{1-\alpha/2}\hat{\sigma}/\sqrt{M}$.

Sample Size Calculation for the Equivalence Test

We want to derive a sample size formula for the equivalence test introduced above under $H_0 : \delta = \delta_0$ and $H_1 : \delta = 0$. Under H_1, $\hat{\delta}$ strongly converges to 0 so that

$$\hat{\sigma}^2 = \frac{1}{M}\sum_{i=1}^{n} \text{var}(\sum_{j=1}^{m_i} d_{ij}) + o_p(1)$$

converges to

$$\sigma^2 = v\{1 + (\bar{\bar{m}}/\bar{m} - 1)\rho\} \tag{8.5}$$

where $\bar{m}$ and $\bar{\bar{m}}$ are the first and second moment of the cluster size (m_i) distribution, $v = \text{var}(d_{ij})$ and $\rho = \text{corr}(d_{ij}, d_{ij'})$ for $j \neq j'$ is the ICC.

Hence, for given M, the power is given as

$$\begin{aligned}
1-\beta &= P\left(\hat{\delta} - z_{1-\alpha/2}\frac{\hat{\sigma}}{\sqrt{M}} < -\delta_0 \text{ and } \hat{\delta} + z_{1-\alpha/2}\frac{\hat{\sigma}}{\sqrt{M}} > \delta_0 \middle| \delta = 0\right)\\
&= P\left(-\delta_0 + z_{1-\alpha/2}\frac{\hat{\sigma}}{\sqrt{M}} < \hat{\delta} < \delta_0 - z_{1-\alpha/2}\frac{\hat{\sigma}}{\sqrt{M}} \middle| \delta = 0\right)\\
&\approx P\left(z_{1-\alpha/2} - \frac{\delta_0\sqrt{M}}{\sigma} < \frac{\hat{\delta}\sqrt{M}}{\sigma} < -z_{1-\alpha/2} + \frac{\delta_0\sqrt{M}}{\sigma} \middle| \delta = 0\right)\\
&= 1 - 2\bar{\Phi}\left(-z_{1-\alpha/2} + \frac{\delta_0\sqrt{M}}{\sigma}\right)
\end{aligned}$$

since $\sqrt{M}\hat{\delta}/\sigma \sim N(0,1)$ under H_1. Hence, we have

$$-z_{1-\alpha/2} + \frac{\delta_0\sqrt{M}}{\sigma} = z_{1-\beta/2}.$$

By solving this equation with respect to the required number of subunits M, we obtain

$$M = \frac{\sigma^2(z_{1-\alpha/2} + z_{1-\beta/2})^2}{\delta_0^2}.$$

Since $M = n\bar{m}$, the required number of patients is given as

$$n = \frac{\sigma^2(z_{1-\alpha/2} + z_{1-\beta/2})^2}{\bar{m}\delta_0^2}. \tag{8.6}$$

Note that, in sample size formula for equivalence tests, $z_{1-\beta}$ replaces $z_{\{1-\beta\}}$ that is used for standard two-sample tests with one-sided alternative hypotheses.

Example

In (8.5), v and ρ are calculated from the differences d_{ij} so that it is difficult to specify them in sample size calculation unless we have pilot data. It is easier to specify the variance and correlation coefficient of the measurements x_{kij} instead.

Let $s^2 = \text{var}(x_{kij})$. Note that

$$v = \text{var}(d_{ij}) = 2s^2(1-\rho_b) \tag{8.7}$$

and, for $j \neq j'$,

$$\begin{aligned}
\rho \times v &= \text{cov}(d_{ij}, d_{ij'}) = \text{cov}(x_{1ij} - x_{2ij}, x_{1ij'} - x_{2ij'})\\
&= s^2(\rho_1 - 2\rho_{12} + \rho_2),
\end{aligned} \tag{8.8}$$

where $\rho_b = \text{corr}(x_{1ij}, x_{2ij})$, $\rho_k = \text{corr}(x_{kij}, x_{kij'})$, and $\rho_{12} = \text{corr}(x_{1ij}, x_{2ij'})$. Assuming that $\rho_1 = \rho_2 (= \rho_k)$, from (8.7) and (8.8), we have

$$\rho = \frac{\rho_1 - 2\rho_{12} + \rho_2}{2(1 - \rho_b)} = \frac{\rho_k - \rho_{12}}{1 - \rho_b}. \tag{8.9}$$

From (8.7) and (8.9), to specify σ^2, we need to specify ρ_b, ρ_k, and ρ_{12} in addition to s^2. To this end, we consider an additive model for measurements

$$x_{kij} = \mu_k + a_k + b_i + c_j + e_{kij}, \tag{8.10}$$

where $\mu_k = E(x_{kij})$ is a constant, and a_k, b_i, c_j, and e_{kij} are independent 0-mean random variables denoting the device-specific error, patient effect, measurement time effect, and pure measurement error, respectively. For c_j, we could consider a time series model, but we assume an exchangeable model for simplicity here. By this model, we have

$$\begin{aligned} s^2\rho_b &= \text{cov}(x_{1ij}, x_{2ij}) = \text{var}(b_i) + \text{var}(c_j), \\ s^2\rho_k &= \text{cov}(x_{kij}, x_{kij'}) = \text{var}(a_k) + \text{var}(b_i), \\ s^2\rho_{12} &= \text{cov}(x_{1ij}, x_{2ij'}) = \text{var}(b_i). \end{aligned} \tag{8.11}$$

It is likely that $\text{var}(e_{kij}) < \min(\text{var}(a_k), \text{var}(c_j), \text{var}(b_i))$. Furthermore, from model (8.10), $s^2 = \text{var}(a_k) + \text{var}(b_i) + \text{var}(c_j) + \text{var}(e_{kij})$. Hence, assuming $\text{var}(a_k) = \text{var}(b_i) = \text{var}(c_j) = 0.3s^2$ and $\text{var}(e_{kij}) = 0.1s^2$, by (8.11), we have $\rho_b = \rho_k = 0.6$, and $\rho_{12} = 0.3$. Plugging these in (9), we have $\rho = 0.75$.

On the other hand, it is known that the variance of body temperature distribution in adults is about $s^2 = 1.25^2$ in Celsius depending on the gender, body location measured, and measurement time. Hence, from (7), $v = 2 \times 1.25^2 \times (1 - 0.6) = 1.25$. We set the equivalence limit at the half of the population standard deviation, i.e., $\delta_0 = 1.25/2 = 0.625$.

Furthermore, we expect $m_i = 50 \sim 90$ measurement pairs per patient. Assuming discrete uniform distribution for cluster sizes, we have $\bar{m} = 70$ and $\bar{\bar{m}} = 5{,}040$. The true cluster distribution is expected to be close to a normal distribution which has a smaller variance than the uniform distribution so that the sample size calculation assuming a discrete uniform distribution will be conservative.

From (8.5), we have $\sigma^2 = 1.25 \times \{1 + (5{,}040/70 - 1) \times 0.75\} = 67.8125$. For $\alpha = 0.05$ and $1 - \beta = 0.85$, we have $z_{1-\alpha/2} = 1.96$ and $z_{1-\beta/2} = 1.44$. Hence, from (8.6), we have

$$n = \frac{67.8125 \times (1.96 + 1.44)^2}{70 \times 0.625^2} = 29.$$

9

Inference of Medians for Paired Survival Data

Paired data have simplest form of clustered data under subunit randomization. There are examples of paired survival times. For example, in a clinical trial conducted to evaluate the influence of HL-A antigens on the survival of allogeneic grafts (defined as the time to rejection of the graft) in burned patients (Batchelor and Hackett 1970), the donor and recipient were matched for ABO blood groups and either closely or poorly matched for HL-A antigens. The survival times of closely matched and poorly matched skin grafts were observed with both types of graft applied to each patient. The objective of the study was to discover whether avoiding severe HL-A incompatibility will extend allograft survival time. The survival times of closely matched graft and poorly matched graft will be correlated for each patient.

Another example is a cancer clinical trial with a crossover design conducted at the Mayo Clinic (Mahood et al. 1991). The trial was designed to test oral cryotherapy for preventing stomatitis in patients receiving chemotherapy that included the drug 5-fluorouracil (5FU). The patients were randomized either to no intervention or to cryotherapy at the time of 5FU administration. Cryotherapy involves the placing of ice chips in the mouth 5 minutes prior to each dose of 5FU and continuously swishing the ice around the mouth for a total of 30 minutes, replenishing the ice chips when necessary. The patients who returned for a second course of chemotherapy with identical drug doses crossed over to the alternative therapy (cryotherapy or control). The response outcome of the study was the time to occurrence of stomatitis. Therefore, each patient had two correlated failure time observations, one from each course of chemotherapy.

Mean survival time is usually not estimable with censoring because the right tail of the survival distribution beyond the maximum censoring time is not observed. As an alternative, median has been a popular measure for summarizing the survival distribution of a group of patients. Methods of calculating confidence intervals for median with possibly censored failure time data have been studied extensively for single groups, e.g., Brookmeyer and Crowley (1982), Efron (1981), Emerson (1982), Reid (1981), Simon and Lee (1981), and Slud et al. (1984).

DOI: 10.1201/9781003221951-9

Wang and Hettmansperger (1990) and Su and Wei (1993) proposed inference methods of median failure times for two independent samples of survival data. Jung and Su (1995) extended the confidence interval method of Su and Wei (1993) method to paired two-sample survival data. We also investigate a statistical testing method of equality of two paired median survival times.

For patient $i(=1, ..., n)$ condition $k(=1, 2)$, let T_{ki} and C_{ki} be the survival time and censoring time, respectively. Under random right censoring, we observe (X_{ki}, δ_{ki}), where $X_{ki} = \min(T_{ki}, C_{ki})$ and $\delta_{ki} = l(T_{ki} \leq C_{ki})$, called an event indicator taking 1 if an event is observed and 0 otherwise. Also, for patient i under condition k, $Y_{ki}(t) = I(X_{ki} \geq t)$ denotes the at-risk process and $N_{ki}(t) = \delta_{ki} I(X_{ki} \leq t)$ denotes the event process, and $Y_k(t) = \sum_{i=1}^n Y_{ki}(t)$ and $N_k(t) = \sum_{i=1}^n N_{ki}(t)$.

Let $S_k(t) = P(T_{ki} \geq t)$ and $\Lambda_k(t) = -\log S_k(t)$ be the marginal survival function and cumulative hazard function, respectively, for the kth condition with median θ_k. Based on $\{(X_{ki}, \delta_{ki}), i = 1, ..., n\}$, $\hat{S}_k(t)$ is estimated by the Kaplan-Meier (1958) estimator, $\hat{S}_k(t)$. The sample median $\hat{\theta}_k$ can be obtained by solving the equation $\hat{S}_k(\theta) = 1/2$ with respect to θ. When there is an interval satisfying this equation, we take the lowest point as the sample median to avoid the ambiguity, although taking any solution does not affect the asymptotic results. Under mild conditions, $\hat{\theta}_k$ is a consistent estimator of θ_k. Furthermore, $\sqrt{n}(\hat{\theta}_1 - \theta_1, \hat{\theta}_2 - \theta_2)$ has an asymptotically normal distribution with mean 0. With matched survival data, the covariance matrix depends on the unknown bivariate density function. In general, however, it is difficult to estimate the density function in the presence of censoring. We overcome this barrier by using an estimating equation method for (θ_1, θ_2).

Statistical Testing on Paired Median Survival Times

We want to test $H_0 : \theta_1 = \theta_2$ against $H_1 : \theta_1 \neq \theta_2$ for a paired survival times. By (9.A3) and (9.A4) of Appendix, $\sqrt{n}\{\hat{S}_1(\theta_1) - 1/2, \hat{S}_2(\theta_2) - 1/2\}^T$ is asymptotically normal with mean 0 and covariance matrix Σ that can be consistently estimated by

$$\hat{\Sigma} = n^{-1} \sum_{i=1}^{n} \hat{\epsilon}_i \hat{\epsilon}_i^T,$$

where $\hat{\epsilon}_i = (\hat{\epsilon}_{1i}, \hat{\epsilon}_{2i})^T$,

$$\begin{aligned} \hat{\epsilon}_{ki} &= -\frac{n}{2} \int_0^{\hat{\theta}_k} Y_k^{-1}(t)\{dN_{ki}(t) - Y_{ki}(t) d\hat{\Lambda}_k(t) \\ &= -\frac{n}{2} \left[\frac{\delta_{ki} I(X_{ki} \leq \hat{\theta}_k)}{\sum_{i'=1}^n I(X_{ki'} \geq X_{ki})} - \sum_{j=1}^{n} \frac{\delta_{kj} I(X_{kj} \leq \hat{\theta}_k \wedge X_{ki})}{\{\sum_{i'=1}^n I(X_{ki'} \geq X_{kj})\}^2} \right] \end{aligned}$$

and $\hat{\Lambda}_k(t) = \int_0^t dN_k(s)/Y_k(s)$ is the Nelson-Aalen (Nelson 1969; Aalen 1978) estimator of $\Lambda_k(t)$.

We consider the quantity

$$W(\theta_1, \theta_2) = n\{\hat{S}_1(\theta_1) - 1/2, \hat{S}_2(\theta_2) - 1/2\}\hat{\Sigma}^{-1}\left\{\begin{array}{c}\hat{S}_1(\theta_1) - 1/2 \\ \hat{S}_2(\theta_2) - 1/2\end{array}\right\}.$$

Appendix shows that, under H_0, $\inf_\theta W(\theta, \theta)$ is asymptotically identical to $(\hat{\theta}_1 - \hat{\theta}_2)^2/\text{var}(\hat{\theta}_1 - \hat{\theta}_2)$, and is distributed as χ_1^2 distribution. Hence, H_0 is rejected with type I error rate α if $\inf_\theta W(\theta, \theta)$ is larger than $\chi^2_{1,1-\alpha}$. Note that, unlike $\hat{\Sigma}$, $\text{var}(\hat{\theta}_1 - \hat{\theta}_2)$ requires estimation of PDFs, which is not quite feasible with censored survival data. So, for statistical testing, we use $\inf_\theta W(\theta, \theta)$ rather than $(\hat{\theta}_1 - \hat{\theta}_2)^2/\text{var}(\hat{\theta}_1 - \hat{\theta}_2)$.

Sample Size for Testing on Paired Median Survival Times

By Appendix, the test statistic $\inf_\theta W(\theta, \theta)$ is identical to

$$\frac{n(\hat{\theta}_1 - \hat{\theta}_2)^2}{s_{11} + s_{22} - 2s_{12}}$$

following χ_1^2 distribution.

Hence, under $H_1 : \theta_1 \neq \theta_2$, the power of $\inf_\theta W(\theta, \theta)$ is

$$1 - \beta = P\left\{\frac{n(\hat{\theta}_1 - \hat{\theta}_2)^2}{s_{11} + s_{22} - 2s_{12}} \geq \chi_{1,1-\alpha}|H_1\right\}$$

$$= P\left\{\frac{\sqrt{n}|\hat{\theta}_1 - \hat{\theta}_2|}{s_{11} + s_{22} - 2s_{12}} \geq z_{1-\alpha/2}|H_1\right\}$$

$$= P\left\{\frac{\sqrt{n}\{(\hat{\theta}_1 - \theta_1) - (\hat{\theta}_2 - \theta_2)\}}{s_{11} + s_{22} - 2s_{12}} \geq z_{1-\alpha/2} - \frac{\sqrt{n}(\theta_1 - \theta_2)}{s_{11} + s_{22} - 2s_{12}}|H_1\right\}$$

Since

$$\frac{\sqrt{n}\{(\hat{\theta}_1 - \theta_1) - (\hat{\theta}_2 - \theta_2)\}}{s_{11} + s_{22} - 2s_{12}}$$

is $N(0, 1)$ under H_1, we have

$$z_{1-\alpha/2} - \frac{\sqrt{n}(\theta_1 - \theta_2)}{s_{11} + s_{22} - 2s_{12}} = -z_{1-\beta}.$$

By solving this equation with respect to n, the required sample size to detect $H_1 : \theta_1 \neq \theta_2$ with power $1 - \beta$ is given as

$$n = \frac{(s_{11} + s_{22} - 2s_{12})(z_{1-\alpha/2} + z_{1-\beta})^2}{(\theta_1 - \theta_2)^2}. \tag{9.1}$$

Now, we derive the explicit form of s_{kk} and s_{12} for a specified bivariate distribution of (T_{1i}, T_{2i}). From Appendix, $s_{kk} = \text{var}(\sqrt{n}(\hat{\theta}_k - \theta_k))$ and $s_{12} = \text{cov}(\sqrt{n}(\hat{\theta}_1 - \theta_1), \sqrt{n}(\hat{\theta}_2 - \theta_2))$. From (9.A1),

$$\sqrt{n}(\hat{\theta}_k - \theta) = \frac{1}{f_k(\theta_k)}\sqrt{n}\{\hat{S}_k(\theta_k) - 1/2\} + o_p(1),$$

where $f_k(t)$ is the PDF of condition k. By (9.A2) of Appendix,

$$\sqrt{n}(\hat{\theta}_k - \theta) = \frac{1}{2f_k(\theta_k)}n^{-1/2}\sum_{i=1}^{n}\int_0^{\theta_k}\frac{1}{y_k(t)}dM_{ki}(t) + o_p(1), \tag{9.2}$$

where $M_{ki}(t) = dN_{ki}(t) - Y_{ki}(t)d\Lambda_k(t)$. Marginally $M_{ki}(t)$ are 0 mean martingales so that, from (9.1),

$$\begin{aligned} s_{kk} &= \frac{1}{f_k(\theta_k)^2}n^{-1}\sum_{i=1}^{n}\int_0^{\theta_k}\frac{1}{y_k(t)^2}Y_{ki}d\Lambda_k(t) \\ &= \frac{1}{f_k(\theta_k)^2}\int_0^{\theta_k}\frac{1}{y_k(t)}d\Lambda_k(t), \end{aligned}$$

where $y_k(t) = S_k(t)G(t)$ is the limit of $n^{-1}Y_k(t)$ and $G(t) = P(C_{ki} \geq t)$.

On the other hand,

$$\begin{aligned} s_{12} &= \text{cov}(\sqrt{n}(\hat{\theta}_1 - \theta_1), \sqrt{n}(\hat{\theta}_2 - \theta_2)) \\ &= \frac{1}{4nf_1(\theta_1)f_2(\theta_2)}\sum_{i=1}^{n}E(\int_0^{\theta_1}\frac{1}{y_1(t)}dM_{1i}(t)\int_0^{\theta_2}\frac{1}{y_2(t)}dM_{2i}(t) \\ &= \frac{1}{4nf_1(\theta_1)f_2(\theta_2)}\sum_{i=1}^{n}\int_0^{\theta_2}\int_0^{\theta_1}\frac{1}{y_1(t_1)y_2(t_2)}E\{dM_{1i}(t_2)dM_{2i}(t_1)\}, \end{aligned}$$

which is asymptotically identical to

$$s_{12} = \frac{1}{4f_1(\theta_1)f_2(\theta_2)}\int_0^{\theta_2}\int_0^{\theta_1}\frac{1}{y_1(t_1)y_2(t_2)}dA(t_1, t_2)$$

by Appendix A of Jung (2008). Here,

$$dA(t_1, t_2) = \{\lambda(t_1, t_2) - \lambda_{1|2}(t_1|t_2)\lambda_2(t_2) - \lambda_{2|1}(t_2|t_1)\lambda_1(t_1) + \lambda_1(t_1)\lambda_2(t_2)\}dt_1dt_2,$$

$\lambda_k(t) = \partial\Lambda_k(t)/\partial t$, $\lambda_{1|2}(t_1|t_2) = -s_1(t_1,t_2)/S(t_1,t_2)$, $S(t_1,t_2) = P(T_{1i} \geq t_1, T_{2i} \geq t_2)$, and $s_1(t_1,t_2) = \partial S(t_1,t_2)/\partial t_1$.

Note that, although the test statistic $\inf_\theta W(\theta,\theta)$ does not require specification of the marginal and joint survival distributions, its sample size formula does.

Confidence Interval of Ratio or Difference of Median Survival Times

Suppose that we are interested in making inferences about $\tau = g(\theta_1,\theta_2)$ for some given function g, such as the ratio θ_2/θ_1 or the difference $\theta_2-\theta_1$. Furthermore, suppose that θ_2 is expressed as a function of τ and θ_1, say $\theta_2 = h(\tau,\theta_1)$. Consider the quantity

$$W(\tau,\theta_1) = \{\hat{S}_1(\theta_1) - 1/2, \hat{S}_2(h(\tau,\theta_1)) - 1/2\}\hat{\Sigma}^{-1}\left\{\begin{array}{c}\hat{S}_1(\theta_1) - 1/2\\ \hat{S}_2(h(\tau,\theta_1)) - 1/2\end{array}\right\}. \tag{9.3}$$

We use $W(\tau,\theta_1)$ for the confidence interval of τ, but it has a nuisance parameter θ_1. We remove the nuisance parameter by taking the infimum of $W(\tau,\theta_1)$ with respect to θ_1. Using similar arguments as in Appendix, we can show that, under $H_0 : \tau = \tau_0$,

$$w(\tau_0) = \inf_{\theta_1} W(\tau_0,\theta_1) \tag{9.4}$$

asymptotically has a chi-square distribution with one degree of freedom. Hence, with significance level α, $H_0 : \tau = \tau_0$ is rejected if $w(\tau_0) > \chi^2_{1,1-\alpha}$, the 100$(1-\alpha)$ percentile of χ^2_1 distribution.

A 100$(1-\alpha)$% confidence interval for τ is given as

$$\{\tau : w(\tau) < \chi^2_{1,1-\alpha}\}. \tag{9.5}$$

The above method is valid for any continuous survival functions S_1 and S_2. Moreover, the testing and confidence methods are non-parametric in the sense that neither the marginal or bivariate distribution of failure times (T_1, T_2) needs to be specified. The censoring distributions can be different between the two condition groups or correlated within each patient.

Real Data Examples

We demonstrate the above method with the skin-graft trial described above. We use the data shown in Woolson and Lachenbruch (1980) in their Table 9.1.

TABLE 9.1

Empirical coverage probability of 95% confidence intervals for $\tau = \theta_2/\theta_1 = 1$ with $\text{corr}(T_1, T_2) = \rho = 0, 0.2, 0.4$, or 0.6 and censoring probabilities of $(0.15, 0.15)$, $(0.15, 0.3)$, or $(0.3, 0.3)$ in two conditions

		Bivariate log-normal case			Bivariate exponential case		
n	ρ	$(0.15, 0.15)$	$(0.15, 0.3)$	$(0.3, 0.3)$	$(0.15, 0.15)$	$(0.15, 0.3)$	$(0.3, 0.3)$
30	0	0.974	0.977	0.976	0.974	0.976	0.976
	0.2	0.980	0.982	0.982	0.980	0.982	0.980
	0.4	0.984	0.988	0.982	0.986	0.986	0.982
	0.6	0.982	0.986	0.982	0.982	0.984	0.986
50	0	0.970	0.971	0.972	0.969	0.971	0.970
	0.2	0.982	0.980	0.980	0.974	0.968	0.966
	0.4	0.982	0.988	0.976	0.976	0.974	0.968
	0.6	0.978	0.976	0.984	0.974	0.980	0.984
100	0	0.959	0.957	0.961	0.966	0.966	0.970
	0.2	0.972	0.966	0.966	0.968	0.962	0.970
	0.4	0.970	0.968	0.972	0.968	0.972	0.970
	0.6	0.972	0.970	0.974	0.972	0.970	0.974
200	0	0.954	0.953	0.954	0.965	0.965	0.963
	0.2	0.951	0.948	0.951	0.964	0.965	0.959
	0.4	0.955	0.948	0.950	0.966	0.963	0.957
	0.6	0.958	0.944	0.950	0.967	0.969	0.972

The data consist of survival times of closely and poorly matched skin grafts of the same patient.

Let θ_1 and θ_2 be the median survival times for poorly ($k = 1$) and closely ($k = 2$) matched, respectively, skin grafts. There are $n = 11$ patients in the trial. Since the paired observations are made from each patient, it is likely that the censoring times of the paired survival times are identical or highly correlated. The Kaplan-Meier curves for the two groups of skin grafts are presented in Figure 9.1. The estimated median survival times are $\hat{\theta}_1 = 21$ and $\hat{\theta}_2 = 29$ days.

We use expressions (9.A3) and (9.A4) to calculate the estimated covariance matrix $\hat{\Sigma}$, and then the confidence interval according to expressions (1), (2), and (3). For the parameter $\tau = \theta_1/\theta_1$, the point estimate is $\hat{\tau} = \hat{\theta}_2/\hat{\theta}_1 = 1.38$, with a 95% confidence interval of $(0.82, 3.75)$. For the parameter $\tau = \tau_2 - \tau_1$, $\hat{\tau} = \hat{\theta}_2 - \hat{\theta}_1 = 8$ days, with a 95% confidence interval of $(-5, 46)$. For testing $H_0 : \theta_1 = \theta_2$, we have p-value $= 0.318$.

For the second example, we apply the method to data from a clinical trial concerning the bioequivalence of an albuterol metered dose inhaler, indicated for acute bronchospasm. The primary objective of this two sequence two-period crossover trial was to compare the effect of a test product ($k = 2$) with a reference product ($k = 1$). Forty patients ($n = 40$) were randomized into either to take the test product first and then the reference or to take these

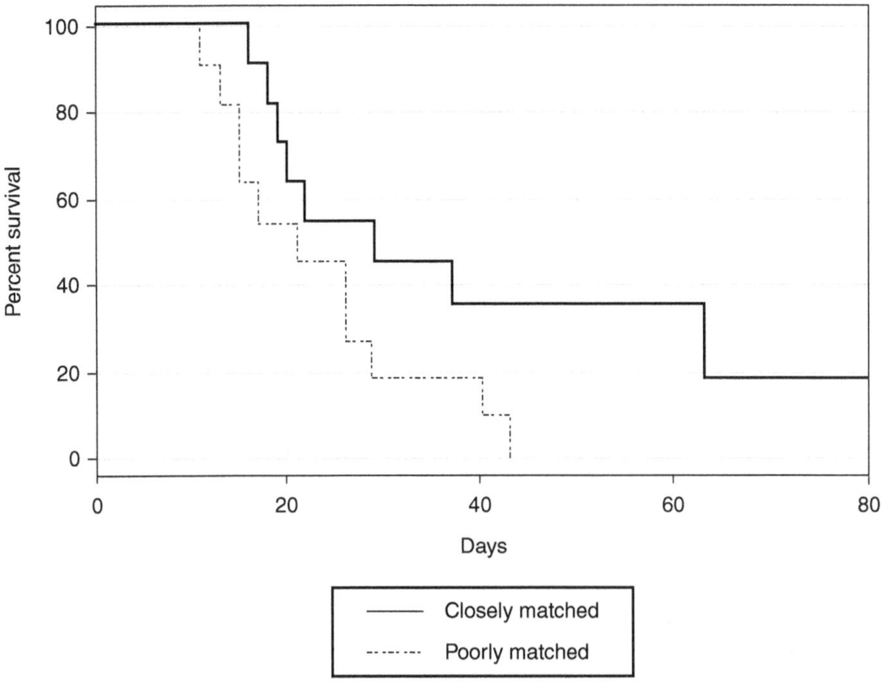

FIGURE 9.1
Survival curves of skin graphs for burn patients that are closely matched and poorly matched.

products in the reverse order. For each patient at each period, the time to response was reported in Table 6 of Liu and Chow (1993). Since a therapeutic response almost always occurs, if at all, within 30 minutes after dosing, the time to response is censored at 30 minutes after the dose administration. Liu and Chow analyzed these data using generalized estimating equations and the proportional hazards model. It is important in a bioequivalence study to calculate the confidence interval for the ratio of the median response times. Under the assumption of no carryover effects (see Liu and Chow 1993), we apply our procedure to compare the median time to response of the two treatments. The Kaplan-Meier survival curves for these two treatments are presented in Figure 9.2. The median response time estimates are $\hat{\theta}_1 = 6.02$ minutes for the reference product and $\hat{\theta}_2 = 8.25$ minutes for the test product. For the parameter $\tau = \theta_2/\theta_1$, the point estimate is $\hat{\tau} = 1.37$, with a 95% confidence interval of $(0.82, 2.38)$. For the parameter $\tau = \theta_2 - \theta_1$, we have $\hat{\tau} = 2.23$ minutes, with a 95% confidence interval of $(-1.21, 7.84)$.

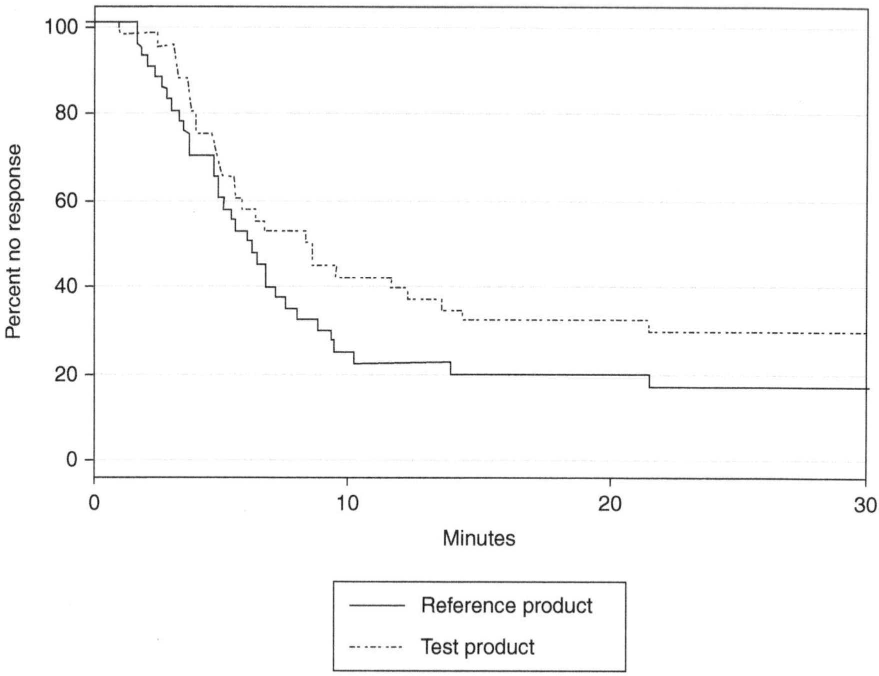

FIGURE 9.2
Time to response for acute bronchospasm patients receiving the test product or the reference product.

Simulation Studies

The method discussed in this section is based on large-sample theory. An extensive simulation study is conducted to investigate the finite-sample performance of the procedure. Simulation results are reported in Table 9.1. The empirical coverage probability of the 95% confidence intervals for $\tau = \theta_2/\theta_1$ is presented for a selection of sample sizes, bivariate survival distributions, and censoring distributions. For survival distributions the bivariate log-normal and a bivariate exponential distributions are generated as follows. Bivariate log-normal random variables are generated by taking an exponential transformation of bivariate normal random variables.

For bivariate exponential distributions, Moran's (1967) algorithm is used. A bivariate exponential distribution is constructed as the joint distribution of $T_1 = (Z_1^2 + Z_2^2)/2$ and $T_2 = (Z_3^2 + Z_4^2)/2$, where (Z_1, Z_3) and (Z_2, Z_4) are mutually independent, but each pair has a bivariate normal distribution with marginal means of 0, variances of 1, and a correlation coefficient of $\sqrt{\rho}$.

It follows that T_l and T_2 have marginally exponential distributions with unit failure rate and that their correlation coefficient is ρ.

Censoring variables were generated as uniformly distributed numbers between 0 and c_k, where c_k for $k = 1, 2$ are chosen to achieve prespecified censoring proportions. The censoring variables for the two treatments are independently generated. For each simulation setting, 1,000 Monte Carlo samples were generated. The method is applied to each sample to construct a 95% confidence interval for $\tau = \theta_2/\theta_1$. An empirical coverage probability is calculated as the proportion of the 1,000 samples whose confidence intervals covering the true value $\tau = 1$.

The results, summarized in Table 9.1, indicate that the large sample approximation to the statistic $w(\tau)$ is fairly satisfactory. The nominal confidence levels are well preserved overall. In small sample cases, however, the method is rather conservative. We also observe that the empirical coverage probabilities approach the nominal level as sample size increases. The simulation results do not seem to depend on the strength of correlation between the two failure time variables.

References

Aalen OO. Nonparametric inference for a family of counting processes. Annals of Statistics 1978; 6: 701–726.

Batchelor JR, Hackett M. HL-A matching in treatment of burned patients with skin allografts. Lancet 1970; 2: 581–583.

Brookmeyer R, Crowley J. A confidence interval for the median survival time. Biometrics 1982; 38: 29–41.

Efron B. Censored data and the bootstrap, Journal of the American Statistical Association 1981; 76: 312–319.

Emerson JD. Nonparametric confidence intervals for the median in the presence of right censoring. Biometrics 1982; 38: 17–27.

Jung SH, Su JQ. Nonparametric estimation for the difference or ratio of median failure times for paired observations. Statistics in Medicine 1995; 14(3): 275–282.

Kaplan EL, Meier P. Nonparametric estimation from incomplete observations. Journal of the American Statistical Association 1958; 53:457–481.

Liu JP, Chow SC. On assessment of bioequivalence for drugs with negligible plasma levels. Biometrical Journal 1993; 35: 109–123.

Mahood DJ, Dose AM, Loprinzi CL, Veeder MH, Athmann, LM, Therneau TM, Sorensen JM, Gainey DK, Mailliard JA, Gusa NL, Finck GK, Johnson C, Goldberg RM. Inhibition of fluorouracil-induced stomatitis by oral cryotherapy. Journal of Clinical Oncology 1991; 9: 449–452.

Moran PAP. Testing for correlation between non-negative variates. Biometrika 1967; 54: 385–394.

Nelson W. Hazard plotting for incomplete failure data. Journal of Quality Technology 1969; 1: 27–52.

Reid N. Estimating the median survival time. Biometrika 1981; 68: 601–608.

Simon R, Lee YJ. Nonparametric confidence limits for survival probabilities and median survival time. Cancer Treatment Reports 1982; 66: 37–42.

Slud EV, Byar DP, Green SB. A comparison of reflected versus test-based confidence interval for the median survival time, based on censored data. Biometrics 1984; 40: 587–600.

Su JQ, Wei LJ. Nonparametric estimation for the difference or ratio of median failure times. Biometrics 1993; 49: 603–608.

Wang JL, Hettmansperger TP. Two-sample inference for median survival times based on one-sample procedures for censored survival data. Journal of the American Statistical Association 1990; 85: 529–536.

Woolson RF, Lachenbruch PA. Rank tests for censored matched pairs. Biometrika 1980; 67: 597–606.

Appendix. Asymptotic distribution of Q

Let $f_k(t) = -\partial S_k(t)/\partial t$ denote the marginal PDF of T_{ki}. Then,

$$\sqrt{n}\{\hat{S}_k(\theta_k) - 1/2\} = f_k(\theta_k)\sqrt{n}(\hat{\theta}_k - \theta_k) + o_p(1). \tag{9.A1}$$

By the marginal martingale representation of the Kaplan-Meier estimator,

$$\sqrt{n}\{\hat{S}_k(\theta_k) - 1/2\} = -\frac{\sqrt{n}}{2}\sum_{i=1}^{n}\int_0^{\theta_k}\frac{1}{Y_k(t)}dM_{ki}(t) + o_p(1), \tag{9.A2}$$

where $M_{ki}(t) = dN_{ki}(t) - Y_{ki}(t)d\Lambda_k(t)$ is marginally a 0-mean martingale.

Since $n^{-l}Y_k(t)$ uniformly converges to $y_k(t) = P(T_{ki} \geq t)P(C_{ki} \geq t)$, (9.A2) is asymptotically identical to

$$-\frac{1}{2\sqrt{n}}\sum_{i=1}^{n}\int_0^{\theta_k}\frac{1}{y_k(t)}dM_{ki}(t).$$

Therefore, $\sqrt{n}\{\hat{S}_1(\theta_1) - 1/2, \hat{S}_1(\theta_2) - 1/2\}$ is asymptotically equivalent to $n^{-1/2}\sum_{i=1}^{n}\epsilon_i$, where $\epsilon_i = (\epsilon_{1i}, \epsilon_{2i})^T$ and

$$\epsilon_{ki} = -\frac{1}{2}\int_0^{\theta_k}\frac{1}{y_k(t)}dM_{ki}(t).$$

Since ϵ_i are IID random vectors with mean 0, from the multivariate central limit theorem, $\sqrt{n}\{\hat{S}_1(\theta_1)-1/2, \hat{S}_2(\theta_2)-1/2\}^T$ is asymptotically normal with mean 0 and covariance matrix Σ that can be consistently estimated by

$$\hat{\Sigma} = \frac{1}{n}\sum_{i=1}^{n}\hat{\epsilon}_i\hat{\epsilon}_i^T, \tag{9.A3}$$

where $\hat{\epsilon}_i = (\hat{\epsilon}_{1i}, \hat{\epsilon}_{2i})^T$ are obtained from $\epsilon_i = (\epsilon_{1i}, \epsilon_{2i})^T$ by replacing θ_k, $y_k(t)$, and $\Lambda_k(t)$ with $\hat{\theta}_k$, $n^{-1}\sum_{i'=1}^{n}Y_{ki'}(t)$, and the Nelson-Aalen (Nelson, 1969;

Aalen, 1978) estimator $\hat{\Lambda}_k(t) = \int_0^t dN_k(s)/Y_k(s)$. That is,

$$\begin{aligned}\hat{\epsilon}_{ki} &= -\frac{n}{2}\int_0^{\hat{\theta}_k} \frac{1}{Y_k(t)} d\hat{M}_{ki}(t) \\ &= -\frac{n}{2}\left[\frac{\delta_{ki} I(X_{ki} \le \hat{\theta}_k)}{\sum_{i'=1}^n I(X_{ki'} \ge X_{ki})} - \sum_{j=1}^n \frac{\delta_{kj} I(X_{kj} \le \hat{\theta}_k \wedge X_{ki})}{\{\sum_{i'=1}^n I(X_{ki'} \ge X_{kj})\}^2}\right], \qquad (9.A4)\end{aligned}$$

where $d\hat{M}_{ki}(t) = dN_{ki}(t) - Y_{ki}(t)d\hat{\Lambda}_k(t)$.

By (9.A1), $\sqrt{n}(\hat{\theta}_1 - \theta, \hat{\theta}_2 - \theta_2)$ is approximately mean 0 and covariance matrix

$$S = \nabla \Sigma \nabla,$$

where ∇ is a 2×2 diagonal matrix with (k,k) component of $f_k(\theta_k)$. Suppose that $\hat{f}_k(t)$ is consistently estimated by $\hat{f}_k(t)$, then $f_k(\theta_k)$ is consistently estimated by $\hat{f}_k(\hat{\theta}_k)$. Let $\hat{\nabla} = \text{diag}(\hat{f}_1(\hat{\theta}_1), \hat{f}_2(\hat{\theta}_2))$. Then, S is consistently estimated by $\hat{S} = \hat{\nabla}\hat{\Sigma}\hat{\nabla}$. Unlike $\hat{\Sigma}$, $\hat{S}$ requires estimation of PDFs, which is not quite feasible with censoring.

Anyway, $W(\theta_1, \theta_2)$ is asymptotically identical to

$$n^{-1}Q(\theta_1, \theta_2) = (\hat{\theta}_1 - \theta_1, \hat{\theta}_2 - \theta_2)\hat{S}^{-1}\begin{pmatrix} \hat{\theta}_1 - \theta_1 \\ \hat{\theta}_2 - \theta_2 \end{pmatrix},$$

so that $\inf_{\theta_1=\theta_2} W(\theta_1, \theta_2)$ is asymptotically identical to $\inf_{\theta_1=\theta_2} Q(\theta_1, \theta_2)$.

Now, we derive the explicit form of $\inf_{\theta_1=\theta_2} Q(\theta_1, \theta_2) = \inf_\theta Q(\theta, \theta)$. Let s_{k_1,k_2} denote the (k_1, k_2)-component of $\hat{S}$. Then, we have

$$\begin{aligned}Q(\theta,\theta) =& \frac{1}{s_{11}s_{22} - s_{12}^2}(\hat{\theta}_1 - \theta, \hat{\theta}_2 - \theta)\begin{pmatrix} s_{22} & -s_{12} \\ -s_{12} & s_{11} \end{pmatrix}\begin{pmatrix} \hat{\theta}_1 - \theta \\ \hat{\theta}_2 - \theta \end{pmatrix} \\ =& \frac{s_{22}(\hat{\theta}_1 - \theta)^2 + s_{11}(\hat{\theta}_2 - \theta)^2 - 2s_{12}(\hat{\theta}_1 - \theta)(\hat{\theta}_2 - \theta)}{s_{11}s_{22} - s_{12}^2} \\ =& \frac{(s_{11} + s_{22} - 2s_{12})\theta^2 - 2\{s_{22}\hat{\theta}_1 + s_{11}\hat{\theta}_2 - s_{12}(\hat{\theta}_1 + \hat{\theta}_2)\}\theta + (s_{22}\hat{\theta}_1^2 + s_{11}\hat{\theta}_2^2 - 2s_{12}\hat{\theta}_1\hat{\theta}_2)}{s_{11}s_{22} - s_{12}^2} \\ =& \frac{1}{s_{11}s_{22} - s_{12}^2}\left[(s_{11} + s_{22} - 2s_{12})\left(\theta - \frac{s_{22}\hat{\theta}_1 + s_{11}\hat{\theta}_2 - s_{12}(\hat{\theta}_1 + \hat{\theta}_2)}{s_{11} + s_{22} - 2s_{12}}\right)^2\right. \\ & \left. - \frac{\{s_{22}\hat{\theta}_1 + s_{11}\hat{\theta}_2 - s_{12}(\hat{\theta}_1 + \hat{\theta}_2)\}^2}{s_{11} + s_{22} - 2s_{12}} + (s_{22}\hat{\theta}_1^2 + s_{11}\hat{\theta}_2^2 - 2s_{12}\hat{\theta}_1\hat{\theta}_2)\right].\end{aligned}$$

Since

$$\frac{s_{11} + s_{22} - 2s_{12}}{s_{11}s_{22} - s_{12}^2} = \frac{E\{(\hat{\theta}_1 - \theta_1) - (\hat{\theta}_2 - \theta_2)\}^2}{\text{var}(\hat{\theta}_1)\text{var}(\hat{\theta}_2)\{1 - \text{corr}(\hat{\theta}_1, \hat{\theta}_2)\}}$$

is larger than or equal to 0, at

$$\theta = \frac{s_{22}\hat{\theta}_1 + s_{11}\hat{\theta}_2 - s_{12}(\hat{\theta}_1 + \hat{\theta}_2)}{s_{11} + s_{22} - 2s_{12}}$$

$Q(\theta, \theta)$ has its minimum

$$\frac{n}{s_{11}s_{22} - s_{12}^2}\left[(s_{22}\hat{\theta}_1^2 + s_{11}\hat{\theta}_2^2 - 2s_{12}\hat{\theta}_1\hat{\theta}_2) - \frac{\{(s_{22} - s_{12})\hat{\theta}_1 + (s_{11} - s_{12})\hat{\theta}_2)\}^2}{s_{11} + s_{22} - 2s_{12}}\right],$$

which is simplified to

$$\frac{\sqrt{n}(\hat{\theta}_1 - \hat{\theta}_2)^2}{s_{11} + s_{22} - 2s_{12}} = \frac{(\hat{\theta}_1 - \hat{\theta}_2)^2}{\mathrm{var}(\hat{\theta}_1 - \hat{\theta}_2)},$$

and has χ_1^2 distribution. Hence, like $\inf_{\theta_1=\theta_2} Q(\theta_1, \theta_2) \sim \chi_1^2$, $\inf_{\theta_1=\theta_2} W(\theta_1, \theta_2)$ has χ_1^2 distribution under $H_0 : \theta_1 = \theta_2$.

10

Rank Tests for Matched Survival Data and Sample Size Calculation

In a clinical trial or an animal study, we may randomize a number of matched subjects, such as twins or litters, to different treatments. The number of treatments equals the number of matched subjects. The intent of matching may be to remove the effect of factors confounded with the treatment effect. Usually matched subjects share common frailties so that they tend to be positively correlated. This results in decrease in the sample size required for testing on the treatment effect. In the context of clustered data, pairs or groups of matched subjects are clusters and matched subjects are subunits. By the study design, subunits are randomized among different treatments.

We assume that the study endpoint is survival time in this chapter. An example of paired survival data is from the skin graft trial for burned patients as we have investigated in Chapter 9. The trial was conducted to evaluate the influence of HL-A antigens on the survival of allogeneic grafts, defined as the time to rejection of graft, in burned patients (Bachelor and Hackett 1970). The donor and recipient were matched for ABO blood groups and either closely and poorly matched for HL-A antigens. The survival times of closely matched and poorly matched skin grafts were observed with both types of graft applied to each patient. The objective was to discover whether avoiding severe HL-A incompatibility will extend the survival time of allograft.

An example of survival data matched for three treatments is from a litter-matched tumorigenesis experiment (Mantel et al. 1977), where three rats in each of 50 female litters were taken and one was randomized into drug-treatment and the other two to controls. The major study objective was to assess whether the time to tumor appearance for the drug-treated group is longer than that for the control group. In this case, animals in a litter share common characteristics so that their times to tumor appearance tend to positively correlated.

In Chapter 9, we used the medians of paired survival times to test on the treatment effect (Jung and Su 1995). In this chapter, we use the weighted rank tests to compare the treatment groups using matched survival times. Numbers of rank tests have been proposed for testing the equality of two survival distributions using independent survival data. Among examples are the Gehan-Wilcoxon test (Gehan 1965), the Prentice-Wilcoxon test (Prentice

DOI: 10.1201/9781003221951-10

1978), the Taron-Ware test (Taron and Ware 1977), and the tests of Harrington and Fleming (1982) class. When two samples are independent, the asymptotic variance of the rank test statistics can be found in Andersen et al. (1982) and Fleming and Harrington (1991).

If matched subjects are randomized into different treatments, the variance of the rank test statistics should be modified to account for possible dependency between the matched survival times. In this chapter, we investigate the rank tests for paired two-sample and matched K-sample tests that were proposed by Jung (1999). We also discuss a sample size method for the paired log-rank tests that presented by Jung (2008).

Weighted Rank Tests for Matched Survival Data

Paired Two-Sample Data Case

Suppose that paired subjects are randomized into two different conditions, such as treatments. Let $\{(T_{1i}, T_{2i}), i = 1, ..., n\}$ be paired survival times with marginal cumulative hazard functions, $\Lambda_1(t)$ and $\Lambda_2(t)$. We want to test the null hypothesis

$$H_0 : \Lambda_1(t) = \Lambda_2(t) \text{ for all } t \geq 0$$

against the alternative hypothesis

$$H_0 : \Lambda_1(t) \neq \Lambda_2(t) \text{ for some } t \geq 0.$$

Since a cumulative hazard function uniquely determines a distribution, H_0 implies that $(T_{1i}, i = 1, ..., n)$ and $(T_{1i}, i = 1, ..., n)$ have the same marginal distributions.

Survival times are subject to censoring due to termination of study or loss to follow-up. Let C_{ki} be the censoring time for the subject who is randomized to condition $k(= 1, 2)$ from pair $i(= 1, ..., n)$. From pair i, we observe $(X_{1i}, X_{2i}, \delta_{1i}, \delta_{2i})$, where $X_{ki} = \min(T_{ki}, C_{ki})$ and $\delta_{ki} = I(T_{ki} \leq C_{ki})$. We assume that $\{(C_{1i}, C_{2i}), i = 1, ..., n\}$ are independent of $\{(T_{1i}, T_{2i}), i = 1, ..., n\}$. C_{1i} and C_{2i} may be correlated or may have different marginal distributions. Let $N_{ki}(t) = \delta_{ki} I(X_{ki} \leq t)$, $Y_{ki}(t) = I(X_{ki} \geq t)$, $N_k(t) = \sum_{i=1}^n N_{ki}(t)$, and $Y_k(t) = \sum_{i=1}^n Y_{ki}(t)$.

Suppose that $H(t)$ is a non-negative bounded predictable process that converges in probability to a bounded left-continuous function $h(t)$ uniformly over $[0, \tau]$, where $\tau = \max\{t : P(X_{1i} \wedge X_{2i} > t) > 0\}$ and $a \wedge b = \min(a, b)$. We consider the class of rank statistics

$$W = \sqrt{n} \int_0^\infty H(t)\{d\hat{\Lambda}_1(t) - d\hat{\Lambda}_2(t)\}, \tag{10.1}$$

where $\hat{\Lambda}_k(t) = \int_0^t Y_k^{-1}(s) dN_k(s)$ is the Nelson-Aalen (Nelson 1969, Aalen 1978) estimator of $\Lambda_k(t)$. The log-rank test (Peto and Peto 1972) uses

$H(t) = n^{-1}Y_1(t)Y_2(t)/\{Y_1(t) + Y_2(t)\}$, the Gehan-Wilcoxon test uses $H(t) = n^{-2}Y_1(t)Y_2(t)$, and the Prentice-Wilcoxon test uses $H(t) = n^{-1}\hat{S}^-(t)Y_1(t)Y_2(t)$, where $\hat{S}^-(t)$ is the left-continuous version of the Kaplan-Meier (1958) estimator in the pooled sample.

Jung (1999) proposed how to calculate the asymptotic normality and the variance of these rank statistics with paired survival data. With possible dependency between paired survival data, Appendix A shows that, under H_0, W is asymptotically normal with mean 0 and variance σ^2 that can be consistently estimated by

$$\hat{\sigma}^2 = \sum_{i=1}^{n} \hat{\epsilon}_i^2,$$

where

$$\begin{aligned}
n^{-1}\hat{\epsilon}_i = & \frac{\delta_{1i}H(X_{1i})}{\sum_{i'=1}^n I(X_{1i'} \geq X_{1i})} \\
& - \sum_{k=1}^{2}\sum_{i'=1}^{n} \frac{\delta_{ki'}I(X_{1i} \geq X_{ki'})H(X_{ki'})}{\{\sum_{j=1}^n I(X_{1j} \geq X_{ki'})\}\{\sum_{k'=1}^2 \sum_{j=1}^n I(X_{k'j} \geq X_{ki'})\}} \\
& - \frac{\delta_{2i}H(X_{2i})}{\sum_{i'=1}^n I(X_{2i'} \geq X_{2i})} \\
& + \sum_{k=1}^{2}\sum_{i'=1}^{n} \frac{\delta_{ki'}I(X_{2i} \geq X_{ki'})H(X_{ki'})}{\{\sum_{j=1}^n I(X_{2j} \geq X_{ki'})\}\{\sum_{k'=1}^2 \sum_{j=1}^n I(X_{k'j} \geq X_{ki'})\}}.
\end{aligned}$$

Hence, we reject H_0 if $|W|/\hat{\sigma} > z_{1-\alpha/2}$.

Matched K-Sample Data Case

More than two treatments may be applied to each subject or the same number of matched subjects. Let $(T_{1i}, ..., T_{Ki})$ be the survival times of K different treatments observed from 'cluster', e.g., litter in the litter-matched animal study, $i(= 1, ..., n)$. For treatment k, $T_{k1}, ..., T_{kn}$ are marginally IID with cumulative hazard function $\Lambda_k(t)$. C_{ki} denotes the censoring time for the subject who is randomized into condition $k(= 1, ..., K)$ from cluster $i(= 1, ..., n)$. From cluster i, we observe $(X_{1i}, \delta_{1i}), ..., (X_{Ki}, \delta_{Ki})$, where $X_{ki} = \min(T_{ki}, C_{ki})$ and $\delta_{ki} = I(T_{ki} \leq C_{ki})$. We assume that $\{(C_{1i}, ..., C_{Ki}), i = 1, ..., n\}$ are independent of $\{(T_{1i}, ..., T_{Ki}), i = 1, ..., n\}$. The censoring times $C_{1i}, ..., C_{Ki}$ in cluster i may be correlated or may have different marginal distributions. Let $N_{ki}(t) = \delta_{ki}I(X_{ki} \leq t)$, $Y_{ki}(t) = I(X_{ki} \geq t)$, $N_k(t) = \sum_{i=1}^n N_{ki}(t)$, $Y_k(t) = \sum_{i=1}^n Y_{ki}(t)$, $N(t) = \sum_{k=1}^K N_k(t)$, and $Y(t) = \sum_{k=1}^K Y_k(t)$.

Suppose that $L(t)$ is a non-negative bounded predictable process that converges in probability to a bounded left-continuous function $\ell(t)$ uniformly

TABLE 10.1

Days of skin graft survival on each burn patient

	Patient										
Match	**1**	**2**	**3**	**4**	**5**	**6**	**7**	**8**	**9**	**10**	**11**
Poor	29	13	15	26	11	17	26	21	43	15	40
Close	37	19	57+	93	16	22	20	18	63	29	60+

+ indicates censoring

over $[0, \tau]$, where $\tau = \max\{t : P(X_{1i} \wedge \cdots \wedge X_{Ki} > t) > 0\}$. For testing $H_0 : \Lambda_1(t) = \cdots = \Lambda_K(t)$ against $H_1 : \Lambda_k(t) \neq \Lambda_{k'}(t)$ for some $1 \leq k < k' \leq K$, we consider the class of rank statistics $\mathbf{W} = (W_1, ..., W_{K-1})^T$ with

$$W_k = \frac{1}{\sqrt{n}} \int_0^\infty Y_k(t)L(t)\{d\hat{\Lambda}_k(t) - d\hat{\Lambda}(t)\}, \tag{10.2}$$

where $\hat{\Lambda}_k(t) = \int_0^t Y_k^{-1}(s)dN_k(s)$ is the Nelson-Aalen (Nelson 1969, Aalen 1978) estimator from group k data and $\hat{\Lambda}(t) = \int_0^t Y^{-1}(s)dN(s)$ is the Nelson-Aalen estimator from the pooled K dependent samples. The log-rank test uses $L(t) = 1$, the Gehan-Wilcoxon test uses $L(t) = n^{-1}Y(t)$, and the Prentice-Wilcoxon test uses $L(t) = \hat{S}^-(t)$, the left-continuous version of the Kaplan-Meier estimator in the pooled K dependent samples. Andersen et al. (1982) proposed to use (10.2) for testing on K independent samples. When $K = 2$, (10.2) is reduced to (10.1).

Appendix B shows that, under H_0, $\mathbf{W}$ is asymptotically normal with mean $\mathbf{0}$ and variance-covariance matrix V that can be consistently estimated under H_0 by

$$\hat{V} = \sum_{i=1}^n \hat{\epsilon}_i \hat{\epsilon}_i^T,$$

where $\hat{\epsilon}_i = (\hat{\epsilon}_{1i}, ..., \hat{\epsilon}_{K-1,i})^T$ and

$$\begin{aligned}
\hat{\epsilon}_{ki} =& \delta_{ki}L(X_{ki}) - \sum_{i'=1}^n \frac{\delta_{ki'}L(X_{ki'})I(X_{ki} \geq X_{ki'})}{\sum_{j=1}^n I(X_{kj} \geq X_{ki'})} \\
&- \sum_{k'=1}^K \frac{\delta_{k'i}L(X_{k'i}) \sum_{i'=1}^n I(X_{ki'} \geq X_{k'i})}{\sum_{l=1}^K \sum_{i'=1}^n I(X_{li'} \geq X_{k'i})} \\
&+ \sum_{k'=1}^K \sum_{i'=1}^n \frac{\delta_{k'i'}L(X_{k'i'})I(X_{k'i} \geq X_{k'i'})\{\sum_{j=1}^n I(X_{kj} \geq X_{k'i'})\}}{\{\sum_{j=1}^n I(X_{k'j} \geq X_{k'i'})\}\{\sum_{l=1}^K \sum_{j=1}^n I(X_{lj} \geq X_{k'i'})\}}.
\end{aligned}$$

We reject H_0 if $Q = \mathbf{W}^T \hat{V}^{-1} \mathbf{W}$ is larger than $\chi^2_{K-1,1-\alpha}$, the $100(1-\alpha)$ percentile of the χ^2 distribution with $K-1$ degrees of freedom.

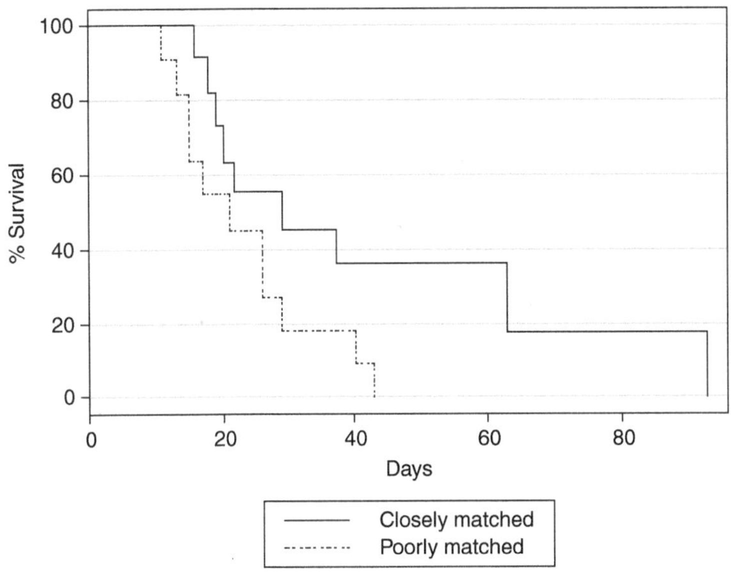

FIGURE 10.1
Survival curves of skin graphs for burn patients that are closely matched and poorly matched.

Real Data Examples

These rank test methods are applied to two sets of real data. The first example is from the skin graft trial that is introduced above. Table 10.1 reports the data taken from Woolson and Lachenbruch (1980). The data consist of survival times, in days, of closely and poorly matched skin grafts on each burn patient. There are $n = 11$ patients in the trial and survival times are censored for two closely matched grafts. For testing the equality of two marginal survival distributions, the standardized test statistics (and two-sided p-values) are -2.503 (0.012) by the log-rank test and -2.142 (0.032) by the Prentice-Wilcoxon test and the Gehan-Wilcoxon test. For this data set, the test statistics by the two Wilcoxon tests happen to be the same. Using the regular variance formula assuming independent two samples, the corresponding test statistics are -2.307 and -1.854, respectively. When using the Wilcoxon tests, we can have a wrong conclusion if we ignore the dependency. The Kaplan-Meier curves for the two skin-graft types are shown in Figure 10.1. We observe that two curves are close at the beginning and split as time passes. This may partially explain the lower significance by the two extensions of Wilcoxon test, which assign more weights to early failure times, than the log-rank test.

The second example is taken from the litter-matched tumorigenesis experiment. For this illustration, the data of $n = 50$ litters of female rats are taken from Table 10.1 of Mantel et al. (1977). The equality of the marginal distributions for three groups, drug, control 1 and control 2, is tested for illustration,

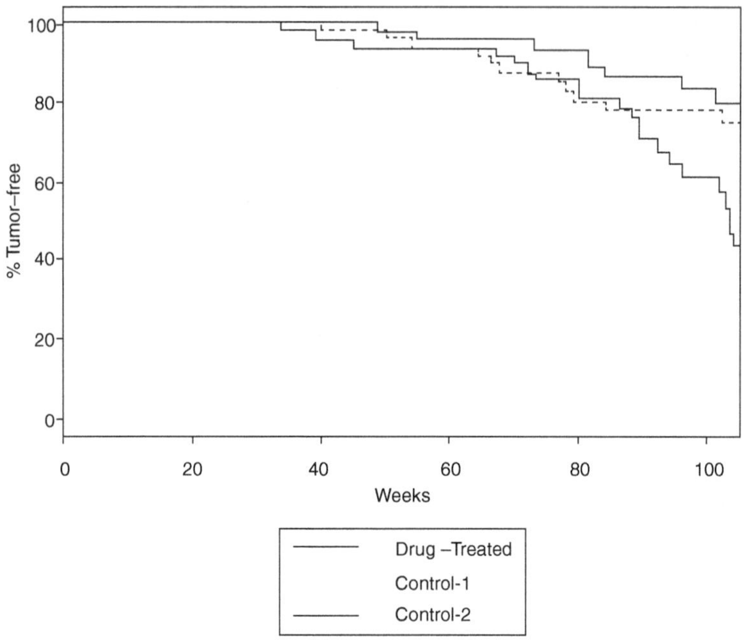

FIGURE 10.2
Time to tumor appearance for litter-matched female rats assigned to drug-treatment, control 1, and control 2.

although the two control groups do not have to be distinguished. Test statistics (W_1, W_2) are $(8.548, -6.286)$, $(14.74, -13.22)$, and $(6.038, -4.971)$ using the log-rank, Prentice-Wilcoxon, and Gehan-Wilcoxon weights, respectively. Their variance-covariance matrices are

$$\begin{pmatrix} 0.1911 & -0.1106 \\ -0.1106 & 0.1573 \end{pmatrix} \begin{pmatrix} 0.8385 & -0.4998 \\ -0.4998 & 0.8178 \end{pmatrix}$$

$$\text{and} \begin{pmatrix} 0.1343 & -0.0780 \\ -0.0780 & 0.1180 \end{pmatrix}$$

giving χ^2 test statistics with 2 degrees of freedom (and p-values), 8.033 (0.018), 5.939 (0.052), and 7.256 (0.026), respectively. The Kaplan-Meier curves of tumor appearance times for the three groups are shown in Figure 10.2. We observe that the three curves are very close until 60 weeks and begin to split after then. This may also explain the lower significance by the two Wilcoxon tests than the log-rank test.

Simulation Studies

The weighted rank tests are based on asymptotic theory. To assess their finite sample properties, simulation studies are carried out. Only the paired sample case $(K = 2)$ is considered here. The rejection probabilities of the log-rank (LR), Prentice-Wilcoxon (PW), and Gehan-Wilcoxon (GW) tests with nominal type I error rate $\alpha = 0.05$ are presented for a selection of sample size and correlation coefficient of bivariate survival distribution. For bivariate survival distributions, we used Moran's algorithm (Moran, 1967), that is, a bivariate exponential distribution is constructed as the joint distribution of $T_1 = (Z_1^2 + Z_2^2)/2$ and $T_2 = (Z_3^2 + Z_4^2)/2$, where (Z_1, Z_3) and (Z_2, Z_4) are mutually independent, but each pair has a bivariate normal distribution with marginal means of 0, variances of 1, and a correlation coefficient of $\sqrt{\rho}$. It follows that T_1 and T_2 have marginally exponential distributions with a hazard rate of 1 each and their correlation coefficient is ρ, denoted as $\mathcal{E}(1, 1, \rho)$. If we want to generate (T_1, T_2) with $\mathcal{E}(\lambda_1, \lambda_2, \rho)$, then we use $T_1 = (Z_1^2 + Z_2^2)/(2\lambda_1)$ and $T_2 = (Z_3^2 + Z_4^2)/(2\lambda_2)$.

We set $\lambda_1 = 1$, $\lambda_2 = 1, 0.75, 0.5$, or 0.25, $\rho = 0, 0.3$, or 0.6, and $n = 10, 20$, or 50. In checking the type I error rate under $H_0 : \lambda_1 = \lambda_2 = 1$, we consider two censoring schemes: $C_k \sim U(0, 3)$ for $k = 1, 2$ for about 30% censoring in each group; $C_1 \sim U(0, 3)$ and $C_2 \sim U(0, 1.5)$ for about 50% censoring in group 2. In power calculations, we consider two censoring schemes, $C_k \sim U(0, 3)$ and $C_k \sim U(0, 3/\lambda_k)$ for $k = 1, 2$. The former gives about 40%, 50%, and 65% censoring in group 2 for $\lambda_2 = 0.75, 0.5$, and 0.25, respectively, and the latter gives about equal (30%) censoring in each group.

For each combination of censoring scheme, ρ, λ_2, and n, 1,000 samples of paired survival data are generated. Rank tests with nominal level $\alpha = 0.05$ are applied to each sample. Empirical rejection probability (ERP) is obtained by the proportion of samples rejecting H_0 among the 1,000 samples.

The results under $H_0 : \lambda_1 = \lambda_2 = 1$ are displayed in Table 10.2. In the equal censoring case (Table 10.2(a)), if the sample size is small ($n = 10$ or 20), the

TABLE 10.2

Empirical type I error probability of rank statistics with $\alpha = 0.05$ under $H_0 : \lambda_1 = \lambda_2 = 1$ using variance estimators reflecting dependency and ignoring dependency (LR = log-rank test, PW = Prentice-Wilcoxon test, GW = Gehan-Wilcoxon test). (a) Equal censoring distribution case: $C_k \sim U(0, 3)$ for about 30% censoring in each group

		Reflecting dependency			**Ignoring dependency**		
ρ	n	**LR**	**PW**	**GW**	**LR**	**PW**	**GW**
0.0	10	0.070	0.050	0.047	0.058	0.056	0.056
	20	0.066	0.048	0.049	0.058	0.052	0.050
	50	0.057	0.044	0.042	0.046	0.046	0.040
0.3	10	0.060	0.043	0.036	0.037	0.039	0.034
	20	0.056	0.043	0.045	0.033	0.032	0.029
	50	0.055	0.046	0.047	0.028	0.031	0.035
0.6	10	0.058	0.035	0.026	0.019	0.018	0.016
	20	0.056	0.037	0.043	0.016	0.010	0.012
	50	0.051	0.042	0.040	0.004	0.004	0.007

TABLE 10.2 (Continued)

(b) Unequal censoring distribution case: $C_1 \sim U(0,3)$ and $C_2 \sim U(0,1.5)$ for about 50% censoring in group 2

		Reflecting dependency			Ignoring dependency		
ρ	n	LR	PW	GW	LR	PW	GW
0.0	10	0.054	0.041	0.034	0.051	0.045	0.050
	20	0.055	0.047	0.040	0.054	0.048	0.046
	50	0.062	0.049	0.048	0.059	0.049	0.051
0.3	10	0.048	0.021	0.027	0.035	0.026	0.026
	20	0.059	0.054	0.053	0.041	0.042	0.039
	50	0.057	0.051	0.055	0.031	0.035	0.036
0.6	10	0.048	0.043	0.036	0.025	0.024	0.021
	20	0.052	0.052	0.043	0.013	0.015	0.013
	50	0.055	0.051	0.044	0.015	0.015	0.015

TABLE 10.3

Empirical power of the rank tests with $\alpha = 0.05$ under $H_1 : \lambda_1 \neq \lambda_2$ ($\lambda_1 = 1$). (a) Equal censoring distribution case: $C_k \sim U(0,3)$ for about 30% censoring when $\lambda_1 = 1$ in group 1, and 40%, 50%, and 65% censoring when $\lambda_2 = 0.75$, 0.5, and 0.25, respectively in group 2

		$n = 10$			$n = 20$			$n = 50$		
ρ	λ_2	LR	PW	GW	LR	PW	GW	LR	PW	GW
0.0	0.75	0.090	0.062	0.052	0.101	0.080	0.068	0.208	0.190	0.176
	0.50	0.173	0.132	0.125	0.364	0.299	0.278	0.739	0.681	0.645
	0.25	0.350	0.279	0.274	0.772	0.716	0.672	0.996	0.996	0.989
0.3	0.75	0.083	0.066	0.045	0.137	0.117	0.102	0.283	0.233	0.209
	0.50	0.224	0.155	0.162	0.417	0.358	0.326	0.814	0.757	0.709
	0.25	0.414	0.344	0.336	0.855	0.802	0.741	1.000	0.999	0.997
0.6	0.75	0.085	0.053	0.048	0.149	0.110	0.113	0.299	0.247	0.245
	0.50	0.211	0.142	0.138	0.527	0.438	0.446	0.904	0.870	0.835
	0.25	0.492	0.402	0.407	0.913	0.857	0.851	1.000	1.000	1.000

log-rank test is slightly anti-conservative under independence ($\rho = 0$) and the Wilcoxon tests are slightly conservative with a high dependency ($\rho = 0.6$). In the unequal censoring case (Table 10.2(b)), if the sample size is small ($n = 10$) and the dependency is low ($\rho = 0.0$ or 0.3), the Prentice- and Gehan-Wilcoxon tests are slightly conservative. For $n = 50$, ERPs of the weighted rank tests are close to the nominal level $\alpha = 0.05$. For comparison, ERPs of the tests ignoring dependence are also reported. They are correct under independence ($\rho = 0$), but are conservative with a positive dependency. As the dependency grows, the conservativeness increases. This happens since the variance estimator ignoring positive dependence overestimates the true variance of a rank test.

ERPs under $H_1 : \lambda_1 \neq \lambda_2$ are displayed in Table 10.3, part (a) in the equal censoring case and part (b) in the unequal censoring case. Note that the equal censoring case has smaller power than the unequal censoring case, since the former has more censoring in group 2 than the latter. When n is large ($n = 50$) and two marginal distributions have a reasonable difference in hazard rates, all three rank tests have good power. The power of the rank tests increases in n, the hazard ratio λ_1/λ_2, and ρ, as was expected. In the bivariate exponential survival distribution case, the two groups have marginally proportional hazards so that the log-rank test is more powerful than the two types of Wilcoxon tests.

Sample Size Calculation for the Weighted Rank Tests with Paired Survival Data

Jung (2007) proposed a simulation-based sample size calculation method for the paired rank tests. A simulation method, however, does not show the explicit relationship between design parameters and the required sample size. Furthermore, if there exists an error in the computer program for simulations, then we will have a wrong sample size. But, it is difficult to validate the computer program for simulations. A closed form sample size formula resolves all of these issues. A formula can be validated using a simulation method. Jung (2008) proposed a closed form of sample size formula for the paired rank tests we have investigated in the section 'Paired Two-Sample Data Case'. We review it in this section.

Gangnon and Kosorok (2004) proposed a sample size formula for the paired rank tests requiring specification of the correlation coefficient between the two parts of rank statistics W, i.e., $\int_0^\infty H(t)d\hat{\Lambda}_1(t)$ and $\int_0^\infty H(t)d\hat{\Lambda}_2(t)$ in (10.1). When a pilot data set is available, one may want to estimate the correlation coefficient from the pilot data to be used for calculating the sample size of the main study. As mentioned by Gangnon and Kosorok (2004), however, the correlation coefficient depends on censoring distribution as well as joint survival distribution. So, estimating it empirically from the pilot data will not separate the contribution of the dependence of paired survival times from that of the censoring. In order to tackle this problem, Jung (2008) expressed the correlation coefficient as a function of specified censoring and joint survival distributions, and derived a practical sample size formula using this expression.

To derive a sample size formula, we have to consider a specific alternative hypothesis H_1 and derive the limiting distribution of the test statistic under H_1. We assume that the distribution of (T_{1i}, T_{2i}) is absolutely continuous. Let $S(t_1, t_2) = P(T_{1i} \geq t_1, T_{2i} \geq t_2)$ and $f(t_1, t_2) = \partial^2 S(t_1, t_2)/\partial t_1 \partial t_2$ denote the joint survivor and probability density functions of (T_{1i}, T_{2i}), respectively. Then, the joint hazard function is given as

$$\lambda(t_1,t_2) = \frac{f(t_1,t_2)}{S(t_1,t_2)}$$

and the conditional hazard function of the subject assigned to treatment 1 at t_1 given that the paired subject assigned to treatment 2 is at risk at t_2 is given as

$$\lambda_{1|2}(t_1|t_2) \equiv \lim_{\epsilon\to 0} P(t_1 \le T_{1i} \le t_1+\epsilon|T_{1i}\ge t_1, T_{2i}\ge t_2) = -\frac{s_1(t_1,t_2)}{S(t_1,t_2)},$$

where $s_1(t_1,t_2) = \partial S(t_1,t_2)/\partial t_1$. We define $\lambda_{2|1}(t_2|t_1)$ and $s_2(t_1,t_2)$ similarly. In addition, we define the joint survivor function for censoring variables $G(t_1,t_2) = P(C_{1i} \ge t_1, C_{2i} \ge t_2)$, and the marginal survivor functions for censoring variable $G_k(t) = P(C_{ki} \ge t)$ and survival variable $S_k(t) = \exp\{-\Lambda_k(t)\}$ for $k = 1, 2$. Then, we obtain following results. See Appendix C for a proof.

Theorem: Under $H_1 : \Lambda_1(t) \ne \Lambda_2(t)$, W is approximately normal with mean $\omega\sqrt{n}$ and variance $\sigma^2 = \sigma_1^2 + \sigma_2^2 - 2\sigma_{12}$, where

$$\omega = \int_0^\infty h(t)\{d\Lambda_1(t) - d\Lambda_2(t)\},$$

$$\sigma_k^2 = \int_0^\infty \frac{h^2(t)}{y_k(t)} d\Lambda_k(t),$$

$$\sigma_{12} = \int_0^\infty \int_0^\infty \frac{h(t_1)h(t_2)}{y_1(t_1)y_2(t_2)} y(t_1,t_2)dA(t_1,t_2),$$

$$dA(t_1,t_2) = \{\lambda(t_1,t_2) - \lambda_{1|2}(t_1|t_2)\lambda_2(t_2) - \lambda_{2|1}(t_2|t_1)\lambda_1(t_1) + \lambda_1(t_1)\lambda_2(t_2)\}dt_1dt_2,$$

$\lambda_k(t) = \Lambda_k(dt)$, and $y(t_1,t_2) = G(t_1,t_2)S(t_1,t_2)$. Assuming that survival times and censoring times are independent, we have $y_k(t) = G_k(t)S_k(t)$. Under a contiguous sequence of models, $\hat\sigma^2 \to \sigma^2$ as $n \to \infty$.

If T_{1i} and T_{2i} are independent, then, for $k \ne k'$, $\lambda_{k|k'}(t_k|t_{k'}) = \lambda_k(t_k)$ so that $\sigma_{12} = 0$ whether C_{1i} and C_{2i} are independent or not. Let $\bar\Phi(\cdot)$ denote the survivor function of the standard normal distribution. By the theorem, for two-sided α, the statistical power for a given n is given as

$$1-\beta = \bar\Phi\left(z_{1-\alpha/2} - \frac{\sqrt{n}|\omega|}{\sigma}\right)$$

and the required sample size for a given power $1-\beta$ is

$$n = \frac{\sigma^2(z_{1-\alpha/2}+z_{1-\beta})^2}{\omega^2}. \quad (10.3)$$

Censoring distribution is decided by accrual and loss to follow-up trend, and additional follow-up period. Note that ω and σ^2 depend on both survival and censoring distributions through $y_k(t)$ and $h(t)$. Gangnon and Kosorok (2004) proposed a formula approximately identical to (10.3), but they treat σ_{12} as an input parameter while Jung (2008) proposed to calculate it from the specified survival and censoring distributions.

A sample size calculation will proceed as follows:

1. Specify $\alpha, \beta, S(t_1, t_2), G(t_1, t_2)$.
2. Calculate ω and σ^2.
3. Calculate the number of pairs n using (10.3).

The statistical power of survival analysis typically depends on the number of events rather than total number of subjects so that one may want to calculate the required number of deaths for a specified alternative hypothesis. Under independent censoring assumption, the probability that a subject assigned to treatment k has no event over the study period is calculated as

$$\mathrm{P}(T_{ki} > C_{ki}) = -\int_0^\infty S_k(t)dG_k(t).$$

Hence, the proportion of subjects to experience an event in treatment k is given as

$$d_k = 1 + \int_0^\infty S_k(t)dG_k(t),$$

and the expected number of subjects experiencing an event is given as $D = n(d_1 + d_2)$.

Sample Size under Some Practical Settings

In this section, we make following assumptions for practical sample size calculations.

(a1) The paired subjects are accrued and censored at the same time, i.e., $G_1 = G_2 (= G)$ and $y(t_1, t_2) = S(t_1, t_2)G(t_1 \vee t_2)$, where $x \vee y = \max(x, y)$.

(a2) Pairs are uniformly accrued during accrual period a and followed during follow-up period b after the completion of accrual.

(a3) We consider the log-rank test:

$$h(t) = \frac{y_1(t)y_2(t)}{y_1(t) + y_2(t)} = \frac{G(t)S_1(t)S_2(t)}{S_1(t) + S_2(t)}.$$

(a4) In order to account for the dependency in survival times within each pair, we consider the positive stable frailty model: for $0 \leq \theta \leq 1$,

$$S(t_1, t_2) = \exp(-[\{-\log S_1(t_1)\}^{1/\theta} + \{-\log S_2(t_2)\}^{1/\theta}]^{\theta}).$$

(a5) We assume marginally exponential survival distributions: $S_k(t) = \exp(-\lambda_k t)$. Combining this with (a4), we have

$$S(t_1, t_2) = \exp[-\{(\lambda_1 t_1)^{1/\theta} + (\lambda_2 t_2)^{1/\theta}\}^{\theta}] \tag{10.4}$$

denoted as $\mathcal{E}(\lambda_1, \lambda_2, \theta)$. (Note that θ is replacing ρ in the previous definition of bivariate exponential distribution.)

Under (a2), assuming no loss to follow-up, the common censoring times $C_1, ..., C_n$ are i.i.d. with $U(b, a+b)$ distribution, i.e.,

$$G(t) = P(C_{ki} \geq t) = I(t < a+b) - \frac{t-b}{a} I(b \leq t < a+b).$$

Under the positive stable frailty model, the dependency between T_1 and T_2 decreases as θ increases from 0 to 1, 0 meaning a complete positive dependency and 1 meaning independence. Now, we derive the relationship between θ and the correlation coefficient ρ of the paired survival times (T_1, T_2) with joint exponential distribution survival function (10.4). From (10.4), $(\tilde{T}_1, \tilde{T}_2) = (\lambda_1 T_1, \lambda_2 T_2)$ have marginally exponential distribution with hazard rates 1 with joint survival function

$$S_0(t_1, t_2) = \exp\{-(t_1^{1/\theta} + t_2^{1/\theta})^{\theta}\}$$

and the same correlation coefficient as (T_1, T_2). Furthermore, by Lemma 2 of Lehmann (1966),

$$E(\tilde{T}_1 \tilde{T}_2) = \int_0^{\infty} \int_0^{\infty} S_0(t_1, t_2) dt_1 dt_2$$

so that we have

$$\rho = \frac{\int_0^{\infty} \int_0^{\infty} S_0(t_1, t_2) dt_1 dt_2 - E(\tilde{T}_1) E(\tilde{T}_2)}{\sqrt{\text{var}(\tilde{T}_1) \text{var}(\tilde{T}_2)}} = \int_0^{\infty} \int_0^{\infty} S_0(t_1, t_2) dt_1 dt_2 - 1 \tag{10.5}$$

By change of variables $u_k = \exp(-t_k)$, we have $dt_k = -u_k^{-1} du_k$ so that we can also calculate the correlation coefficient by

$$\rho = \int_0^1 \int_0^1 S_u(u_1, u_2)/(u_1 u_2) du_1 du_2 - 1 \tag{10.6}$$

where

$$S_u(u_1, u_2) = \exp[-\{(-\log u_1)^{1/\theta} + (-\log u_2)^{1/\theta}\}^\theta]$$

for $0 \le u_1, u_2 \le 1$. We calculate the double integrals in (10.5) and (10.6) using a numerical method.

For the exponential marginal survival and uniform common censoring distributions, the expected number of events is given as $D = n(d_1 + d_2)$ with

$$d_k = 1 - \frac{\exp(-b\lambda_k)}{a\lambda_k}\{1 - \exp(-a\lambda_k)\}.$$

Under these settings, sample size is calculated as follows:

1. Specify $(\alpha, \beta, \lambda_1, \lambda_2, \theta, a, b)$.
2. Calculate ω and σ^2. (See Appendix D.)
3. Calculate the number of pairs n using (10.3).

When Accrual Rate Is Given Instead of Accrual Period

For formula (10.3), we assume that accrual period is specified together with other design parameters. However, it is more natural to specify accrual rate based on the number of patients who have visited the clinics participating in the trial recently. Suppose that accrual rate r is given together with $(\alpha, \beta, \lambda_1, \lambda_2, \theta, b)$ in this section. In this case, accrual period a is an output variable together with n. For example, under uniform accrual with a constant rate r, we have

$$n = a \times r. \tag{10.7}$$

Given other input variables, $\sigma^2 = \sigma^2(a)$ and $\omega = \omega(a)$ in formula (10.3) are functions of a. From (10.3) and (10.4), we have

$$a \times r = \frac{\sigma^2(a)(z_{1-\alpha/2} + z_{1-\beta})^2}{\omega(a)^2}.$$

We solve this equation with respect to a using numerical methods, and obtain the required sample size, $n = a^* \times r$, where a^* is the solution to the equation.

When Historical Data Are Available with Both of the Paired Subjects Treated by the Same Treatment

When historical data are available, we usually estimate the design parameters to be used in designing a new study from them. Often in this case, both of the paired subjects in the historical data are treated by the control treatment which is a current standard therapy. From such historical data, we can

TABLE 10.4

Sample size (and, empirical type I error and power) under each design setting with $\alpha = 0.05$, $\lambda_1 = 0.5$ and $a = 3$

λ_2	$1-\beta$	b	$\theta = 0.3$	$\theta = 0.6$	$\theta = 0.9$
0.35	0.8	0	78 (0.046,0.845)	161 (0.052,0.816)	259 (0.048,0.812)
		2	45 (0.042,0.861)	95 (0.052,0.819)	151 (0.047,0.821)
	0.9	0	105 (0.047,0.937)	215 (0.044,0.910)	347 (0.049,0.902)
		2	60 (0.042,0.939)	127 (0.055,0.914)	203 (0.049,0.910)
0.3	0.8	0	48 (0.043,0.822)	87 (0.048,0.822)	136 (0.050,0.807)
		2	28 (0.040,0.900)	51 (0.053,0.837)	79 (0.052,0.829)
	0.9	0	65 (0.042,0.961)	117 (0.053,0.928)	183 (0.050,0.919)
		2	38 (0.042,0.971)	69 (0.051,0.927)	106 (0.055,0.919)

estimate the marginal survival distribution for the control treatment and the correlation coefficient of the paired survival variables using the maximum likelihood method. Assuming a positive stable frailty model and exponential marginal distributions, the correlation coefficient is free of the marginal hazard rates so that its estimate will be a good estimate for a new randomized study although the paired subjects may have different marginal survival distributions. The marginal survival distribution for the experimental treatment can be chosen based on a clinically significant difference from the control treatment.

Simulation Studies

The sample size formula is based on large sample theories and a nearby alternative hypothesis approximation. To evaluate the performance of the formula under finite sample and fixed alternative hypothesis, some simulations are conducted. In the first set of simulations, we specify an accrual period. We set $\alpha = 0.05$; $1-\beta = 0.8$ or 0.9; $\lambda_1 = 0.5$, $\lambda_2 = 0.35$ or 0.3; $a = 3$; $b = 0$ or 2; $\theta = 0.3, 0.6$, or 0.9. With $b = 0$, we assume that the data analysis is conducted as soon as the last patient is accrued.

Under the positive stable frailty model, the paired survival times are generated by generating T_1 from $S_1(t) = \exp(-\lambda_1 t)$ and then, given $T_1 = t_1$, generating T_2 by solving $S_{2|1}(t_2|t_1) = u$ with respect to t_2, where

$$S_{2|1}(t_2|t_1) = -\frac{s_1(t_1, t_2)}{f_1(t_1)}$$

$f_k(t) = \lambda_k \exp(-\lambda_k t)$ and u is a $U(0,1)$ random number.

In the simulations, sample size n is calculated using (10.3) under each design setting, and then $B = 5{,}000$ simulation samples of size n are generated from the same setting. The log-rank test is applied to each simulation sample, and an empirical power is obtained as the proportion of simulation samples

TABLE 10.5

Sample size (and, empirical type I error and power): sample sizes are calculated under the positive stable frailty model as in Table 10.1, but empirical type I errors and powers are calculated under the true survival distribution following Moran's model (1967)

λ_2	$1-\beta$	b	$\theta = 0.3(\rho = 0.803)$	$\theta = 0.6(\rho = 0.449)$	$\theta = 0.9(\rho = 0.103)$
0.35	0.8	0	78 (0.044,0.651)	161 (0.048,0.697)	259 (0.049,0.787)
		2	45 (0.048,0.761)	95 (0.047,0.768)	151 (0.054,0.806)
	0.9	0	105 (0.051,0.792)	215 (0.054,0.817)	347 (0.055,0.895)
		2	60 (0.047,0.893)	127 (0.052,0.878)	203 (0.050,0.904)
0.3	0.8	0	48 (0.048,0.698)	87 (0.046,0.720)	136 (0.056,0.787)
		2	28 (0.043,0.828)	51 (0.064,0.792)	79 (0.052,0.820)
	0.9	0	65 (0.043,0.828)	117 (0.051,0.832)	183 (0.053,0.894)
		2	38 (0.045,0.935)	69 (0.053,0.900)	106 (0.048,0.917)

for which H_0 is rejected with $\alpha = 0.05$. For the groups with the hazard rate $0.5, 0.35$, and 0.3, the censoring probabilities are about 52%, 62%, and 66%, respectively, with $b = 0$, and 19%, 31%, and 36%, respectively, with $b = 2$. Table 10.4 reports the simulation results. Note that sample size increases in θ and $1 - \beta$, and decreases in hazard ratio λ_1/λ_2 and b. With a high dependency ($\theta = 0.3$), the estimated sample size is relatively small and the empirical power is larger than the nominal $1 - \beta$ level. It is more so with $\lambda_2 = 0.3$ because of the larger hazard ratio and the smaller required sample size. Because the calculated sample sizes in these cases are small, the increase in sample size from the one for an accurate power will be rather small. For example, when $(1 - \beta, \lambda_2, \theta, b) = (0.8, 0.3, 0.3, 2)$, through simulations we found that approximately $n = 22$ provides an empirical power close to $1 - \beta = 0.8$, which is smaller than the size from our formula $n = 28$ only by 6. Otherwise, the empirical power is close to the nominal one.

We also evaluate the performance of the paired log-rank test by checking the empirical type I error under $H_0 : \lambda_1 = \lambda_2 = 0.5$ with the sample size and other parameters fixed at the same values as above. Empirical type I error rates, reported in Table 10.4, are close to the nominal level, $\alpha = 0.05$ overall.

In the second simulation study, we address the sensitivity of the sample sizes on the misspecification of the joint survival distribution. Sample sizes are calculated under the positive stable frailty model at the same design settings as above, but the simulation data are generated from Moran's (1967) model, i.e., $T_1 = (Z_1^2 + Z_2^2)/(2\lambda_1)$ and $T_2 = (Z_3^2 + Z_4^2)/(2\lambda_2)$, where (Z_1, Z_3) and (Z_2, Z_4) are mutually independent random vectors, but each pair has a bivariate normal distribution with marginal means of 0, variances of 1, and a correlation coefficient of $\sqrt{\rho}$. Then, T_k are marginally exponential with hazard rates λ_k and $\text{corr}(T_1, T_2) = \rho$. Since the probability density function of Moran's bivariate exponential distribution is expressed as a sum of infinitely many functions, we cannot use it for sample size calculations.

Using a numerical method, we can show that $\theta = 0.3$, 0.6, and 0.9 for the positive stable frailty model correspond to $\rho = 0.803$, 0.449, and 0.103, respectively. The simulation results are reported in Table 10.5. As in Table 10.4, the empirical type I error rates are close to the nominal $\alpha = 0.05$. If the dependency is high, i.e., $\theta = 0.3$ ($\rho = 0.803$) or $\theta = 0.6$ ($\rho = 0.449$), and there is no additional follow-up after the completion of accrual, i.e., $b = 0$, then the calculated sample sizes tend to be underpowered. However, with a low dependency like $\theta = 0.9$ ($\rho = 0.103$) or an additional follow-up of $b = 2$, the empirical power is close to the nominal power. The impact of censoring on the statistical power for these paired survival models can be examined by checking how their dependency changes over time span.

In order to investigate how the follow-up period influences on the correlation of paired censored data from the positive stable frailty model, 100,000 paired survival times are generated from the joint distribution with $\theta = 0.3$ ($\rho = 0.803$) and $(\lambda_1, \lambda_2) = (0.5, 0.35)$, and the conditional correlation coefficient $\rho_{t_0} = \text{corr}(T_1, T_2 | T_1 \vee T_2 \leq t_0)$ is estimated from the paired observations whose maximum value is smaller than t_0. By ρ_{t_0}, we can examine how the dependency between paired survival times changes for different choice of study period $t_0 = a + b$.

Figure 10.3 displays the conditional correlation coefficients for various t_0 values. The conditional correlation coefficients are similarly estimated from the Moran's model with $\rho = \rho_\infty = 0.803$ and $(\lambda_1, \lambda_2) = (0.5, 0.35)$. From Figure 10.3, we observe that, for the Moran's model, the conditional correlation coefficient is close to 0 for small paired survival times, and monotonely increases to the overall correlation coefficient level $\rho = 0.803$ as t_0 increases. However, for the positive stable frailty model, ρ_{t_0} is very stable over the whole span of t_0 values. Hence, if the true survival distribution follows the Moran's model, then with a short follow-up, e.g., $b = 0$, the correlation between the paired censored data will be much lower than ρ, and the sample size calculated under the positive stable frailty model will be much underpowered. On the other hand, the dependency of the paired censored data from the positive stable frailty model is not much influenced by censoring so that the difference in required sample size between the two survival models decreases with an additional follow-up ($b = 2$). Figure 10.3 also displays the conditional correlation coefficients for the two joint survival models under a weaker correlation, $\rho = 0.103$ ($\theta = 0.9$). Note that the conditional correlation coefficients are similar between the two models under the weaker correlation. As a result, we observe from Table 10.5 that the sample sizes calculated under the positive stable frailty model are very accurate for the Moran's model even without an additional follow-up, $b = 0$, in this case.

Examples

Suppose we want to design a paired randomization study of the influence of HL-A antigens on the survival of allogeneic grafts in burned patients that was

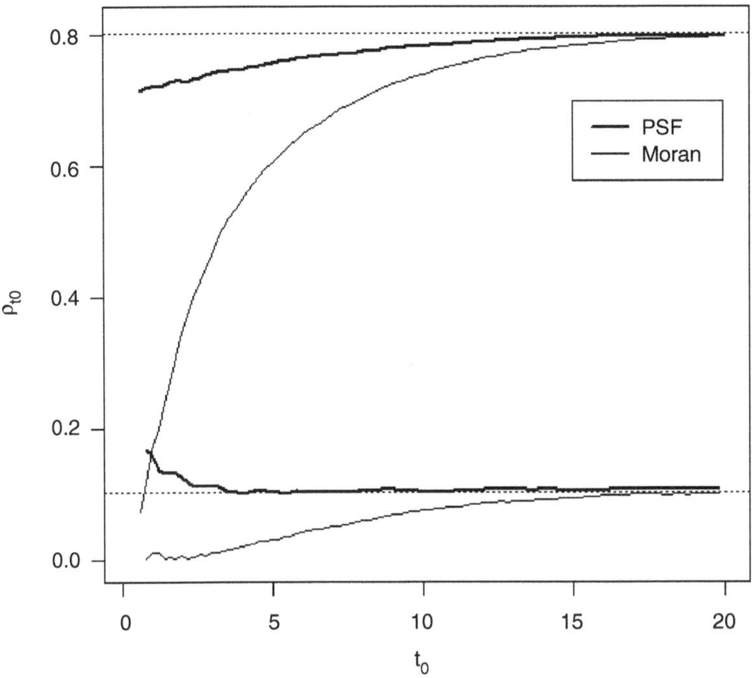

FIGURE 10.3
Conditional correlation coefficient, ρ_t, for the positive stable frailty (PSF) model and Moran model. The upper two curves are for $\rho = 0.803$ ($\theta = 0.3$ for PSF), and the lower two curves are for $\rho = 0.103$ ($\theta = 0.9$ for PSF).

discussed in the section 'Weighted Rank Tests for Matched Survival Data'. Data from Bachelor and Hackett (1970) are reported in Table 10.1, and will be used as pilot data here. The maximum likelihood estimates based on the positive stable frailty model are $\hat{\lambda}_1 = 0.043$ per day for the poor match group, $\hat{\lambda}_2 = 0.025$ per day for close match group, and $\hat{\theta} = 0.33$ ($\hat{\rho} = 0.77$). For the design of a prospective study, we assume $(\lambda_1, \lambda_2, \theta) = (0.04, 0.03, 0.35)$. We also set $\alpha = 0.05$, $1 - \beta = 0.9$, an accrual rate of $r = 10$ patients per month, and an additional follow-up of $b = 2$ months. Under these design settings, the required sample size is $n = 79$ pairs, with $D = 155$ expected events from the two treatment groups. The empirical power for this sample size is obtained as 0.929 from 5,000 simulations.

Early Treatment Diabetic Retinopathy Study (ETDRS Research Group 1991) accrued 3,711 patients with non-proliferative or early-proliferative diabetic retinopathy in both eyes for over 5 years. For each patient, one eye was randomized into photocoagulation and the other into no treatment, and the time from registration to severe visual loss or vitrectomy was observed from each eye. Suppose that we want to design a paired randomization study using our formula. From the resulting data, we observe $\hat{\lambda}_1 = 0.021$ and $\hat{\lambda}_2 = 0.012$. For the design of a prospective study, we assume these estimates are the true parameter values. If we set $\alpha = 0.05$, $1 - \beta = 0.9$, an annual accrual rate of $r = 700$ patients, and an additional follow-up of $b = 2$ years, then we need $n = 595$ patients ($D = 47$, $a = 0.85$ years) if $\theta = 0.3$, $n = 918$ patients ($D = 79$, $a = 1.32$ years) if $\theta = 0.6$, and $n = 1310$ patients ($D = 124$, $a = 1.87$ years) if $\theta = 0.9$. The empirical powers from 5,000 simulations are 0.946 with $\theta = 0.3$, 0.920 with $\theta = 0.6$, and 0.905 with $\theta = 0.9$. It seems that the original study is overpowered for a specified difference of $\lambda_1 = 0.021$ vs. $\lambda_2 = 0.012$ over a wide range of correlation levels.

Discussion

We have discussed weighted rank test statistics for paired survival data and matched K sample survival data that were proposed by Jung (1999). We also have investigated the sample size formula for the paired rank tests that was presented by Jung (2008). Although we have not discussed the sample size calculation of the rank test statistics for K matched survival data, it can be easily derived by extending Jung and Hui's (2008) sample size method proposed for K independent samples and Jung's (2008) method of paired two samples.

We have assumed only administrative censoring, but no loss to follow-up. However, if some loss to follow-up is expected for a new study, we can easily reflect it in the sample size calculation. Let's consider the case where paired subjects are accrued and censored at the same time. For pair i, let $\tilde{C}_i$ denote the censoring variable defined by administrative censoring, and E_i the censoring variable defined by loss to follow-up. Then, the censoring variable incorporating both administrative censoring and loss to follow-up is defined by $C_i = \min(\tilde{C}_i, E_i)$. If the distribution of loss to follow-up is independent of the accrual time (i.e., $\tilde{C}_i$ and E_i are independent), then the survivor function for the common censoring variable is obtained as $G(t) = P(\tilde{C}_i \geq t)P(E_i \geq t)$. For example, if we assume $\tilde{C}_i \sim U(b, a+b)$ as in (a2) and exponential loss to follow-up distribution with rate ν, then we have

$$G(t) = \begin{cases} \exp(-\nu t) & \text{if } t < b \\ \{1 - (t-b)/a\}\exp(-\nu t) & \text{if } b \leq t < a+b \\ 0 & \text{otherwise} \end{cases}$$

For example, let's consider a case with $(\lambda_1, \lambda_2, \theta, \alpha, 1-\beta) = (0.5, 0.3, 0.9, 0.05, 0.9)$. From Table 10.4, we need $n = 106$ pairs with administrative censoring only specified by $(a, b) = (3, 2)$. Suppose that we expect additional censoring due to loss to follow-up following an exponential distribution with $\nu = 0.1$. Then, by using the general formulas given in Appendix C, we need a slightly larger sample size of $n = 121$ pairs due to the additional censoring. By simulations, the empirical power was obtained as 0.918 which is close to the nominal $1 - \beta = 0.9$.

On the other hand, if one wants to assume that paired subjects have independent loss to follow-up times E_{1i} and E_{2i} which are also independent of the common administrative censoring time $\tilde{C}_i$, then the joint survivor function for paired censoring times, $C_{ki} = \min(\tilde{C}_i, E_{ki})$ for $k = 1, 2$, is obtained $G(t_1, t_2) = P(\tilde{C}_i \geq t_1 \vee t_2)P(E_{1i} \geq t_1)P(E_{2i} \geq t_2)$. These variations in censoring mechanism can be easily incorporated in the formula.

We have considered the positive stable frailty model with marginally exponential distributions to model the paired survival times. Exponential distributions have been widely used to model independent survival distributions in the design stage of a project, e.g., Schoenfeld (1983) and Yateman and Skene (1992). However, we can use other marginal distributions, such as Weibull, to construct a joint distribution model. We can use other models to specify the joint distribution of the paired survival times too. We chose the positive stable frailty model with exponential distributions since it was easy to calculate the joint and conditional hazard functions and to generate the bivariate random numbers for simulations. We observed from simulations that the choice of a joint survival model has some impact in the sample size calculation or power, especially depending on the trend of the correlation between paired observations over different choice of study period. However, with a reasonable study period, the impact was shown to be minimal. If we have pilot data, we may choose a model that seems to be best fitting the data. Shih (1998) proposes a goodness-of-fit test for the Clayton's (1998) model. Wang and Wells (2000) propose a goodness-of-fit method for a family of more general joint survival models, called Archimedean copula. The latter requires estimation of the joint survivor function, which can be unstable under censoring.

References

Aalen OO. Nonparametric inference for a family of counting processes. Annals of Statistics 1978; 6: 701–726.

Andersen PK, Borgan O, Gill RD, Kidding N. Linear nonparametric tests for comparison of counting processes with application to censored survival data (with discussion). International Statistical Review 1982; 50: 219–258.

Batchelor JR, Hackett M. HL-A matching in treatment of burned patients with skin allografts. Lancet 1970; 2: 581–583.

Calyton DG. A model for association in bivariate life tables and its application to epidemiological studies of familial tendency in chronic disease incidence. Biometrika 1998; 65: 141–151.

ETDRS Research Group. Early photocoagulation for diabetic retinopathy. ETDRS Report Number 9. Ophthalmology 1991; 98: 766–785.

Fleming TR, Harrington DP. Counting Processes and Survival Analysis. Wiley: New York, 1991.

Gangnon RE, Kosorok MR. Sample size formula for clustered survival data using weighted log-rank statistics. Biometrika 2004; 91: 263–275.

Gehan EA. A generalized Wilcoxon test for comparing arbitrarily single censored samples. Biometrika 1965; 52: 203–223.

Harrington DP, Fleming TR. A class of rank test procedures for censored survival data. Biometrika 1982; 69: 133–143.

Jung SH. Rank tests for matched survival data. Lifetime Data Analysis 1999; 5: 67–79.

Jung SH. Sample size calculation for paired survival data: a simulation method, Journal of Statistical Computation and Simulation 2007; 78: 85–92.

Jung SH. Sample size calculation for the weighted rank statistics with paired survival data. Statistics in Medicine 2008; 27: 3350–3365.

Jung SH, Hui S. Sample size calculations to compare K different survival distributions. Lifetime Data Analysis 2002; 8: 361–373.

Jung SH, Su JQ. Nonparametric estimation for the difference or ratio of median failure times for paired observations. Statistics in Medicine 1995; 14(3): 275–382.

Kaplan EL, Meier P. Nonparametric estimator from incomplete observations. Journal of the American Statistical Association 1958; 53: 457–481.

Lee EW, Wei LJ, Ying Z. Linear regression analysis for highly stratified failure time data. Journal of the American Statistical Association 1993; 88: 557–565.

Lehmann EL. Some concepts of dependence. Annals of Mathematical Statistics 1966; 37: 1137–1153.

Mantel N, Bohidar NR, Ciminera JL. Mantel-Haenszel analyses of litter-matched time-to-response data, with modifications for recovery of interlitter information. Cancer Research 1977; 37: 3863–3868.

Moran PAP. Testing for correlation between non-negative variates. Biometrika 1967; 54: 385–394.

Murray S. Nonparametric rank-based methods for group sequential monitoring of paired censored survival data. Biometrics 2000; 56: 984–990.

Nelson W. Hazard plotting for incomplete failure data. Journal of Quality Technology 1969; 1: 27–52.

Peto R, Peto J. Asymptotically efficient rank invariant test procedures (with discussion). Journal of the Royal Statistical Society. Series A 1972; 135: 185–206.

Prentice RL. Linear rank tests with right censored data. Biometrika 1978; 65: 167–179.

Schoenfeld DA. Sample size formula for the proportional hazards regression model. Biometrics 1983; 39:499–503.

Shih JH. A goodness-of-fit test for association in a bivariate survival model. Biometrika 1998; 85: 189–200.

Tarone RE, Ware J. On distribution-free tests for equality of survival distributions. Biometrika 1977; 64: 156–160.

Wang W, Wells MT. Model selection and semiparametric inference for bivariate failure-time data. Journal of the American Statistical Association 2000; 95: 62–72.

Woolson RF, Lachenbruch PA. Rank tests for censored matched pairs. Biometrika 1980; 67: 597–606.

Yateman NA, Skene AM. Sample size for proportional hazards survival studies with arbitrary patient entry and loss to follow-up distributions. Statistics in Medicine 1992; 11: 1103–1113.

Ying Z, Wei LJ. The Kaplan-Meier estimate for dependent failure time observations. Journal of Multivariate Analysis 1994; 50: 17–29.

Appendix A. Asymptotic normality of W under H_0

By the definition of W and $\hat{\Lambda}_k(t)$, we have

$$
\begin{aligned}
W =& \sqrt{n}\int_0^\infty H(t)\left\{\frac{dN_1(t)}{Y_1(t)} - \frac{dN_2(t)}{Y_2(t)}\right\} \\
=& \sqrt{n}\int_0^\infty \frac{H(t)}{Y_1(t)}\{dN_1(t) - Y_1(t)d\Lambda_1(t)\} \\
& - \sqrt{n}\int_0^\infty \frac{H(t)}{Y_2(t)}\{dN_2(t) - Y_2(t)d\Lambda_2(t)\} + \omega\sqrt{n}.
\end{aligned}
$$

Here

$$\omega = \int_0^\infty H(t)\{d\Lambda_1(t) - d\Lambda_2(t)\}, \tag{10.A1}$$

which is 0 under H_0. Let $M_{ki}(t) = N_{ki}(t) - \int_0^t Y_{ki}(s)d\Lambda_k(s)$ and $M_k(t) = \sum_{i=1}^n M_{ki}(t)$.

Under H_0, we have

$$W = \sqrt{n}\int_0^\infty \frac{H(t)}{Y_1(t)}dM_1(t) - \sqrt{n}\int_0^\infty \frac{H(t)}{Y_2(t)}dM_2(t)$$

$$= \frac{1}{\sqrt{n}}\sum_{i=1}^n\left\{\int_0^\infty \frac{H(t)}{n^{-1}Y_1(t)}dM_{1i}(t) - \int_0^\infty \frac{H(t)}{n^{-1}Y_2(t)}dM_{2i}(t)\right. .$$

Let $h(t)$ and $y_k(t)$ be the limit of $H(t)$ and $n^{-1}Y_k(t)$ for $k = 1, 2$, respectively. Refer to Ying and Wei (1994) for the uniform convergence of Kaplan-Meier estimator and Nelson's estimator based on correlated survival data.

We then can show by arguments similar to Appendix A of Lee, Wei, and Ying (1993) that

$$\frac{1}{\sqrt{n}}\sum_{i=1}^n\int_0^\infty \frac{H(t)}{n^{-1}Y_k(t)}dM_{ki}(t)$$

and

$$\frac{1}{\sqrt{n}}\sum_{i=1}^n\int_0^\infty \frac{h(t)}{y_k(t)}dM_{ki}(t)$$

are asymptotically equivalent. Hence, under H_0, W is asymptotically equivalent to

$$W^* = \frac{1}{\sqrt{n}}\sum_{i=1}^n \epsilon_i.$$

where

$$\epsilon_i = \int_0^\infty \frac{h(t)}{y_1(t)}dM_{1i}(t) - \int_0^\infty \frac{h(t)}{y_2(t)}dM_{2i}(t).$$

Since $h(t)$ and $y_k(t)$ are deterministic functions and $M_{ki}(t)$ are 0-mean processes, $\epsilon_1, ..., \epsilon_n$ are independent 0-mean random variables. By the standard central limit theorem for sum of independent random variables, W^* converges to a normal distribution with mean 0 and variance σ^2 that can be consistently estimated by

$$\hat{\sigma}^2 = \frac{1}{n}\sum_{i=1}^{n}\hat{\epsilon}_i^2,$$

where $\hat{\epsilon}_i$ are obtained from ϵ_i by replacing $h(t)$, $y_k(t)$, and $\Lambda_k(t)$ with $H(t)$, $n^{-1}Y_k(t)$, and $\hat{\Lambda}(t) = \int_0^t \{Y_1(t) + Y_2(t)\}^{-1}(t)d\{N_1(t) + N_2(t)\}$ the Nelson-Aalen estimator from the pooled paired two samples, respectively.

Appendix B. Asymptotic normality of $\mathbf{W} = (W_1, ..., W_{K-1})^T$ under H_0

Let $N_{\cdot i}(t) = \sum_{k=1}^K N_{ki}(t)$, $N_k(t) = \sum_{i=1}^n N_{ki}(t)$, $N(t) = \sum_{k=1}^K \sum_{i=1}^n N_{ki}(t)$, $Y_{\cdot i}(t) = \sum_{k=1}^K Y_{ki}(t)$, $Y_k(t) = \sum_{i=1}^n Y_{ki}(t)$, $Y(t) = \sum_{k=1}^K \sum_{i=1}^n Y_{ki}(t)$, $M_{ki}(t) = N_{ki}(t) - \int_0^t Y_{ki}(s)d\Lambda_k(s)$, $M_{\cdot i}(t) = \sum_{k=1}^K M_{ki}(t)$, $M_k(t) = \sum_{i=1}^n M_{ki}(t)$, and $M(t) = \sum_{k=1}^K \sum_{i=1}^n M_{ki}(t)$.

By the definition of $\hat{\Lambda}_k(t)$ and $\hat{\Lambda}(t)$,

$$\begin{aligned} W_k =& \frac{1}{\sqrt{n}}\int_0^\infty Y_k(t)L(t)\left\{\frac{dN_k(t)}{Y_k(t)} - \frac{dN(t)}{Y(t)}\right\} \\ =& \frac{1}{\sqrt{n}}\int_0^\infty L(t)dM_k(t) - \frac{1}{\sqrt{n}}\int_0^\infty L(t)\frac{Y_k(t)}{Y(t)}dM(t) + \omega_k\sqrt{n}, \end{aligned}$$

where $\omega_k = \int_0^\infty n^{-1}Y_k(t)L(t)\{d\Lambda_k(t) - d\Lambda(t)\}$ which is 0 under $H_0 : \Lambda_1(t) = \cdots = \Lambda_K(t)(= \Lambda(t))$.

Under H_0, we have

$$W_k = \frac{1}{\sqrt{n}}\sum_{i=1}^n\int_0^\infty L(t)dM_{ki}(t) - \frac{1}{\sqrt{n}}\sum_{i=1}^n\int_0^\infty L(t)\frac{n^{-1}Y_k(t)}{n^{-1}Y(t)}dM_{\cdot i}(t). \tag{10.A2}$$

Also, by arguments similar to Appendix A of Lee, Wei, and Ying (1993), we can show that (10.A2) is asymptotically equivalent to

$$\frac{1}{\sqrt{n}}\sum_{i=1}^n\int_0^\infty \ell(t)dM_{ki}(t) - \frac{1}{\sqrt{n}}\sum_{i=1}^n\int_0^\infty \ell(t)\frac{y_k(t)}{y(t)}dM_{\cdot i}(t),$$

where $y_k(t)$ and $\ell(t)$ are the limits of $n^{-1}Y_k(t)$ and $L(t)$, respectively, and $y(t) = \sum_{k=1}^K y_k(t)$.

Hence, under H_0, **W** is asymptotically equivalent to $\mathbf{W}^* = n^{-1/2}\sum_{i=1}^n \epsilon_i$ with $\epsilon_i = (\epsilon_{1i}, ..., \epsilon_{K-1,i})^T$ and

$$\epsilon_{ki} = \int_0^\infty \ell(t)dM_{ki}(t) - \int_0^\infty \ell(t)\frac{y_k(t)}{y(t)}dM_{\cdot i}(t).$$

Since $\ell(t)$ and $y_k(t)$ are deterministic functions and $M_{ki}(t)$ are 0-mean processes, $\epsilon_1, ..., \epsilon_n$ are independent 0-mean random vectors. By the multivariate central limit theorem, **W** converges to a multivariate normal distribution with mean 0 and variance-covariance matrix V that can be consistently estimated by

$$\hat{V} = \frac{1}{n}\sum_{i=1}^n \hat{\epsilon}_i\hat{\epsilon}_i^T,$$

where $\hat{\epsilon}_i = (\hat{\epsilon}_{1i}, ..., \hat{\epsilon}_{K-1,i})^T$ and $\hat{\epsilon}_{ki}$ are obtained from ϵ_{ki} by replacing $\ell(t)$, $y_k(t)$, and $\Lambda_k(t)$ with $L(t)$, $n^{-1}Y_k(t)$, and $\hat{\Lambda}(t) = \int_0^t Y^{-1}(t)dN(t)$ the Nelson-Aalen estimator from the pooled matched K samples, respectively.

Appendix C. Limiting Distribution of the Paired Log-Rank Test under H_1

In Appendix A, we derived the asymptotic normality of weighted rank statistics under H_0. In this appendix, we derive the limiting distribution of the paired log-rank test under H_1.

By the definition of W,

$$\begin{aligned} W =& \sqrt{n}\sum_{i=1}^n\{\int_0^\infty \frac{H(t)}{Y_1(t)}dM_{1i}(t) - \int_0^\infty \frac{H(t)}{Y_2(t)}dM_{2i}(t)\} \\ &+ \sqrt{n}\int_0^\infty H(t)\{d\Lambda_1(t) - d\Lambda_2(t)\}. \end{aligned}$$

Let $\tau = \max\{t : S_1(t)S_2(t)G(t) > 0\}$. As $n \to \infty$, $n^{-1}Y_k(t)$ and $H(t)$ uniformly converge to $y_k(t)$ and $h(t)$ in $[0, \tau]$, respectively so that we have

$$W = \frac{1}{\sqrt{n}}\sum_{i=1}^n(\epsilon_{1i} - \epsilon_{2i}) + \sqrt{n}\int_0^\infty h(t)\{d\Lambda_1(t) - d\Lambda_2(t)\} + o_p(1),$$

where $\epsilon_{ki} = \int_0^\infty y_k(t)^{-1}h(t)dM_{ki}(t)$. Since, $\{\epsilon_{1i} - \epsilon_{2i}, i = 1, ..., n\}$ are independent random variables with mean 0, by the central limit theorem, W is approximately normal with mean $\sqrt{n}\omega$, where $\omega = \int_0^\infty h(t)\{d\Lambda_1(t) - d\Lambda_2(t)\}$. Its variance is expressed as $\sigma^2 = \sigma_1^2 + \sigma_2^2 - 2\sigma_{12}$ with

$$\sigma_k^2 = \frac{1}{n}\sum_{i=1}^n \text{var}(\epsilon_{ki}) = \int_0^\infty \frac{h^2(t)}{y_k(t)}d\Lambda_k(t)$$

and

$$\sigma_{12} = \frac{1}{n}\sum_{i=1}^{n}\text{cov}(\epsilon_{1i}, \epsilon_{2i}) = \frac{1}{n}\sum_{i=1}^{n}\int_0^\infty\int_0^\infty \frac{h(t_1)h(t_2)}{y_1(t_1)y_2(t_2)}E\{dM_{1i}(t_1)dM_{2i}(t_2)\}.$$

By the lemma given below, $\{dM_{1i}(t_1)dM_{2i}(t_2) - Y_{1i}(t_1)Y_{2i}(t_2)dA(t_1,t_2), i = 1,...,n\}$ are independent random variables with mean 0. Hence, we have

$$\begin{aligned}\sigma_{12} &= \frac{1}{n}\sum_{i=1}^{n}\int_0^\infty\int_0^\infty \frac{h(t_1)h(t_2)}{y_1(t_1)y_2(t_2)}E\{Y_{1i}(t_1)Y_{2i}(t_2)\}dA(t_1,t_2)\\ &= \int_0^\infty\int_0^\infty \frac{h(t_1)h(t_2)}{y_1(t_1)y_2(t_2)}y(t_1,t_2)dA(t_1,t_2).\end{aligned}$$

By definition,

$$\begin{aligned}\hat{\sigma}^2 =& n\sum_{i=1}^{n}[\int_0^\infty \frac{H(t)}{Y_1(t)}\{dN_{1i}(t) - Y_{1i}(t)d\hat{\Lambda}(t)\}\\ &- \int_0^\infty \frac{H(t)}{Y_2(t)}\{dN_{2i}(t) - Y_{2i}(t)d\hat{\Lambda}(t)\}]^2\\ =& n\sum_{i=1}^{n}[\int_0^\infty \frac{H(t)}{Y_1(t)}dM_{1i}(t) - \int_0^\infty \frac{H(t)}{Y_2(t)}dM_{2i}(t)\\ &+ \int_0^\infty \frac{H(t)}{Y_1(t)}Y_{1i}(t)\{d\Lambda_1(t) - d\hat{\Lambda}(t)\}\\ &- \int_0^\infty \frac{H(t)}{Y_2(t)}Y_{2i}(t)\{d\Lambda_2(t) - d\hat{\Lambda}(t)\}]^2.\end{aligned}$$

By the uniform convergence of $n^{-1}Y_k(t)$ and $Y_k(t)^{-1}dN_k(t)$ to $y_k(t)$ and $d\Lambda_k(t)$, respectively, $d\hat{\Lambda}(t) = \{Y_1(t) + Y_2(t)\}^{-1}\{dN_1(t) + dN_2(t)\}$ uniformly converges to $\{y_1(t) + y_2(t)\}^{-1}\{y_1(t)d\Lambda_1(t) + y_2(t)d\Lambda_2(t)\}$ in $[0, \tau]$ so that we have

$$\hat{\sigma}^2 = \frac{1}{n}\sum_{i=1}^{n}(\epsilon_{1i} + \epsilon_{1i} + \eta_i)^2 + o_p(1).$$

Here,

$$\eta_i = \int_0^\infty \frac{h(t)}{y_1(t) + y_2(t)}\{Y_{1i}(t)\frac{y_2(t)}{y_1(t)} + Y_{2i}(t)\frac{y_1(t)}{y_2(t)}\}\{d\Lambda_1(t) - d\Lambda_2(t)\}$$

are negligible under a contiguous sequence of models. Hence, $\hat{\sigma}^2 = n^{-1}\sum_{i=1}^{n}(\epsilon_{1i} + \epsilon_{1i})^2 + o_p(1)$ converges to σ^2.

Lemma: For $i = 1,...,n$, $dM_{1i}(t_1)dM_{2i}(t_2) - Y_{1i}(t_1)Y_{2i}(t_2)dA(t_1,t_2)$ are independent 0-mean random variables.

Proof: The independence of the random variables is granted by the independence of n pairs. For each k, $M_{ki}(t)$ marginally is a 0-mean martingale with respect to the filtration $\{\mathcal{F}_t : t \geq 0\}$ where $\mathcal{F}_t = \sigma\{N_{ki}(s), N_{ki}^c(s) : 0 \leq s \leq t, i = 1, ..., n_k\}$ and $N_{ki}^c(t) = (1 - \delta_{ki})I(X_{ki} \leq t)$. However, with a general dependency between paired survival times, M_{ki} is not a martingale over the joint probability space so that we cannot use the martingale theory to derive the covariance of $dM_{1i}(t_1)$ and $dM_{2i}(t_2)$. Instead, we take a direct approach using the basic assumptions and formulations for joint survival distributions. By definition,

$$\begin{aligned} dM_{1i}(t_1)dM_{2i}(t_2) &= dN_{1i}(t_1)dN_{2i}(t_2) - Y_{2i}(t_2)\lambda_2(t_2)dN_{1i}(t_1)dt_2 \\ &\quad - Y_{1i}(t_1)\lambda_1(t_1)dt_1 dN_{2i}(t_2) + Y_{1i}(t_1)Y_{2i}(t_2)\lambda_1(t_1)\lambda_2(t_2)dt_1 dt_2. \end{aligned} \quad (10.A3)$$

We want to calculate the expected value of (10.A3) by

$$E\{dM_{1i}(t_1)dM_{2i}(t_2)\} = E[E\{dM_{1i}(t_1)dM_{2i}(t_2)|Y_{1i}(t_1)Y_{2i}(t_2)\}].$$

From the first term in the righthand side of (10.A3), we have

$$\begin{aligned} & E\{dN_{1i}(t_1)dN_{2i}(t_2)|Y_{1i}(t_1)Y_{2i}(t_2)\} \\ & = Y_{1i}(t_1)Y_{2i}(t_2)P(t_1 \leq X_{1i} < t_1 + dt_1, t_2 \leq X_{2i} < t_2 + dt_2, \delta_{1i} = 1, \\ & \delta_{2i} = 1 | X_{1i} \geq t_1, X_{2i} \geq t_2) \\ & = Y_{1i}(t_1)Y_{2i}(t_2) \\ & \quad \times \frac{P(t_1 \leq T_{1i} < t_1 + dt_1, t_2 \leq T_{2i} < t_2 + dt_2, T_{1i} < C_{1i}, T_{2i} < C_{2i})}{P(X_{1i} \geq t_1, X_{2i} \geq t_2)} \\ & \equiv Y_{1i}(t_1)Y_{2i}(t_2) \times \frac{B_1}{B_2}. \end{aligned} \quad (10.A4)$$

The second equality in (10.A2) holds by assuming that, for each subject, censoring and event do not occur at the same time. If the event time is tied with the censoring, then we assume that the censoring has occurred right after the event. The independent censoring assumption yields

$$B_2 = S(t_1, t_2)G(t_1, t_2). \quad (10.A5)$$

For B_1, we have

$$\begin{aligned} & P(t_1 \leq T_{1i} < t_1 + dt_1, t_2 \leq T_{2i} < t_2 + dt_2, C_{1i} \geq t_1 + dt_1, C_{2i} \geq t_2 + dt_2) \leq B_1 \\ & \leq P(t_1 \leq T_{1i} < t_1 + dt_1, t_2 \leq T_{2i} < t_2 + dt_2, C_{1i} \geq t_1, C_{2i} \geq t_2), \end{aligned}$$

which can be expressed as

$$\begin{aligned} & P(t_1 \leq T_{1i} < t_1 + dt_1, t_2 \leq T_{2i} < t_2 + dt_2)G(t_1 + dt_1, t_2 + dt_2) \leq B_1 \\ & \leq P(t_1 \leq T_{1i} < t_1 + dt_1, t_2 \leq T_{2i} < t_2 + dt_2)G(t_1, t_2) \end{aligned}$$

under the independent censoring assumption. In addition, assuming that the censoring variables are continuous and ignoring the negligible error terms as $dt_1, dt_2 \to 0$, we have

$$B_1 = P(t_1 \le T_{1i} < t_1 + dt_1, t_2 \le T_{2i} < t_2 + dt_2)G(t_1, t_2). \tag{10.A6}$$

Combining (10.A4)–(10.A6), we obtain

$$\begin{aligned} &E\{dN_{1i}(t_1)dN_{2i}(t_2)|Y_{1i}(t_1)Y_{2i}(t_2)\} \\ &= Y_{1i}(t_1)Y_{2i}(t_2)P(t_1 \le T_{1i} < t_1 + dt_1, t_2 \le T_{2i} < t_2 + dt_2|T_{1i} \ge t_1, T_{2i} \ge t_2) \\ &= Y_{1i}(t_1)Y_{2i}(t_2)\lambda(t_1, t_2)dt_1dt_2, \end{aligned}$$

and

$$E\{dN_{1i}(t_1)dN_{2i}(t_2)\} = \lambda(t_1, t_2)dt_1dt_2E\{Y_{1i}(t_1)Y_{2i}(t_2)\}. \tag{10.A7}$$

Similarly, from the second term of (10.A3), we have

$$E\{Y_{2i}(t_2)dN_{1i}(t_1)|Y_{1i}(t_1)Y_{2i}(t_2)\} = Y_{1i}(t_1)Y_{2i}(t_2)\lambda_{1|2}(t_1|t_2)dt_1,$$

so that

$$E\{Y_{2i}(t_2)dN_{1i}(t_1)\} = \lambda_{1|2}(t_1|t_2)dt_1E\{Y_{1i}(t_1)Y_{2i}(t_2)\}. \tag{10.A8}$$

Also, for the third term of (10.A1), we have

$$E\{Y_{1i}(t_1)dN_{2i}(t_2)\} = \lambda_{2|1}(t_2|t_1)dt_2E\{Y_{1i}(t_1)Y_{2i}(t_2)\}. \tag{10.A9}$$

Hence, from (10.A3) and (10.A7)–(10.A9),

$$\{dM_{1i}(t_1)dM_{2i}(t_2) - Y_{1i}(t_1)Y_{2i}(t_2)dA(t_1, t_2), i = 1, ..., n\}$$

are independent random variables with mean 0, where

$$\begin{aligned} dA(t_1, t_2) =&\{\lambda(t_1, t_2) - \lambda_{1|2}(t_1|t_2)\lambda_2(t_2) - \lambda_1(t_1)\lambda_{2|1}(t_2|t_1) \\ &+ \lambda_1(t_1)\lambda_2(t_2)\}dt_1dt_2. \end{aligned}$$

Murray (2000) introduces a similar expression,

$$\begin{aligned} d\tilde{A}(t_1, t_2) =&\{\tilde{\lambda}(t_1, t_2) - \tilde{\lambda}_{1|2}(t_1|t_2)\tilde{\lambda}_2(t_2) - \tilde{\lambda}_1(t_1)\tilde{\lambda}_{2|1}(t_2|t_1) \\ &+ \tilde{\lambda}_1(t_1)\tilde{\lambda}_2(t_2)\}dt_1dt_2, \end{aligned}$$

where

$$\begin{aligned} \tilde{\lambda}_k(t) &= \lim_{dt \to 0} P(t \le X_{ki} < t + dt, \delta_{ki} = 1|X_{ki} \ge t), \\ \tilde{\lambda}(t_1, t_2) &= \lim_{dt_1 \to 0} \lim_{dt_2 \to 0} P(t_1 \le X_{1i} < t_1 + dt_1, t_2 \le X_{2i} < t_2 + dt_2, \delta_{1i}\delta_{2i} \\ &=1|X_{1i} \ge t_1, X_{2i} \ge t_2), \end{aligned}$$

and for $k \neq k' \in \{1, 2\}$,

$$\tilde{\lambda}_{k|k'}(t) = \lim_{dt_k \to 0} P(t_k \leq X_{ki} < t_k + dt_k, \delta_{ki} = 1 | X_{ki} \geq t_k, X_{k'i} \geq t_{k'}).$$

Note that these expressions depend on both the joint survival and censoring distributions. This lemma shows that they can be expressed in terms of the joint survival distribution only under some reasonable assumption.

Appendix D. Calculation of ω and σ^2 under some practical settings

Under the common uniform censoring assumption,

$$G(t) = I(t < a + b) - \frac{t - b}{a} I(b \leq t < a + b).$$

Also, for the log-rank test and under the marginal exponential distributions with $\lambda_k(t) = \lambda_k$, we have

$$h(t) = G(t) \frac{e^{-(\lambda_1 + \lambda_2)t}}{e^{-\lambda_1 t} + e^{-\lambda_2 t}}.$$

Further, with the positive stable frailty model, we have

$$\begin{aligned}
S(t_1, t_2) &= \exp[-\{(\lambda_1 t_1)^{1/\theta} + (\lambda_2 t_2)^{1/\theta}\}^\theta], \\
s_k(t_1, t_2) &= -\lambda_k (\lambda_k t_k)^{1/\theta - 1} \{(\lambda_1 t_1)^{1/\theta} + (\lambda_2 t_2)^{1/\theta}\}^{\theta - 1} S(t_1, t_2), \\
f(t_1, t_2) &= \lambda_1 \lambda_2 (\lambda_1 t_1)^{1/\theta - 1} (\lambda_2 t_2)^{1/\theta - 1} \exp[-\{(\lambda_1 t_1)^{1/\theta} + (\lambda_2 t_2)^{1/\theta}\}^\theta] \\
&\quad \times \{(\lambda_1 t_1)^{1/\theta} + (\lambda_2 t_2)^{1/\theta}\}^{\theta - 2} \left[\{(\lambda_1 t_1)^{1/\theta} + (\lambda_2 t_2)^{1/\theta}\}^\theta + \frac{1 - \theta}{\theta} \right], \\
\lambda(t_1, t_2) &= \lambda_1 \lambda_2 (\lambda_1 \lambda_2 t_1 t_2)^{1/\theta - 1} \{(\lambda_1 t_1)^{1/\theta} \\
&\quad + (\lambda_2 t_2)^{1/\theta}\}^{\theta - 2} [\{(\lambda_1 t_1)^{1/\theta} + (\lambda_2 t_2)^{1/\theta}\}^\theta + \frac{1 - \theta}{\theta}]
\end{aligned}$$

and, for $k \neq k' \in \{1, 2\}$,

$$\lambda_{k|k'}(t_k | t_{k'}) = \lambda_k (\lambda_k t_k)^{1/\theta - 1} \{(\lambda_1 t_1)^{1/\theta} + (\lambda_2 t_2)^{1/\theta}\}^{\theta - 1}.$$

Hence, using the formulas given in the section 'Sample Size Calculation for the Weighted Rank Tests with Paired Survival Data', we obtain

$$\omega = (\lambda_1 - \lambda_2) \left\{ \int_0^{a+b} \frac{e^{-(\lambda_1 + \lambda_2)t}}{e^{-\lambda_1 t} + e^{-\lambda_2 t}} dt - \frac{1}{a} \int_b^{a+b} \frac{(t - b) e^{-(\lambda_1 + \lambda_2)t}}{e^{-\lambda_1 t} + e^{-\lambda_2 t}} dt \right\}$$

and $\sigma^2 = \sigma_1^2 + \sigma_2^2 - 2\sigma_{12}$, where, for $k \neq k' \in \{1, 2\}$,

$$\sigma_k^2 = \lambda_k \left\{ \int_0^{a+b} \frac{e^{-(\lambda_k+2\lambda_{k'})t}}{(e^{-\lambda_1 t} + e^{-\lambda_2 t})^2} dt - \frac{1}{a} \int_b^{a+b} \frac{(t-b)e^{-(\lambda_k+2\lambda_{k'})t}}{(e^{-\lambda_1 t} + e^{-\lambda_2 t})^2} dt \right\},$$

$$\sigma_{12} = \int_0^{a+b} \int_0^{a+b} \frac{S(t_1,t_2)G(t_1 \vee t_2)e^{-\lambda_2 t_1 - \lambda_1 t_2}}{(e^{-\lambda_1 t_1} + e^{-\lambda_2 t_1})(e^{-\lambda_1 t_2} + e^{-\lambda_2 t_2})} dA(t_1,t_2),$$

and

$$dA(t_1,t_2) = \{\lambda(t_1,t_2) - \lambda_2\lambda_{1|2}(t_1|t_2) - \lambda_1\lambda_{2|1}(t_2|t_1) + \lambda_1\lambda_2\} dt_1 dt_2.$$

11

Rank Tests for Clustered Survival Data and Sample Size Calculation under Cluster Randomization

A cluster randomization trial (CRT) randomizes clusters between intervention arms, and an outcome variable is observed from each subunit. In this case, the subunits of each cluster share common frailties so that their observations of the outcome variable tend to be positively correlated while those from different clusters are independent. Some CRTs have a time to event as their primary endpoint, and the usual study objective is to compare the marginal survival distributions between intervention arms. For example, in an otology study (Howie and Schwartz 1983; Teele et al. 1989), 78 children suffering from otitis media in the ears received ventilating tubes as a surgical intervention. Children were randomized into either no treatment or a post-surgery treatment when the medical therapy failed. They were regularly followed to check if the tube of each ear was functioning or not. One of the study aims was to determine if the post-surgery treatment extends the functioning time of ventilating tubes or not. In this study, children are clusters and ears are subunits. The number of subunits in each cluster, called cluster size, is fixed at two in this example.

In a dentistry study, children (clusters) with carious lesions in the teeth (subunits) are enrolled when the teeth are restored, and randomized into one of four treatment groups when one of the restored teeth shows evidence of demineralization, a sign that can lead to secondary caries. The outcome variable for this study is the time that each tooth remains free of secondary caries. Teeth that do not develop caries will be censored at the last exam.

In another example, Harper et.al. (2015) conducted a CRT to study interventions for reducing unintended pregnancy. They performed the study in 40 clinics across United States, of which 20 clinics were randomly assigned to receive a specialized training on intrauterine devices or progestin implants and the other 20 clinics to receive a standard care. Each clinic recruited women who were attending family planning or abortion care visits and had no intention of pregnancy in the following 12 months. One of the study endpoints was the time to unintended pregnancy during the follow-up period.

DOI: 10.1201/9781003221951-11

In this study, clinics are clusters and women are subunits. Note that cluster size is variable in this study, unlike in the otology study.

For independent survival data, weighted rank tests have been widely used as nonparametric methods to compare the survival distributions between treatment groups. Among the popular weighted rank statistics are the log-rank test (Peto and Peto 1972), Gehan-Wilcoxon test (Gehan 1965), Prentice-Wilcoxon (Prentice 1978), Tarone-Ware (1977) test and the tests of Harrington and Fleming's (1982) class. For the asymptotic distributions of the weighted rank tests, readers may refer to Andersen et al. (1982) and Fleming and Harrington (1991). Sample size calculation for the log-rank test with independent survival data has been studied by various investigators including George and Desu (1974), Schoenfeld (1983), Freedman (1982), Lakatos (1988), and Lakatos and Lan (1992).

In this chapter, we assume that cluster sizes are possibly random and the number of clusters is large for asymptotic theories. At first, we discuss the weighted rank tests to compare the marginal survival distributions between two treatment arms for CRTs and extend it to comparison of K treatment arms as proposed by Jung and Jeong (2003). And then, we also discuss the sample size calculation method of the rank statistics for two-sample comparisons as proposed by Li and Jung (2020).

Sample size calculation is a critical component in designing of clinical trials. Xie and Waksman (2003) derived a sample size formula for marginal proportional hazards regression (Lee et al. 1992) with a treatment indicator as the only covariate which is identical to the clustered log-rank test (Jung and Jeong, 2003) that we are considering in this chapter. Their formula inflates the Freedman's (1982) formula by a design effect which involves an intracluster correlation coefficient (ICC). They proposed to use the correlation coefficient of the censoring indicators of clusters as the ICC without much rational. They noticed that the sample size depends on the first and second moments of cluster size distribution, but they assumed that its variance was negligible. Our simulation study shows that their sample size formula is not very accurate, especially when cluster sizes are widely dispersed.

Gangnon and Kosorok (2004) proposed a sample size formula for the clustered log-rank test. Their method requires specification of the correlation coefficient between marginal martingales within each cluster that depends on censoring distribution as well as joint survival distribution. Since they did not provide the functional form of these design parameters, we cannot use their formula even when we know the censoring distribution and the joint survival distribution. Furthermore, at a design stage, the censoring distribution is specified by the expected accrual period and additional follow-up period, and accrual period is one of output parameters, like sample size so that we cannot use their formula when designing a CRT.

There are some existing sample size calculation methods associated with different statistical tests for clustered survival data. Hayes and Bennett (1999) proposed a sample size formula for comparing observed person-years rates in CRTs using an unpaired t-test. Jahn-Eimermacher et al. (2013) assumed a parametric gamma frailty model to modify the Hayes and Bennett formula. They tested the performance of their formula with a Wald test of shared frailty model. Manatunga and Chen (2000) also proposed a sample size formula by assuming a parametric model with exponential marginal distribution. Their derivation is based on the asymptotic normality of maximum likelihood estimator of the hazard rate. These methods either do not accurately reflect variable cluster size or the associated testing methods are overly parametric. We consider it is irrelevant to compare sample size formulas developed for different statistical tests, therefore in this chapter we do not focus on comparing with these methods.

In this chapter, we investigate the closed form sample size formula for clustered weighted rank tests for two-sample comparison of marginal survival distributions as introduced above.

Weighted Rank Tests for Clustered Survival Data

At first, we derive test statistics for two-sample test and extend them to K-sample test with $K \geq 3$. Suppose that n_k clusters are randomized into arm $k(= 1, ..., K)$. For cluster $i(= 1, ..., n_k)$ in treatment k, let m_{ki} be the number of subunits, called cluster size, and $(T_{kij}, j = 1, ..., m_{ki})$ be their survival times. We assume that subunits within each cluster have a common marginal survival distribution with cumulative hazard function $\Lambda_k(t)$ and survival function $S_k(t) = \exp\{-\Lambda_k(t)\}$. We do not specify the marginal and joint distribution functions for statistical testing, although we would have to for sample size calculation as will be discussed later.

Because of early termination of study or loss to follow-up, survival times may not be observed. Let C_{kij} be the censoring time with survival function G(t) that is associated with survival time T_{kij}. From the subunits in cluster i of treatment k, we observe $\{(X_{kij}, \delta_{kij}), j = 1, ..., m_{ki}\}$, where $X_{kij} = \min(T_{kij}, C_{kij})$ and $\delta_{kij} = I(T_{kij} \leq C_{kij})$. We assume that $(C_{kij}, j = 1, ..., m_{ki})$ are independent of $(T_{kij}, j = 1, ..., m_{ki})$. Censoring times may be correlated within each cluster (as in the case of common censoring within each cluster) and may have different distributions in different treatment groups. We assume that the maximum cluster size is bounded, and asymptotic theories are applied to large number of clusters. Define event processes $N_{kij}(t) = \delta_{kij}I(X_{kij} \leq t)$, $N_{ki}(t) = \sum_{j=1}^{m_{ki}} N_{kij}(t)$, $N_k(t) = \sum_{i=1}^{n_k} N_{ki}(t)$, and $N(t) = \sum_{k=1}^{K} N_k(t)$, and at-risk processes $Y_{kij}(t) = I(X_{kij} \geq t)$, $Y_{ki}(t) = \sum_{j=1}^{m_{ki}} Y_{kij}(t)$, $Y_k(t) = \sum_{i=1}^{n_k} Y_{ki}(t)$, and $Y(t) = \sum_{k=1}^{K} Y_k(t)$.

Two-Sample Case ($K = 2$)

We want to test if two treatment arms have the same marginal survival distributions or not, i.e.,

$$H_0 : \Lambda_1(t) = \Lambda_2(t) \text{ for all } t \geq 0$$

against

$$H_1 : \Lambda_1(t) \neq \Lambda_2(t) \text{ for some } t \geq 0.$$

Suppose that $H(t)$ is a non-negative bounded predictable process that converges in probability to a bounded left-continuous function $h(t)$ uniformly over $[0, \eta]$, where $\eta = \max\{t : S_1(t)S_2(t)G(t) > 0\}$, the minimum of the upper limits of the supports of survival and censoring distributions. We consider the class of rank statistics

$$W = \sqrt{n} \int_0^\infty H(t)\{d\hat{\Lambda}_1(t) - d\hat{\Lambda}_2(t)\}, \tag{11.1}$$

where $n = n_1 + n_2$, $\hat{\Lambda}_k(t) = \int_0^t Y_k^{-1}(s)dN_k(s)$ is the Nelson-Aalen (Nelson 1969; Aalen 1978) estimator based on the clustered survival data. By Ying and Wei (1994), $\hat{\Lambda}_k(t)$ uniformly converges to $\Lambda_k(t)$.

We use $H(t) = n^{-1}Y_1(t)Y_2(t)/Y(t)$ for the log-rank statistic (Peto and Peto, 1972), $H(t) = n^{-2}Y_1(t)Y_2(t)$ for the Gehan-Wilcoxon test, and $H(t) = n^{-1}\hat{S}^-(t)Y_1(t)Y_2(t)/Y(t)$ for the Prentice-Wilcoxon test, where $Y(t) = Y_1(t) + Y_2(t)$ and $\hat{S}^-(t)$ is the left-continuous version of the Kaplan-Meier (1958) estimate in the pooled sample

$$\{(X_{kij}, \delta_{kij}), 1 \leq j \leq m_{ki}, 1 \leq i \leq n_k, k = 1, 2\}.$$

When subunits within clusters are independent, readers may refer to Gill (1980) or Fleming and Harrington (1991) for the asymptotic normality of W and its variance estimator. With possible dependency within clusters, however, the estimator is inappropriate. In Appendix A we show that, under H_0, W is asymptotically normal with mean 0 and variance σ^2 that can be consistently estimated by $\hat{\sigma}^2$ as given in (11.A3), i.e.,

$$\hat{\sigma}^2 = \frac{1}{n}\sum_{i=1}^{n_1} \hat{\varepsilon}_{1i}^2 + \frac{1}{n}\sum_{i=1}^{n_2} \hat{\varepsilon}_{2i}^2,$$

where

$$n^{-1}\hat{\varepsilon}_{ki} = \sum_{j=1}^{m_{ki}} \frac{\delta_{kij} H(X_{kij})}{Y_k(X_{kij})} - \sum_{k'=1}^{2}\sum_{i'=1}^{n_{k'}}\sum_{j'=1}^{m_{k'i'}} \frac{\delta_{k'i'j'} Y_{ki}(X_{k'i'j'}) H(X_{k'i'j'})}{Y_k(X_{k'i'j'}) Y(X_{k'i'j'})}.$$

Specifically, for the log-rank test,

$$\hat{\varepsilon}_{ki} = \sum_{j=1}^{m_{ki}} \frac{\delta_{kij} Y_{3-k}(X_{kij})}{Y(X_{kij})} - \sum_{k'=1}^{2}\sum_{i'=1}^{n_{k'}}\sum_{j'=1}^{m_{k'i'}} \frac{\delta_{k'i'j'} Y_{ki}(X_{k'i'j'}) Y_{3-k}(X_{k'i'j'})}{Y(X_{k'i'j'})^2}.$$

Based on these results, we reject H_0 when the absolute value of $W/\hat{\sigma}$ is larger than $z_{1-\alpha/2}$. Stedman et al. (2011) developed a SAS macro for the clustered log-rank test. Our log-rank statistic is asymptotically equivalent to the partial score test of Lee, Wei and Amato (1992) based on the marginal Cox regression model with a binary covariate distinguishing two arms. The log-rank and the Prentice-Wilcoxon tests are special cases of Lee, Wei, and Ying (1993).

Extension To K Sample Cases

Now, we consider comparing more than two treatment groups with cluster randomization. Let $L(t)$ be a non-negative bounded predictable process that converges in probability to a bounded left-continuous function $\ell(t)$ uniformly over $[0, \eta]$, where $\eta = \max\{t : G(t)\prod_{k=1}^{K} S_k(t) > 0\}$. For testing $H_0 : \Lambda_1(t) = \cdots = \Lambda_K(t)$, we consider the vector of test statistics $\boldsymbol{W} = (W_1, ..., W_{K-1})^T$ with

$$W_k = \frac{1}{\sqrt{n}} \int_0^{\infty} Y_k(t)L(t)\{d\hat{\Lambda}_k(t) - d\hat{\Lambda}(t)\}, \tag{11.2}$$

where $n = \sum_{k=1}^{K} n_k$ and $\hat{\Lambda}(t) = \int_0^t Y^{-1}(s)dN(s)$ is the pooled Nelson's estimate from the K samples that is uniformly convergent to the common cumulative hazard function $\Lambda(t)$ under H_0 by Ying and Wei (1994).

Andersen et al. (1982) proposed to use (11.2) for testing K samples using independent survival data. The log-rank statistic uses $L(t) = 1$, the Gehan-Wilcoxon test uses $L(t) = n^{-1}Y(t)$, and the Prentice-Wilcoxon test uses $L(t) = \hat{S}^{-}(t)$, the pooled Kaplan-Meier estimate from the K clustered samples. When $K = 2$, (11.2) is reduced to (11.1).

In Appendix B we show that, under H_0, $\boldsymbol{W}$ is asymptotically normal with mean 0 and variance-covariance matrix V, which can be consistently estimated under H_0 by $\hat{V}$ as given in (11.A4). Hence, we reject H_0 when $Q = \boldsymbol{W}^T\hat{V}^{-1}\boldsymbol{W}$ is larger than $\chi^2_{K-1,\alpha}$, the $100(1-\alpha)$ percentile of a χ^2 distribution with $K-1$ degrees of freedom.

Simulation Studies

The methods discussed above are based on asymptotic theory. To assess their finite sample size performance, simulation studies are carried out for the two-sample ($K = 2$) tests.

The rejection probabilities of the log-rank (LR), Gehan-Wilcoxon (GW), and Prentice-Wilcoxon (PW) tests with nominal level $\alpha = 0.05$ are presented for a selection of sample size and ICC of clustered survival times under cluster randomization.

TABLE 11.1

Empirical type I error probabilities of $\alpha = 0.05$ tests under $H_0 : \lambda_1 = \lambda_2 = 1$ and 30% of censoring by the new method and the standard method ignoring dependency

		New method			Ignoring dependency		
ϕ	n_k	LR	GW	PW	LR	GW	PW
0.0	10	0.055	0.054	0.056	0.052	0.047	0.050
	30	0.063	0.059	0.058	0.059	0.058	0.060
	50	0.053	0.052	0.053	0.048	0.050	0.049
0.3	10	0.070	0.056	0.056	0.198	0.174	0.185
	30	0.059	0.050	0.051	0.191	0.173	0.179
	50	0.058	0.052	0.051	0.193	0.168	0.178
0.6	10	0.077	0.060	0.063	0.323	0.301	0.303
	30	0.061	0.053	0.056	0.310	0.306	0.308
	50	0.056	0.053	0.053	0.306	0.304	0.307

$\phi = \text{corr}(T_{kij}, T_{kij'})$

At first, cluster sizes m_{ki} are independently generated from a discrete uniform distribution between 1 and 10. Given cluster size m_{ki}, clustered survival times are generated by modifying Moran's (1967) algorithm. Let $(U_1, ..., U_{m_{ki}})$ and $(V_1, ..., V_{m_{ki}})$ be IID normal random vectors with marginally 0 mean and unit variance, and exchangeable structure with correlation coefficient $\sqrt{\phi}$. Define $T_{kij} = (U_j^2 + V_j^2)/(2\lambda_k)$. Then, $T_{ki1}, ..., T_{kim_{ki}}$ are random variables that have marginally exponential distributions with failure rates λ_k and exchangeable structure with correlation coefficient ϕ.

We set $\lambda_1 = 1$; $\lambda_2 = 1, 0.75, 0.5$, or 0.25; $\phi = 0, 0.3$, or 0.6; $n_1 = n_2 = 10$, 30, or 50. In checking the type I error probability under $H_0 : \lambda_1 = \lambda_2 = 1$, censoring variables are generated from IID $U(0, c_1)$ with c_1 chosen for 30% censoring overall. In checking power, censoring variables are generated from IID $U(0, c_1)$ or $U(c_0, c_0 + c_1)$ with c_0 chosen for 10% or 20% censoring in group 1 by $U(c_0, c_0 + c_1)$.

For each combination of ϕ, λ_2, and n_k, 5,000 samples of clustered survival data

$$\{(X_{kij}, \delta_{kij}), 1 \leq j \leq m_{ki}, 1 \leq i \leq n_k, k = 1, 2\}$$

are generated. Rank tests with nominal level $\alpha = 0.05$ are applied to each sample. Empirical rejection probability (ERP) is obtained by the proportion of samples rejecting H_0 among the 5,000 samples.

The results under $H_0 : \lambda_1 = \lambda_2 = 1$ are displayed in Table 11.1. If the sample size is small ($n_k = 10$ or 30), our test statistics, especially LR, are slightly anticonservative. Otherwise, they have ERP's close to the nominal level. For comparison, ERP's of the tests ignoring dependency are also reported. They are correct under independence ($\phi = 0$), but are anti-conservative

TABLE 11.2

Empirical rejection probabilities of the new tests with $\alpha = 0.05$ under $H_a : \lambda_1 \neq \lambda_2$ ($\lambda_1 = 1$)

Censoring			30%			20%			10%		
ϕ	λ_2	n_k	LR	GW	PW	LR	GW	PW	LR	GW	PW
0.0	0.8	10	0.160	0.135	0.140	0.180	0.142	0.151	0.199	0.161	0.160
		30	0.376	0.301	0.331	0.429	0.352	0.376	0.481	0.389	0.396
		50	0.555	0.469	0.502	0.618	0.524	0.549	0.689	0.588	0.596
	0.6	10	0.517	0.415	0.460	0.572	0.472	0.501	0.643	0.543	0.556
		30	0.943	0.888	0.917	0.967	0.927	0.941	0.985	0.963	0.966
		50	0.996	0.985	0.991	0.998	0.995	0.997	1.000	0.998	0.998
	0.4	10	0.910	0.838	0.873	0.944	0.897	0.915	0.975	0.946	0.953
		30	1.000	1.000	1.000	1.000	1.000	1.000	1.000	1.000	1.000
		50	1.000	1.000	1.000	1.000	1.000	1.000	1.000	1.000	1.000
0.3	0.8	10	0.123	0.096	0.099	0.132	0.102	0.107	0.142	0.110	0.111
		30	0.207	0.173	0.184	0.213	0.187	0.195	0.239	0.203	0.207
		50	0.305	0.254	0.271	0.319	0.271	0.281	0.336	0.292	0.295
	0.6	10	0.318	0.243	0.264	0.346	0.279	0.292	0.397	0.314	0.321
		30	0.690	0.606	0.644	0.720	0.647	0.669	0.766	0.696	0.703
		50	0.891	0.835	0.859	0.908	0.855	0.873	0.931	0.893	0.897
	0.4	10	0.683	0.574	0.620	0.719	0.627	0.658	0.795	0.700	0.718
		30	0.990	0.974	0.983	0.992	0.984	0.988	0.996	0.990	0.992
		50	1.000	0.999	1.000	1.000	1.000	1.000	1.000	1.000	1.000
0.6	0.8	10	0.112	0.082	0.091	0.117	0.090	0.093	0.126	0.091	0.092
		30	0.157	0.127	0.135	0.174	0.143	0.150	0.180	0.140	0.141
		50	0.211	0.172	0.187	0.226	0.185	0.194	0.246	0.203	0.206
	0.6	10	0.239	0.173	0.189	0.248	0.186	0.204	0.280	0.202	0.207
		30	0.500	0.403	0.439	0.523	0.434	0.456	0.570	0.483	0.493
		50	0.704	0.609	0.648	0.738	0.652	0.677	0.784	0.705	0.713
	0.4	10	0.516	0.395	0.444	0.556	0.430	0.474	0.611	0.501	0.526
		30	0.923	0.861	0.894	0.940	0.887	0.911	0.957	0.920	0.928
		50	0.993	0.976	0.984	0.996	0.987	0.990	0.997	0.992	0.993

$\phi = \text{corr}(T_{kij}, T_{kij'})$

under dependence ($\phi = 0.3$ or 0.6). As the dependency grows, the anti-conservativeness increases since the variance estimator ignoring positive ICC underestimates the true variance of rank tests.

ERP's when $\lambda_1 > \lambda_2$ are displayed in Table 11.2. As expected, the power of the rank tests increases as n_k or the hazard ratio $\Delta = \lambda_1/\lambda_2$ increases, or ϕ or censoring proportion decreases. All three tests have good power if n_k is large ($n_k = 50$) and two marginal distributions have a reasonable difference in hazard rates ($\lambda_2 \leq 0.6$). Note that the power is very sensitive to ICC, ϕ. Under the simulation settings, the marginal survival distributions in two groups have proportional hazards so that the log-rank test has a higher power than the two types of Wilcoxon tests.

TABLE 11.3

Empirical rejection probabilities of the log-rank test (LR) and the penalized likelihood test (PL) with $\alpha = 0.05$ under $H_0 : \lambda_1 = \lambda_2 = 0.1$ and $H_a : \lambda_1 = 0.1, \lambda_2 = 0.07$ when random frailty model is (a) correctly specified or (b) erroneously specified (i.e., Moran's model is the true model)

		(a) Frailty model			(b) Moran model		
	$\phi =$	0.1	0.25	0.4	0.1	0.25	0.4
H_0	LR	0.059	0.056	0.059	0.062	0.065	0.063
	PL	0.058	0.058	0.058	0.063	0.065	0.058
H_a	LR	0.554	0.437	0.298	0.596	0.532	0.456
	PL	0.552	0.451	0.326	0.609	0.534	0.475

$\phi = \text{corr}(T_{kij}, T_{kij'})$

We also compare the weighted rank tests with tests based on parametric distributions, such as frailty models. Splus implements a hypothesis testing that applies the penalized likelihood approach to random frailty models, see pp. 253–256 of Therneau and Grambsch (2000) for example. We compare the log-rank test with the penalized likelihood test (PL) through simulations in two cases: (a) when the random frailty model is correctly specified, but two groups have non-proportional hazards (gamma-exponential frailty model); (b) when two groups have proportional hazards, but the random frailty model is erroneously specified (Moran's model). In each of 5,000 simulation samples, we allocate $n_k = 40$ clusters to two groups and cluster sizes m_{ki} are generated from a discrete uniform distribution between 1 and 5.

At first, we generate the clustered survival times from the gamma-exponential frailty models, where survival variables $T_{kij} (j = 1, ..., m_{ki})$ have an exponential distribution with hazard rate $u\theta_k$ given the shared frailty u and the frailty has $\Gamma(\gamma, 1/\gamma)$ distribution with variance $1/\gamma$. Under this model, the ICC, $\phi = \text{corr}(T_{kij}, T_{kij'})$ for $j \neq j'$, is given as $1/\gamma$ $(\gamma > 2)$. We set $\phi = 0.1$, 0.25, or 0.4 (i.e., $\gamma = 10$, 4, or 2.5, respectively) and determine θ_k so that the marginal survival expectation, $E(T_{kij}) = \gamma/\{\theta_k(\gamma - 1)\}$, equals $1/\lambda_k$.

Censoring variables are generated from $U(0, a)$, where a is chosen for about 20% censoring in a group with $\lambda_k = 0.1$ and about 30% censoring in a group with $\lambda_k = 0.07$. Simulation results are summarized in Table 11.3(a). Under $H_0 : \lambda_1 = \lambda_2 = 0.1$, both tests are slightly anticonservative. Under $H_1 : \lambda_1 = 0.1, \lambda_2 = 0.07$, the log-rank test is as powerful as the penalized likelihood test with low intracluster correlation $(\phi = 0.1)$, but the former becomes slightly less powerful than the latter as the dependency increases. Under the gamma-exponential random frailty model, the marginal hazard functions

$$\tilde{\lambda}_k(t) = \theta_k/(1 + \theta_k t/\gamma) \tag{11.3}$$

are not proportional, but our non-parametric LR is comparable to the parametric PL in power. In fact, PL tests $\theta_1 = \theta_2$ rather than $\tilde{\lambda}_1(t) = \tilde{\lambda}_2(t)$ so that it does not detect the difference in marginal hazards $\tilde{\lambda}_k(t)$ if $\theta_1 = \theta_2$ but two groups have different intracluster correlation, i.e., $\gamma_1 \neq \gamma_2$.

Second, we generate the clustered survival times using the modified Moran's algorithm as described above. We set ϕ at 0.1, 0.25, or 0.4. Censoring times are generated from the uniform distribution used in the simulations based on gamma frailty models. Simulation results are summarized in Table 11.3(b). Under $H_0 : \lambda_1 = \lambda_2 = 0.1$, both tests are about equally anti-conservative. Although the Moran's algorithm does not generate a gamma frailty model, PL based on gamma frailty assumption performs well. Under $H_1 : \lambda_1 = 0.1, \lambda_2 = 0.07$, LR is as powerful as PL if $\phi = 0.1$ or 0.25, but is slightly less powerful if $\phi = 0.4$. We observed similar results with constant cluster sizes, such as $m_{ki} = 2$.

Real Example

The weighted rank tests are applied to the otology data introduced above to determine if two treatment groups have equal survival distributions or not. Table 11.4 reports the data set taken from Le (1997). In this data set, all children contributed observations from both ears so that $m_{ki} = 2$. Marginal survival curves for two groups are estimated using Kaplan-Meier (1958) method and displayed in Figure 11.1. For the clustered rank tests, test statistic $W/\hat{\sigma}$ (two-sided p-value) are 1.927 (.054) by LR, 1.781 (.075) by GW, and 1.789 (.074) by the PW. On the other hand, the standard rank test statistics

TABLE 11.4

Survival of ventilating tubes for 78 children with otitis media. The paired survival times (in months) are for right and left ears respectively, and censoring times are marked with + sign

(i) Control group ($n_1 = 38$)
(3.1,4.8+), (12.7,6.0), (3.1,6.4), (8.5,12.7), (9.1,9.1), (0.5,5.1), (18.1,15.0), (6.0,6.0), (6.4,6.4), (4.4+,1.3), (12.8,12.8), (8.8,8.8), (2.8+,2.8+), (9.3,27.1), (6.1,6.1), (17.9,20.9), (9.3,3.1), (2.9,1.0), (9.1,9.1), (5.8,9.3), (2.9,1.1), (6.2,9.2), (1.1+,1.1+), (6.0,10.7), (6.2,6.2), (9.3,19.3+), (0.8,0.8), (13.3,13.3), (0.8,8.1), (3.0,15.8), (9.4,9.4), (3.1,3.1), (7.6,10.1), (5.5,5.5), (0.7,0.7), (7.0,7.0), (11.7,3.1), (14.3,3.2)
(ii) Treatment group ($n_2 = 40$)
(11.9,8.8), (15.4,9.2), (9.3,9.3), (15.0,0.9), (15.0,11.9), (17.8,12.2), (5.9,8.7), (8.9,12.6), (0.6,5.7), (6.0,9.4), (14.6,9.0), (12.1,2.9), (3.0,3.0), (24.9,8.7), (5.2,9.0), (24.3,18.8), (15.2,12.5), (33.0,12.1), (13.1,0.7), (6.1,17.1+), (9.5,3.4), (15.1,17.8), (5.8,5.8), (0.6,3.0), (2.8,1.6), (6.2,9.0), (8.7,3.4), (20.9+,3.4), (9.2,6.0), (6.4,14.3+), (8.8,8.8), (18.5,13.3), (12.2,12.2), (12.5+,8.8), (8.5,21.7), (1.8,20.7), (6.2,9.0), (9.7,11.1+), (6.0,6.0), (8.7,8.7)

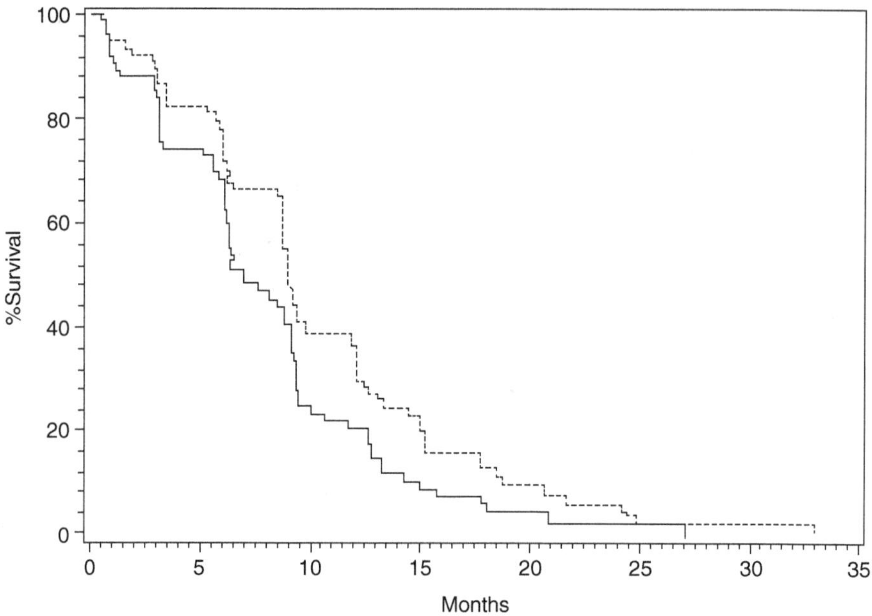

FIGURE 11.1
Survival of ventilating tubes. Solid line for control group and dotted line for treatment group.

ignoring dependency give 2.073 (.038) by LR, 2.035 (.042) by GW, and 2.041 (.041) by PW. We observe that ignoring dependency inflate the significance level because of clustering effect. Le and Lindgren (1996) observe similar comparisons.

We apply PL implemented in Splus to the otology study data, and obtain two-sided p-value 0.028, which is much more significant than the testing results from our rank tests. In fact, PL tests if two groups have the same conditional hazard rates, i.e., $H_0 : \theta_1 = \theta_2$ in model (11.3), given shared frailty. If two groups have equal frailty distribution, i.e., $\gamma_1 = \gamma_2$ in model (11.3), then this is the same as testing the equivalence of two marginal hazards, i.e., $H_0 : \lambda_1 = \lambda_2$, as we intended. However, if two groups have different frailty distributions, then PL does not test the equivalence of two marginal hazards. In other words, PL can give a small p-value if two groups have different intracluster correlation level (i.e., different frailty distributions) even when two marginal survival curves look alike, for example when two curves cross with similar medians. In this data set, the estimated ICCs using Lin and Ying's (1993) approach are $\hat{\phi}_1 = 0.50$ for the control group and $\hat{\phi}_2 = 0.12$ for the treatment group. The high significance by PL may result from the discrepancy in ICC between the two groups.

Sample Size Calculation of the Log-Rank Test for Two-Arm CRTs

Jung (2007) proposed a simulation-based sample size calculation method of the two-sample ($K = 2$) rank tests for CRTs as investigated above. A simulation method, however, does not show the explicit relationship between design parameters and the required sample size. Furthermore, if there exists errors in the computer program for simulations, we will have a wrong sample size. But, it is not always easy to identify and correct all programming errors. Most of all, it is impossible to validate a simulation-based sample size method without another sample size calculation method. A closed-form sample size formula resolves these issues. A formula can be validated through simulations. We will investigate Li and Jung's (2020) closed-form sample size formula of the log-rank tests for CRTs. It can be easily modified for other weighted rank tests.

The sample size of a CRT usually means the number of clusters, rather than the total number of subunits. The cluster sizes of a CRT can be either fixed as in Howie's study or random as in Harper's trial or the dental trial introduced above. Even when the cluster size is random, its distribution can be pre-specified based on some historical information. For example, in Harper's trial, cluster sizes can be estimated by the expected accrual rate of each member clinic and accrual period of the trial.

Let $p_k = n_k/n$ denote the allocation proportion for arm k ($p_1 + p_2 = 1$), and $\bar{m} = E(m_{ki})$ and $\bar{\bar{m}} = E(m_{ki}^2)$ denote the first and second moments, respectively, of the distribution of cluster sizes. If the cluster sizes are constant $m_{ki} = m$, then we have $\bar{m} = m$ and $\bar{\bar{m}} = m^2$.

In clustered data, we assume that the outcomes of subunits within each cluster have exchangeable correlation structure. Suppose that, for arm k, subunits have marginal survival function $S_k(t)$, marginal hazard function $\lambda_k(t) = \partial\Lambda_k(t)/\partial t$, bivariate joint survival function

$$S_k(t_1, t_2) = P(T_{kij} \geq t_1, T_{kij'} \geq t_2)$$

and joint probability density function $f_k(t_1, t_2) = \partial^2 S_k(t_1, t_2)/\partial t_1 \partial t_2$. Further, we define the joint hazard function

$$\lambda_k(t_1, t_2) = f_k(t_1, t_2)/S_k(t_1, t_2)$$

and two conditional hazard functions

$$\lambda_{k(1|2)}(t_1, t_2) = \lim_{\epsilon \to 0} \frac{P(t_1 \leq T_{kij} < t_1 + \epsilon, T_{kij'} \geq t_2)}{P(T_{kij} \geq t_1, T_{kij'} \geq t_2)} = -\frac{\partial S_k(t_1, t_2)/\partial t_1}{S_k(t_1, t_2)}$$

and

$$\lambda_{k(2|1)}(t_1, t_2) = \lim_{\epsilon \to 0} \frac{P(T_{kij} \geq t_1, t_2 \leq T_{kij'} < t_2 + \epsilon)}{P(T_{kij} \geq t_1, T_{kij'} \geq t_2)} = -\frac{\partial S_k(t_1, t_2)/\partial t_2}{S_k(t_1, t_2)}$$

for $j \neq j'$.

In sample size calculation, we have to specify the censoring distribution based on the accrual and follow-up pattern of subunits and clusters. The censoring times may be possibly correlated between subunits of each cluster. For example, if clusters are censored, then the subunits in each cluster will have the same censoring time. Let $G(t) = P(C_{kij} \geq t)$ and $G(t_1, t_2) = P(C_{kij} \geq t_1, C_{kij'} \geq t_2)$ for $j \neq j'$ denote the marginal and bivariate survival functions, respectively, of a censoring distribution.

By Appendix C, under H_1, the log-rank statistic W in (11.1) is approximately normal with mean $\omega\sqrt{n}$ and variance

$$\sigma^2 = p_1\{\bar{m}\sigma_{11}^2 + (\bar{\bar{m}} - \bar{m})\sigma_{12}\} + p_2\{\bar{m}\sigma_{21}^2 + (\bar{\bar{m}} - \bar{m})\sigma_{22}\},$$

where

$$\omega = p_1 p_2 \bar{m} \int_0^\infty \frac{S_1(t)S_2(t)G(t)}{p_1S_1(t) + p_2S_2(t)}\{d\Lambda_1(t) - d\Lambda_2(t)\}$$

$$\sigma_{k1}^2 = p_{3-k}^2 \int_0^\infty \frac{S_{3-k}^2(t)S_k(t)G(t)}{\{p_1S_1(t) + p_2S_2(t)\}^2} d\Lambda_k(t)$$

$$\sigma_{k2} = p_{3-k}^2 \int_0^\infty \int_0^\infty \frac{S_{3-k}(t_1)S_{3-k}(t_2)S_k(t_1,t_2)G(t_1,t_2)}{\{p_1S_1(t_1) + p_2S_2(t_1)\}\{p_1S_1(t_2) + p_2S_2(t_2)\}} dA_k(t_1,t_2)$$

and

$$\begin{aligned} dA_k(t_1,t_2) =& \{\lambda_k(t_1,t_2) - \lambda_{k(1|2)}(t_1,t_2)\lambda_k(t_2) - \lambda_{k(2|1)}(t_1,t_2)\lambda_k(t_1) \\ &+ \lambda_k(t_1)\lambda_k(t_2)\}dt_1dt_2 \end{aligned}$$

Without giving this explicit form, Gangnon and Kosorok (2004) require specification of σ_{k2} as an input parameter in sample size calculation.

Also by Appendix C, the variance estimator $\hat{\sigma}^2$ converges to σ^2. Hence, for a given sample size n, the power is given as

$$1 - \beta = P\left(|\frac{W}{\hat{\sigma}}| > z_{1-\alpha/2}\middle| H_1\right) \approx P\left(\frac{W - \omega\sqrt{n}}{\sigma} > z_{1-\alpha/2} - \frac{\omega\sqrt{n}}{\sigma}\middle| H_1\right) \quad (11.4)$$

Since $(W - \omega\sqrt{n})/\sigma$ is a $N(0,1)$ random variable under H_1, from (11.4), we have

$$1 - \beta = \bar{\Phi}\left(z_{1-\alpha/2} - \frac{p_1p_2\bar{m}\tilde{\omega}\sqrt{n}}{\sigma}\right), \quad (11.5)$$

where $\bar{\Phi}(t)$ is the survival function for the standard normal distribution and

$$\tilde{\omega} = \frac{\omega}{p_1p_2\bar{m}} = \int_0^\infty \frac{S_1(t)S_2(t)G(t)}{p_1S_1(t) + p_2S_2(t)}\{d\Lambda_1(t) - d\Lambda_2(t)\}.$$

By solving (11.5) with respect to n, we have the sample size (i.e., required number of clusters) formula

$$n = \frac{\sigma^2(z_{1-\alpha/2} + z_{1-\beta})^2}{(\bar{m}p_1p_2\tilde{\omega})^2}. \tag{11.6}$$

Since $\tilde{\omega}$ and σ_{k1}^2 depend only on the marginal survival and censoring distributions and σ_{k2}^2 depends only on the marginal and bivariate survival and censoring distributions, the power of the log-rank test depends only on the marginal and bivariate survival and censoring distributions. So, a sample size calculation requires specification of the first two dimensional distributions of clustered survival and censoring times even when the cluster sizes are larger than two. From (11.6), we find that we need a large number of clusters n if the average cluster size $\bar{m}$ is small and the variance of cluster size distribution $\bar{\bar{m}} - \bar{m}^2$ is large. Note that $\rho_k = \sigma_{k2}/\sigma_{k1}^2$ is an ICC of clustered survival times. The sample size also increases in this ICC.

We simplify sample size (11.6) under nearby alternative hypothesis where $\Delta - 1 \approx \log\Delta$ for the hazard ratio $\Delta = \lambda_1/\lambda_2$. Appendix D shows that our sample size formula (11.6) can be simplified to

$$n = \frac{(z_{1-\alpha/2} + z_{1-\beta})^2}{\bar{m}dp_1p_2(\log\Delta)^2}\text{IF}, \tag{11.7}$$

where $\text{IF} = 1 + (\bar{\bar{m}}/\bar{m} - 1)\rho$, $\rho = (p_1c_1 + p_2c_2)/(p_1d_1 + p_2d_2)$,

$$c_k = \int_0^\infty \int_0^\infty S_k(t_1, t_2)G(t_1, t_2)dA_k(t_1, t_2)$$

and $d_k = -\int_0^\infty G(t)dS_k(t)$ is the probability that a subunit in arm k has an event.

In (11.7), $M = \bar{m}n$ is the total number of subunits, and, by Schoenfeld (1983),

$$D_0 = \frac{(z_{1-\alpha/2} + z_{1-\beta})^2}{p_1p_2(\log\Delta)^2}$$

is the required number of events when subunits are independent. Hence, IF is the inflation factor of required sample size to adjust for intracluster correlation.

In the following subsections, we propose some practical models for survival and censoring distributions to be used in sample size calculations. We also discuss sample size calculation when accrual rate, instead of accrual period, is given.

Specification of Survival Distribution

Exponential distributions have been widely used for modeling survival distributions in sample size calculation of real clinical trials. For exponential distributions, there exists a 1-to-1 relationship among hazard rate, median, and survival probability at a time point so that they are fully specified by any one of these parameters. So, when designing a new trial, it is easy to specify the survival distribution for the control arm based on an estimate of any of these parameters from a previous study. So, in designing a CRT also, we propose to use an exponential distribution with hazard rate λ_k marginally for each subunit in arm k.

We consider using a copula to model the joint survival distribution among subunits of each cluster. With exponential marginal survival distributions, the bivariate survival function of arm k using Clayton and Cuzick's (1985) frailty model is given by

$$S_k(t_1, t_2) = \{\exp(\lambda_k t_1/\theta) + \exp(\lambda_k t_2/\theta) - 1\}^{-\theta},$$

where $\theta = 1/(2\tau) - 1/2$ and $\tau \in [0, 1]$ is the Kendall's tau with 0 meaning no relationship and 1 meaning a perfect relationship between paired survival times. For this joint survival distribution, we have the joint hazard function

$$\lambda_k(t_1, t_2) = \frac{\lambda_k^2(1 + 1/\theta)e^{(t_1+t_2)\lambda_k/\theta}}{(e^{\lambda_k t_1/\theta} + e^{\lambda_k t_2/\theta} - 1)^2}$$

and two conditional hazard functions

$$\lambda_{k(1|2)}(t_1, t_2) = \frac{\lambda_k e^{\lambda_k t_1/\theta}}{e^{\lambda_k t_1/\theta} + e^{\lambda_k t_2/\theta} - 1},$$

$$\lambda_{k(2|1)}(t_1, t_2) = \frac{\lambda_k e^{\lambda_k t_2/\theta}}{e^{\lambda_k t_1/\theta} + e^{\lambda_k t_2/\theta} - 1}.$$

Hence, we have

$$dA_k(t_1, t_2) = \lambda_k^2 \left\{ \frac{(1 + 1/\theta)e^{(t_1+t_2)\lambda_k/\theta}}{(e^{\lambda_k t_1/\theta} + e^{\lambda_k t_2/\theta} - 1)^2} - \frac{e^{\lambda_k t_1/\theta} + e^{\lambda_k t_2/\theta}}{e^{\lambda_k t_1/\theta} + e^{\lambda_k t_2/\theta} - 1} + 1 \right\} \tag{11.8}$$

$dt_1 dt_2$.

Specification of Censoring Distribution

In a CRT, the censoring distribution of subunits is determined by the accrual and follow-up patterns of clusters and subunits. We investigate censoring distributions appropriate for the two CRTs that are discussed above. In the otology study, patients (clusters) are recruited during an accrual period a and the both ears (subunits) of each patient are accrued at the time of patient accrual. In this case, if there exists administrative censoring only or loss to follow-up occurs only when patients are missing, then all subunits in each cluster have the same censoring time. We call this a 'common censoring case'.

On the other hand, in the Harper's trial, all clinics (clusters) are recruited when the study opens and the women (subunits) are independently accrued to each clinic over an accrual period. In this case, the censoring times are independent among subunits whether they belong to the same clinics or not. We call this an 'independent censoring case'.

(i) Common Censoring Case
If all subunits of each cluster have a common censoring time, i.e., $C_{kij} = C_{ki}$, then we have $G(t_1, t_2) = P(C_{ki} \geq t_1, C_{ki} \geq t_2) = G(t_1 \vee t_2)$, where $t_1 \vee t_2$ denotes the maximum of t_1 and t_2. Note that the bivariate censoring distribution is specified by the marginal censoring distribution. Furthermore, if clusters are accrued at a constant rate for a period of a and followed for an additional period of b after the completion of accrual, then, with administrative censoring only, censoring variable C_{ki} has $U(b, a+b)$ distribution, i.e.,

$$G(t) = I(t < a+b) - \frac{t-b}{a} I(b \leq t < a+b).$$

(ii) Independent Censoring Case
If all clusters are recruited before study opens and the subunits of each cluster are independently accrued during an accrual period, then the censoring times are independent among subunits so that we have $G(t_1, t_2) = G(t_1)G(t_2)$. As in the common censoring case, we need to specify only the marginal distribution for censoring. If subunits of each cluster are accrued at a constant rate for period a and followed for an additional period of b after the completion of accrual, then, with administrative censoring only, censoring times C_{kij} are IID $U(b, a+b)$. Note that the marginal censoring distribution is identical to that of common censoring case.

Sample Size Calculation under Practical Design Settings

Let's consider a sample size calculation assuming multivariate exponential survival distributions using Clayton and Cuzick's (1985) frailty model and the two censoring (or accrual) patterns just discussed. In order to calculate a sample size using (11.6), we need to calculate $\bar{m}$, $\bar{\bar{m}}$, ω, σ_{k1}^2, and σ_{k2}^2 for a given survival distribution and a censoring distribution that is defined by an assumed accrual pattern. Since the two accrual patterns discussed in the section 'Specification of Censoring Distribution' result in the same marginal censoring distribution and $\tilde{\omega}$ and σ_{k1}^2 depend only on the marginal censoring distribution, we derive them commonly for the both accrual patterns. From

Appendix E, we have

$$\tilde{\omega} =(\lambda_1 - \lambda_2)\left\{\int_0^{a+b} \frac{e^{-(\lambda_1-\lambda_2)t}}{(p_1e^{-\lambda_1 t}+p_2e^{-\lambda_2 t})^2}dt - \frac{1}{a}\int_b^{a+b} \frac{(t-b)e^{-(\lambda_1-\lambda_2)t}}{(p_1e^{-\lambda_1 t}+p_2e^{-\lambda_2 t})^2}dt\right\}, \tag{11.9}$$

$$\sigma_{k1}^2 =p_{3-k}^2\lambda_k\left\{\int_0^{a+b} \frac{e^{-(\lambda_k+2\lambda_{3-k})t}}{(p_1e^{-\lambda_1 t}+p_2e^{-\lambda_2 t})^2}dt - \frac{1}{a}\int_b^{a+b} \frac{(t-b)e^{-(\lambda_k+2\lambda_{3-k})t}}{(p_1e^{-\lambda_1 t}+p_2e^{-\lambda_2 t})^2}dt\right\}. \tag{11.10}$$

The integrals in these formulas and those in the following subsections can be calculated using a numerical integration method.

Unlike $(\tilde{\omega}, \sigma_{k1}^2)$, $(\bar{m}, \bar{\bar{m}}, \sigma_{k2})$ are different between the censoring patterns.

(i) Common Censoring Case

Let $q(m)$ denote the probability mass function of the cluster size distribution that can be estimated from historical data. Then, the first and second moments of cluster size distribution are calculated by $\bar{m} = \sum_m m \times q(m)$ and $\bar{\bar{m}} = \sum_m m^2 \times q(m)$, respectively. Also, by Appendix E, we have

$$\sigma_{k2} = p_{3-k}^2 \int_0^{a+b}\int_0^{a+b} \frac{e^{-\lambda_{3-k}(t_1+t_2)}(e^{\lambda_k t_1/\theta}+e^{\lambda_k t_2/\theta}-1)^{-\theta}}{(p_1e^{-\lambda_1 t_1}+p_2e^{-\lambda_2 t_1})(p_1e^{-\lambda_1 t_2}+p_2e^{-\lambda_2 t_2})} \times(1-a^{-1}[t_1 \vee t_2 - b]_+)dA_k(t_1,t_2), \tag{11.11}$$

where $[t]_+ = t \times I(t \geq 0)$ and $dA_k(t_1, t_2)$ is given in (11.8).

(ii) Independent Censoring Case

In the Harper's trial, the cluster size of each clinic will be estimated by its accrual rate and a selected accrual period. Suppose that clinics will have variable patient volumes so that the expected accrual rate is different among clinics. For clinic (cluster) i with an expected accrual rate r_i, the expected cluster size will be $m_i = a \times r_i$ for a given accrual period a. Let $\bar{r}$ and $\bar{\bar{r}}$ denote the first and second moments of the accrual rate distribution, respectively. Then, given an accrual period a, the first and second moments of cluster size distribution will be estimated by $\bar{m} = a\bar{r}$ and $\bar{\bar{m}} = a^2\bar{\bar{r}}$, respectively. Also, by Appendix E, we have

$$\sigma_{k2} = p_{3-k}^2 \int_0^{a+b}\int_0^{a+b} \frac{e^{-\lambda_{3-k}(t_1+t_2)}(e^{\lambda_k t_1/\theta}+e^{\lambda_k t_2/\theta}-1)^{-\theta}}{(p_1e^{-\lambda_1 t_1}+p_2e^{-\lambda_2 t_1})(p_1e^{-\lambda_1 t_2}+p_2e^{-\lambda_2 t_2})} \times(1-a^{-1}[t_1 - b]_+)(1-a^{-1}[t_2 - b]_+)dA_k(t_1,t_2), \tag{11.12}$$

where $dA_k(t_1, t_2)$ is given in (11.8).

Sample Size Calculation for given Accrual Rate instead of Accrual Period

So far, we have calculated sample sizes given an accrual period a. In practice, however, it is easier to specify the accrual rate, rather than accrual period, based on the number of eligible patients who have visited the study institutions recently for both of the otology trial and Harper's trial. Note that patients are clusters in the otology trial and subunits in Harper's trial. As such, given an accrual rate, sample size calculation procedure is slightly different between the common censoring case and the independent censoring case. For the common censoring case, the cluster sizes are free of accrual period, whereas, for the independent censoring case, the cluster size increases in accrual period. In this section, we present sample size calculation methods under the design settings of the section 'Sample Size Calculation under Practical Design Settings'. From the formulas derived in Appendix E we know that $\tilde{\omega} = \tilde{\omega}(a)$, $\sigma_{k1}^2 = \sigma_{k1}^2(a)$, and $\sigma_{k2} = \sigma_{k1}^2(a)$ are all functions of the unknown accrual period a.

(i) Common Censoring Case
Using (11.9–11.11), we calculate the variance of the test statistic W, $\sigma^2 = \sigma^2(a) = p_1\{\bar{m}\sigma_{11}^2(a) + (\bar{\bar{m}} - \bar{m})\sigma_{12}(a)\} + p_2\{\bar{m}\sigma_{21}^2(a) + (\bar{\bar{m}} - \bar{m})\sigma_{22}(a)\}$ as a function of accrual period a. Given an accrual rate of clusters r and an accrual period a, we have $n \approx a \times r$ under a uniform accrual trend. Hence, by replacing n with its approximation $a \times r$, (11.6) is expressed as an equation on a

$$a \times r = \frac{\sigma^2(a)(z_{1-\alpha/2} + z_{1-\beta})^2}{\{\bar{m}p_1p_2\tilde{\omega}(a)\}^2}, \tag{11.13}$$

We can solve (11.13) using a numerical method, such as the bisection method. Let $a = a^*$ denote the solution to (11.13), then the required sample size is given as $n = a^* \times r$.

(ii) Independent Censoring Case
In an independent censoring case, suppose that the participating clinics (i.e., clusters) in Harper's trial have different patient volumes so that the accrual rate of patients (subunits) is varying among clinics. Let $\bar{r}$ and $\bar{\bar{r}}$ denote the first and second moments, respectively, of the distribution of accrual rates among clinics. Given an accrual period a and a distribution of accrual rates, we have $\bar{m} = a\bar{r}$ and $\bar{\bar{m}} = a^2\bar{\bar{r}}$. Combining this with (11.9), (11.10), and (11.12), σ^2 as a function of accrual period a is expressed as

$$\sigma^2(a) = a[p_1\{\bar{r}\sigma_{11}^2(a) + (a\bar{\bar{r}} - \bar{r})\sigma_{12}(a)\} + p_2\{\bar{r}\sigma_{21}^2(a) + (a\bar{\bar{r}} - \bar{r})\sigma_{22}(a)\}].$$

Hence, given an accrual period a, the required number of clusters is calculated by

$$n = [p_1\{\bar{r}\sigma_{11}^2(a) + (a\bar{\bar{r}} - \bar{r})\sigma_{12}(a)\} + p_2\{\bar{r}\sigma_{21}^2(a) + (a\bar{\bar{r}} - \bar{r})\sigma_{22}(a)\}] \times \frac{(z_{1-\alpha/2} + z_{1-\beta})^2}{a\{\bar{r}p_1p_2\tilde{\omega}(a)\}^2}. \quad (11.14)$$

Sometimes, one may want to calculate the required accrual period a when the number of clusters n is fixed in advance. In this case, for given n, the required accrual period is obtained by solving (11.14) with respect to a. For the solution $a = a^*$ to equation (11.14), the resulting number of subunits is given as $M = n \times \bar{r} \times a^*$.

Simulation Studies

Our sample size formulas are derived using large sample theories. We conduct simulations to evaluate the finite sample performance of our proposed sample size formulas.

Suppose that, for arm k, clustered survival times $(T_1, ..., T_m)$ have the Clayton and Cuzick's (1985) model with exponential marginal distributions whose joint survival function is given as

$$S_k(t_1, ..., t_m) = \left\{\sum_{j=1}^{m} \exp(\lambda_k t_j/\theta) - (m-1)\right\}^{-\theta},$$

where $\theta = 1/2(1/\tau - 1) > 0$. For this distribution, the conditional survival function of T_j given $T_1 = t_1, ..., T_{j-1} = t_{j-1}$ is

$$S_k(t_j|t_1, ..., t_{j-1}) = \frac{\partial^{j-1}S_k(t_1, ..., t_j)}{\partial t_1 \cdots \partial t_{j-1}} \Big/ \frac{\partial^{j-1}S_k(t_1, ..., t_{j-1})}{\partial t_1 \cdots \partial t_{j-1}}$$

$$= \left\{\frac{\sum_{j'=1}^{j} e^{\lambda_k t_{j'}/\theta} - (j-1)}{\sum_{j'=1}^{j-1} e^{\lambda_k t_{j'}/\theta} - (j-2)}\right\}^{-\theta-j+1}.$$

For IID $U(0,1)$ random variables $u_1, .., u_m$, survival times $(T_1, ..., T_m) = (t_1, ..., t_m)$ for a cluster in arm k are sequentially generated by solving the equations $u_1 = S_k(t_1) = \exp(-\lambda_k t_1)$ and $u_j = S_k(t_j|t_1, ..., t_{j-1})$ for $j = 2, ..., m$ with respect to $(t_1, ..., t_m)$. That is, for $j = 1, ..., m$, we have

$$t_j = \frac{\theta}{\lambda_k} \log\{j - 1 - e_{j-1} + (e_{j-1} - j + 2)u_j^{-1/(\theta+j-1)}\},$$

where $e_0 = 0$ and $e_j = e_{j-1} + \exp(\lambda_k t_j/\theta)$ for $j = 1, ..., m-1$.

In this simulation study, we assume that all subunits of each cluster are accrued at the same time, and cluster sizes are fixed at $m = 11$, or random with a discrete uniform distribution between 9 and 13, denoted as $U(9,13)$ or a discrete uniform distribution between 2 and 20, denoted as $U(2,20)$. Note that these three cluster size distributions have the same mean $\bar{m} = 11$, but different variances $\bar{\bar{m}} - \bar{m}^2 = 0$, 2, and 30, respectively. We set $\alpha = 0.05$; $1-\beta = 0.8, 0.85$, or 0.9; $p_1 = p_2 = 1/2$ for balanced allocation; $\Delta = \lambda_1/\lambda_2 = 1.4, 1.6$, or 1.8; median survival for arm 1 at 7 months, i.e., $\lambda_1 = 7^{-1}\log 2$ per month; Kendall's $\tau = 0.3$ or 0.6; $b = 1$ year: $r = 100$ clusters per year.

At first, we calculate the required sample size n using (11.6) or (11.7) under a design setting of $(\alpha, 1-\beta, \lambda_1, \lambda_2, \tau, p_1, r, b, \bar{m}, \bar{\bar{m}})$. Once a sample size is calculated, we generate 5,000 samples of survival data for arm 1 and 2 with size n using the design parameter values specified for the sample size calculation. We apply the clustered log-rank test to each simulated sample using two-sided $\alpha = 0.05$. We estimate an empirical power, $1-\hat{\beta}$, by the proportion of simulation samples rejecting H_0 among the 5,000 simulation samples. If the empirical power is close to the nominal power $1-\beta$, then we will conclude that the calculated sample size is accurate. In order to evaluate the finite sample property of the clustered log-rank test, we calculate an empirical type I error rate, $\hat{\alpha}$, by generating 5,000 simulation samples of size n under the same design setting specified for the sample size calculation, but with λ_2 set at λ_1 to generate clustered survival data under H_0.

Table 11.5 reports calculated sample size, and empirical type I error rate and power under the various design settings. Required sample size decreases in hazard ratio Δ and increases in $1-\beta$, τ, and the variance of cluster size distribution. We observe that both of our proposed formulas return similar sample sizes and their empirical powers are close to the nominal powers. Empirical type I error rate $\hat{\alpha}$ is close to the nominal level $\alpha = 0.05$ for most of the simulation settings too.

Freedman (1982) proposed a sample size formula for the standard log-rank test with independent survival data with balanced allocation,

$$M = \frac{2(z_{1-\alpha/2} + z_{1-\beta})^2(1+\Delta)^2}{(1-\Delta)^2(d_1+d_2)},$$

where d_k is the probability of having an event for subunits in arm k. When M subunits consist of n clusters, Xie and Waksman (2003) proposed to calculate the required number of clusters by

$$n = \frac{M}{\bar{m}}\{1 + (\bar{m}-1)\rho_0\}, \tag{11.15}$$

where ρ_0 is the correlation coefficient of event indicators δ_{kij} and $\delta_{kij'}$ for $j \neq j'$. Since $M/\bar{m}$ is the expected number of clusters, $1 + (\bar{m}-1)\rho_0$ is an inflation factor to adjust for intracluster correlation. They assume that the variance of cluster size distribution is negligible so that their inflation factor depends only on the first moment of the cluster size distribution, while IF in (11.7) depends on the first and second moments. Furthermore, the correlation

TABLE 11.5

Simulation results: Each cell reports $n(\hat{\alpha}, 1 - \hat{\beta})$, where n denotes the sample size calculated by equation (11.6) or (11.7), and $\hat{\alpha}$ and $1 - \hat{\beta}$) empirical type I error rate and power, respectively

			$m = 11$		$m \sim U(9, 13)$		$m \sim U(2, 20)$	
$1 - \beta$	τ	Δ	By (11.6)	By (11.7)	By (11.6)	By (11.7)	By (11.6)	By (11.7)
0.8	0.3	1.4	182 (0.057,0.806)	180 (0.054,0.811)	185 (0.051,0.819)	183 (0.057,0.809)	222 (0.054,0.812)	220 (0.059,0.802)
		1.6	99 (0.049,0.820)	95 (0.054,0.800)	100 (0.057,0.817)	97 (0.059,0.813)	120 (0.054,0.819)	116 (0.057,0.808)
		1.8	67 (0.056,0.832)	63 (0.061,0.805)	68 (0.059,0.822)	64 (0.063,0.797)	81 (0.059,0.835)	76 (0.057,0.801)
	0.6	1.4	275 (0.056,0.800)	277 (0.056,0.805)	279 (0.056,0.807)	282 (0.053,0.797)	336 (0.061,0.813)	340 (0.060,0.804)
		1.6	153 (0.052,0.812)	152 (0.068,0.808)	155 (0.055,0.812)	154 (0.055,0.819)	186 (0.059,0.814)	186 (0.060,0.816)
		1.8	105 (0.061,0.823)	102 (0.058,0.801)	107 (0.052,0.817)	104 (0.062,0.814)	128 (0.059,0.826)	125 (0.059,0.805)
0.85	0.3	1.4	208 (0.059,0.859)	205 (0.057,0.855)	211 (0.057,0.860)	209 (0.055,0.856)	253 (0.064,0.863)	249 (0.061,0.865)
		1.6	113 (0.060,0.864)	108 (0.055,0.844)	114 (0.058,0.863)	110 (0.054,0.850)	137 (0.054,0.873)	128 (0.054,0.856)
		1.8	77 (0.060,0.875)	71 (0.054,0.850)	78 (0.054,0.879)	72 (0.058,0.851)	93 (0.057,0.888)	82 (0.058,0.858)
	0.6	1.4	312 (0.058,0.852)	314 (0.056,0.852)	317 (0.063,0.852)	319 (0.052,0.859)	382 (0.057,0.849)	378 (0.053,0.850)
		1.6	174 (0.056,0.859)	172 (0.061,0.847)	176 (0.055,0.867)	175 (0.057,0.857)	211 (0.057,0.863)	201 (0.057,0.851)
		1.8	119 (0.061,0.865)	116 (0.057,0.847)	121 (0.060,0.866)	118 (0.059,0.860)	145 (0.059,0.880)	132 (0.057,0.848)
0.9	0.3	1.4	242 (0.059,0.907)	240 (0.054,0.904)	246 (0.055,0.904)	243 (0.059,0.904)	296 (0.059,0.905)	294 (0.060,0.904)
		1.6	131 (0.054,0.911)	126 (0.053,0.905)	133 (0.054,0.919)	128 (0.057,0.899)	160 (0.054,0.915)	154 (0.055,0.891)
		1.8	89 (0.059,0.915)	83 (0.063,0.894)	90 (0.056,0.922)	84 (0.059,0.906)	108 (0.054,0.917)	101 (0.063,0.903)
	0.6	1.4	363 (0.059,0.906)	364 (0.056,0.900)	368 (0.057,0.908)	370 (0.059,0.903)	445 (0.054,0.904)	448 (0.051,0.908)
		1.6	201 (0.052,0.911)	199 (0.054,0.916)	204 (0.058,0.912)	202 (0.057,0.906)	245 (0.060,0.910)	243 (0.059,0.907)
		1.8	138 (0.055,0.916)	134 (0.057,0.901)	140 (0.054,0.916)	136 (0.058,0.904)	168 (0.065,0.912)	164 (0.065,0.906)

coefficients ρ and ρ_0 are different between the two inflation factors. Note that ρ_0 depends on both survival and censoring distributions so that it will be difficult to specify its value at the time of sample size calculation.

We compare our sample size with those of Xie and Waksman's (2003) under various design settings. To evaluate the accuracy of the calculated sample sizes, we also calculate the empirical power of these sample sizes for the clustered log-rank test using simulated data. We consider a balanced allocation case $p_1 = p_2 = 1/2$, and exponential marginal distributions with median survival time of 7 months for the control arm ($k = 1$). To model the joint survival distribution, we use Clayton and Cuzick's copula with Kendall's $\tau = 0.1, 0.3,$ 0.5, or 0.7. Hazard ratio $\Delta = \lambda_1/\lambda_2$ is set at 1.3. We use an accrual period of $a = 1$ or 2 years, and a follow-up period of $b = 0.3$ or 1.2 years for a censoring probability of about 9% to 41% in the control arm. We also consider $(\alpha, 1 - \beta) = (0.05, 0.8)$ and a cluster size distribution of discrete (a) $U(9, 13)$ or (b) $U(2, 20)$. For the Xie and Waksman's formula, ρ_0 is calculated using the specified survival and censoring distributions.

Figures 11.2 (a) and (b) summarize the sample sizes and empirical powers for our formula (11.6) and Xie and Waksman's formula (11.15) under the design settings. Under each design setting, an empirical power is calculated from 5,000 simulation samples of the calculated sample size. For the simulation settings, our sample sizes are correctly powered overall. Note that Xie and Waksman's sample sizes are identical between Figure 11.1(a) and (b) since the two cluster size distributions have the same mean $\bar{m} = 11$ while they have different variances. Xie and Waksman's sample sizes are much underpowered except when the intracluster correlation is low (i.e., $\tau = 0.1$) and censoring is high (i.e., $b = 0.3$). This bias in power is much amplified with a large variance of cluster size distribution, i.e., $m \sim U(2, 20)$. With a high censoring and a low intracluster correlation, Xie and Waksman's sample sizes tend to be overpowered, except for $(a, b) = (1, 0.3)$ and $m \sim U(2, 20)$. Overall, Xie and Waksman's sample size formula does not seem to be appropriately powered for the clustered log-rank test.

Examples

Our sample size formula (11.6) is applied to design some real study examples.

Example 1: We apply the proposed sample size formula to design the otology study example that is introduced in the beginning of this chapter. Manatunga and Chen (2000) proposed a parametric model and calculated sample size for the study. Their method is based on the maximum likelihood estimator of the hazard ratio Δ of exponential distributions. In this study, the number of ears (subunits) per child (cluster) is constant, $m = 2$. With input parameters of $\alpha = 0.05$, $1 - \beta = 0.9$, $\lambda_1 = 7^{-1} \log 2$ per month, $\Delta = 1/0.7$, $\theta = 0.56$, $m_i = m = 2$, $a = 2.5$ years, $b = 1.5$ years, and $p_1 = 0.5$, their method yields 340 clusters (patients) in total. For the same input parameter

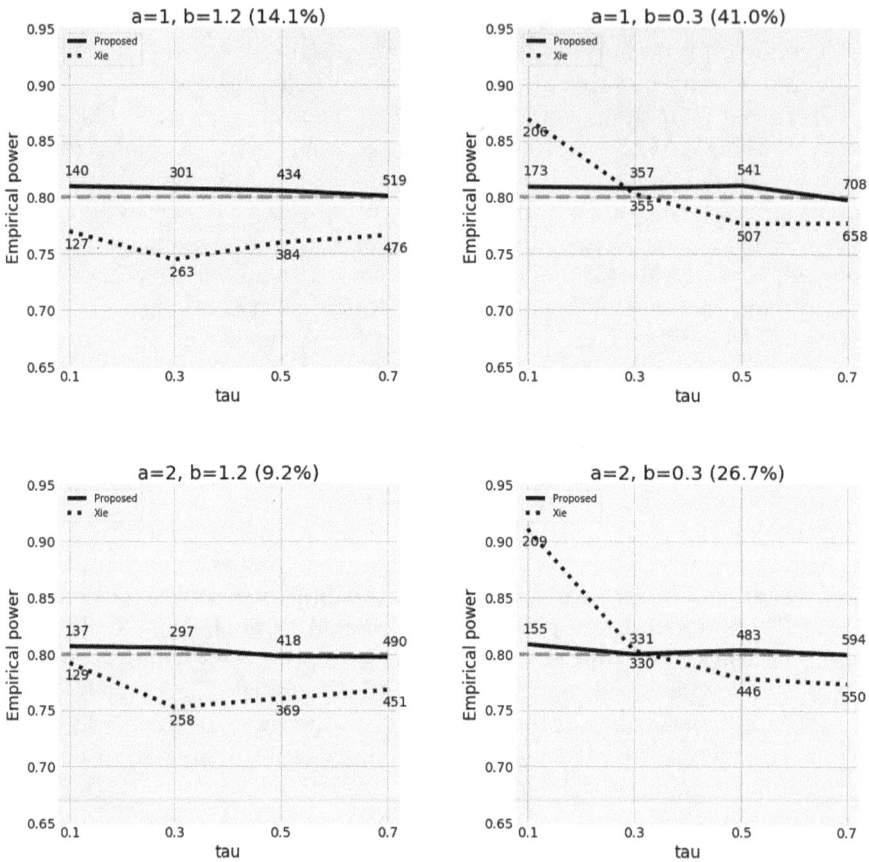

FIGURE 11.2
Sample size (marked above polygonal lines) and empirical power (y-axis) for the proposed method and Xie and Waksman 15 method with $a = 1$ or 2, $b = 0.3$ or 1.2 (censoring proportion presented in the parenthesis); $\tau = 0.1, 0.3, 0.5$, or 0.7; $(\alpha, 1-\beta) = (0.05, 0.8)$. (a) $U(9, 13)$ of cluster size distribution.

values and assuming Clayton and Cuzick's copula with marginal exponential distributions, the log-rank test for clustered data requires 333 clusters by our sample size formula. From 5,000 simulation samples, our sample size is shown to have an empirical power of 0.903 which is close to the nominal level $1-\beta = 0.9$.

We can specify an accrual rate instead of an accrual period. If the accrual rate is $r = 50$ patients per year, with other design parameters unchanged, the log-rank test for clustered data requires an accrual period $a = 6.3$ years for a total sample size of $n = 316$. If the accrual rate is $r = 100$ per year, then the required accrual period will be $a = 3.27$ years for $n = 327$ clusters.

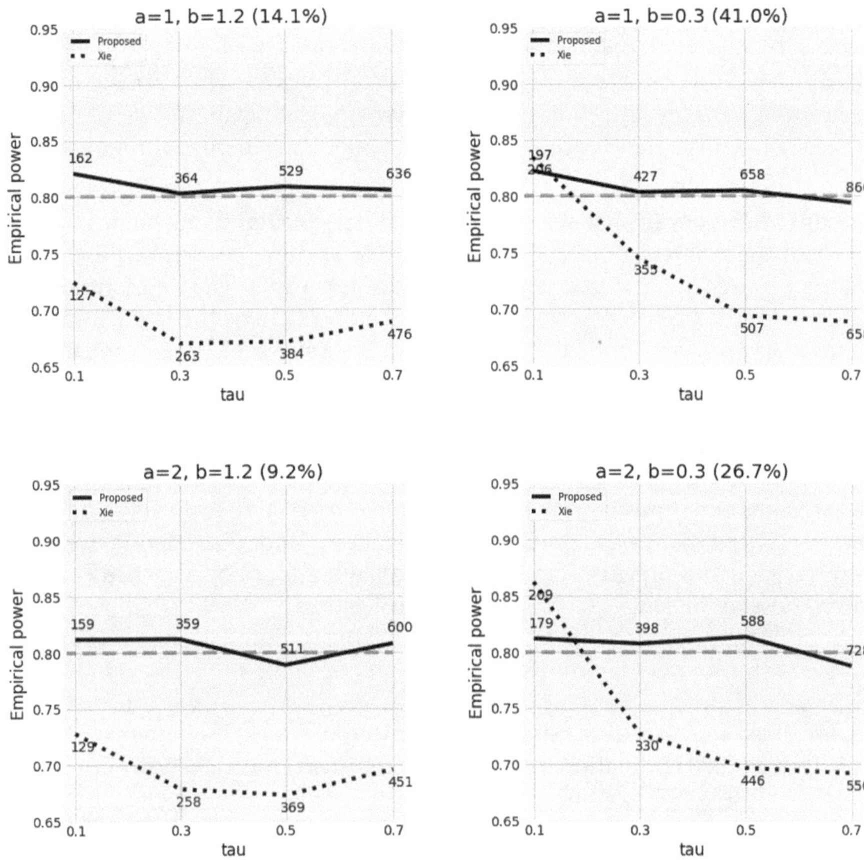

FIGURE 11.2 (Continued)
(b) $U(2, 20)$ of cluster size distribution.

Example 2: We consider the example in Xie and Waksman (2003). Suppose that we design a clinical trial to compare a topical agent with vehicle in treating diabetic foot ulcers. Each patient (cluster) has a variable number of ulcers (subunits), m_i, when enrolled in the study and all of them will be treated. The primary endpoint is time to complete healing for each ulcer. Patients are randomly assigned to the two treatment arms with a balanced allocation, i.e., $p_1 = p_2 = 1/2$. From some previous studies, the median times to heal in the treatment and the vehicle arms were approximately 122 and 200 days, respectively. Assuming exponential marginal distributions, this corresponds to a hazard ratio of $\Delta = 1.64(= 200/122)$. We use the Clayton and Cuzick's copula model with Kendall's $\tau = 0.5$ for joint survival distributions. Suppose that there are an average of $\bar{m} = 11$ ulcers per patient with a cluster size distribution of $U(9, 13)$ or $U(2, 20)$. We consider an accrual period of $a = 280$ days and a follow-up period of $b = 160$ days to result in about 28% censoring. For $(\alpha, 1-\beta) = (0.05, 0.9)$, we need $n = 181$ patients under $U(9, 13)$ cluster size distribution and $n = 221$ patients under $U(2, 20)$ cluster size distribution. We need more patients if the variance of cluster size distribution is large. Under the design setting, the formula by Xie and Waksman (2003) gives $n = 163$ for any cluster size distribution with mean $\bar{m} = 11$.

Example 3: Suppose that we design the Harper's trial using time to pregnancy as the primary outcome. We want to determine the intervention effect among women who attend the family planning visits. The 12-month pregnancy rate for the control arm is approximately 0.2, and the hazard ratio is about $\Delta = \lambda_1/\lambda_2 = 1/0.6$. As in the original Harper's trial, we assume that all clinics (clusters) start to recruit women (subunits) from the beginning so that subunits have independent censoring times unlike the previous examples. Since clinics usually have different patient volumes, the expected accrual rate will vary among clinics. Suppose that the yearly accrual rate is 100, 150, or 200 with an equal probability of 1/3 among clinics so that we have $\bar{r} = 150$ and $\bar{\bar{r}} = 24{,}166.67$. We use the Clayton and Cuzick's copula to model the joint survival distribution with Kendall's $\tau = 0.05$ which corresponds to a Pearson correlation coefficient of 0.067 in the control group.

At first, suppose that we want to complete the required accrual within $a = 0.2$ years (for an average number of women per clinic $\bar{m} = 150 \times 0.2 = 30$) with an additional follow-up period of $b = 1$ year as in the original trial. Under these assumptions, we need $n = 51$ clinics for 90% power with $\alpha = 0.05$. Using 5,000 simulation samples, we obtain an empirical power of 0.898, which is close to the nominal $1 - \beta = 0.9$.

Now, suppose that, as in the original trial, a total of $n = 40$ (20 per arm) clinics participate in the new trial and we want to calculate the required accrual period for the study. Using the same design parameter values, other than the accrual period, we need $a = 0.3$ years for 90% of power. In this case, the average number of women per clinic will be $\bar{m} = \bar{r} \times a = 150 \times 0.3 = 45$.

Appendix A. Asymptotic Normality of W under H_0

By the definition of W and $\hat{\Lambda}_k$, under $H_0 : \Lambda_1(t) = \Lambda_2(t)$, we have

$$W = \sqrt{n}\int_0^\infty \frac{H(t)}{Y_1(t)}\{dN_1(t) - Y_1(t)d\Lambda_1(t)\} - \sqrt{n}\int_0^\infty \frac{H(t)}{Y_2(t)}\{dN_2(t) - Y_2(t)d\Lambda_2(t)\}.$$

Let $M_{kij}(t) = N_{kij}(t) - \int_0^t Y_{kij}(s)d\Lambda_k(s)$ and $M_{ki}(t) = \sum_{j=1}^{m_{ki}} M_{kij}(t)$. Then

$$W = \frac{1}{\sqrt{n}}\sum_{i=1}^{n_1}\int_0^\infty \frac{H(t)}{n^{-1}Y_1(t)}dM_{1i}(t) - \frac{1}{\sqrt{n}}\sum_{i=1}^{n_2}\int_0^\infty \frac{H(t)}{n^{-1}Y_2(t)}dM_{2i}(t). \tag{11.A1}$$

Let, for group k, $\bar{m}$ be the mean cluster size and $y_k(t) = \bar{m}p_k P(T_k \geq t)P(C_k \geq t) = \bar{m}p_k S_k(t)G(t)$ be the limit of $Y_k(t)/n$. Readers may refer to Ying and Wei (1994) for the uniform convergence of Kaplan-Meier (1958) estimator and Nelson's estimator based on correlated survival data. By Ying and Wei (1994), $n^{-1/2}\sum_{i=1}^{n_k} M_{ki}(t)$ converges weakly to a Gaussian process $U_k(t)$. Since $nH(t)/Y_k(t)$ is of bounded variation that is convergent to $h(t)/y_k(t)$, as in Lee, Wei and Ying (1993), we can show that

$$W_k = \frac{1}{\sqrt{n}}\sum_{i=1}^{n_k}\int_0^\infty \frac{H(t)}{n^{-1}Y_k(t)}dM_{ki}(t)$$

in (11.A1) and

$$W_k^* = \frac{1}{\sqrt{n}}\sum_{i=1}^{n_k}\int_0^\infty \frac{h(t)}{y_k(t)}dM_{ki}(t)$$

converge a.s. to the same limit $\int_0^\infty h(t)/\{p_k y_k(t)\}dU_k(t)$ for $k = 1, 2$. By the standard central limit theorem for sum of independent random variables, W_k^* (also W_k) converges to a normal distribution with mean 0 and variance

$$\sigma_k^2 = \lim_{n\to\infty}\frac{1}{n}\sum_{i=1}^{n_k}\{\int_0^\infty \frac{h(t)}{y_k(t)}dM_{ki}(t)\}^2. \tag{11.A2}$$

Because of independence of two treatment groups, W is asymptotically normal with mean 0 and variance $\sigma^2 = \sigma_1^2 + \sigma_2^2$ that can be consistently estimated by replacing $h(t)$, $y_k(t)$, and $\Lambda_k(t)$ with $H(t)$, $n^{-1}Y_k(t)$, and $\hat{\Lambda}(t) = \int_0^t Y(s)^{-1}dN(s)$, respectively in (11.A2), where $N(t) = N_1(t) + N_2(t)$. That is, σ^2 is consistently estimated by

$$\hat{\sigma}^2 = \frac{1}{n}\sum_{i=1}^{n_1}\hat{\varepsilon}_{1i}^2 + \frac{1}{n}\sum_{i=1}^{n_2}\hat{\varepsilon}_{2i}^2, \tag{11.A3}$$

where

$$n^{-1}\hat{\varepsilon}_{ki} = \sum_{j=1}^{m_{ki}}\int_0^\infty \frac{H(t)}{Y_k(t)}\{dN_{kij}(t) - Y_{kij}(t)d\hat{\Lambda}(t)\}$$

$$= \sum_{j=1}^{m_{ki}}\frac{\delta_{kij}H(X_{kij})}{Y_k(X_{kij})} - \sum_{k'=1}^{2}\sum_{i'=1}^{n_{k'}}\sum_{j'=1}^{m_{k'i'}}\frac{\delta_{k'i'j'}Y_{ki}(X_{k'i'j'})H(X_{k'i'j'})}{Y_k(X_{k'i'j'})Y(X_{k'i'j'})}.$$

For example, for the log-rank test,

$$\hat{\varepsilon}_{ki} = \sum_{j=1}^{m_{ki}}\frac{\delta_{kij}Y_{3-k}(X_{kij})}{Y(X_{kij})} - \sum_{k'=1}^{2}\sum_{i'=1}^{n_{k'}}\sum_{j'=1}^{m_{k'i'}}\frac{\delta_{k'i'j'}Y_{ki}(X_{k'i'j'})Y_{3-k}(X_{k'i'j'})}{Y(X_{k'i'j'})^2}.$$

Appendix B. Asymptotic Normality of $\boldsymbol{W} = (W_1, ..., W_{K-1})^T$ under H_0

Let $M(t) = \sum_{k=1}^{K} M_k(t)$, $M_k(t) = \sum_{i=1}^{n_k} M_{ki}(t)$ and $M_{ki}(t) = N_{ki}(t) - \int_0^t Y_{ki}(s)d\Lambda_k(s)$. By the definition of $\hat{\Lambda}_k$ and $\hat{\Lambda}$, under $H_0 : \Lambda_1 = \cdots = \Lambda_K (= \Lambda)$, we have

$$W_k = \frac{1}{\sqrt{n}} \int_0^\infty Y_k(t)L(t) \left\{ \frac{dN_k(t)}{Y_k(t)} - \frac{dN(t)}{Y(t)} \right\}$$

$$= \frac{1}{\sqrt{n}} \int_0^\infty L(t)dM_k(t) - \frac{1}{\sqrt{n}} \int_0^\infty L(t)\frac{Y_k(t)}{Y(t)}dM(t).$$

So, we have

$$W_k = \frac{1}{\sqrt{n}} \sum_{i=1}^{n_k} \int_0^\infty L(t)dM_{ki}(t) - \frac{1}{\sqrt{n}} \sum_{l=1}^{K} \sum_{i=1}^{n_l} \int_0^\infty L(t)\frac{Y_k(t)}{Y(t)}dM_{li}(t)$$

$$= \frac{1}{\sqrt{n}} \sum_{k'=1}^{K} \sum_{i=1}^{n_{k'}} \int_0^\infty L(t) \left\{ \delta_{k,k'} - \frac{n^{-1}Y_k(t)}{n^{-1}Y(t)} \right\} dM_{k'i}(t),$$

where $\delta_{k,k'} = I(k = k')$ for the indicator function $I(\cdot)$.

Let $y_k(t)$ and $\ell(t)$ be the limits of $n^{-1}Y_k(t)$ and $L(t)$, respectively, and $y(t) = \sum_{k=1}^{K} y_k(t)$. By arguments similar to Appendix A, we can show that the asymptotic distribution of $\boldsymbol{W}$ is equal to that of $\boldsymbol{W}^* = n^{-1/2} \sum_{k=1}^{K} \sum_{i=1}^{n_k} \boldsymbol{\varepsilon}_{ki}$ with $\boldsymbol{\varepsilon}_{ki} = (\varepsilon_{1ki}, ..., \varepsilon_{K-1,ki})^T$ and

$$\varepsilon_{kk'i} = \int_0^\infty \ell(t)\{\delta_{k,k'} - \frac{y_k(t)}{y(t)}\}dM_{k'i}(t).$$

By the multivariate central limit theorem for sum of independent random vectors, $\boldsymbol{W}^*$ (also $\boldsymbol{W}$) converges to a normal distribution with mean 0 and variance-covariance matrix

$$V = \lim_{n \to \infty} \frac{1}{n} \sum_{k=1}^{K} \sum_{i=1}^{n_k} \boldsymbol{\varepsilon}_{ki} \boldsymbol{\varepsilon}_{ki}^T.$$

A consistent estimate of V is given as

$$\hat{V} = \frac{1}{n} \sum_{k=1}^{K} \sum_{i=1}^{n_k} \hat{\boldsymbol{\varepsilon}}_{ki} \hat{\boldsymbol{\varepsilon}}_{ki}^T, \tag{11.A4}$$

where $\hat{\boldsymbol{\varepsilon}}_{ki} = (\hat{\varepsilon}_{1ki}, ..., \hat{\varepsilon}_{K-1,ki})^T$ are obtained from $\boldsymbol{\varepsilon}_{ki}$ by replacing $y_k(t)$, $\ell(t)$, and $\Lambda_k(t)$ with $n^{-1}Y_k(t)$, $L(t)$, and $\hat{\Lambda}(t) = \int_0^t Y(s)^{-1}dN(s)$, respectively, that is

$$\hat{\varepsilon}_{kli} = \sum_{j=1}^{m_{li}} \delta_{lij} L(X_{lij}) \left\{ \delta_{k,l} - \frac{Y_k(X_{lij})}{Y(X_{lij})} \right\}$$

$$- \sum_{k'=1}^{K} \sum_{i'=1}^{n_{k'}} \sum_{j'=1}^{m_{k'i'}} \delta_{k'i'j'} L(X_{k'i'j'}) \left\{ \delta_{k,l} - \frac{Y_k(X_{k'i'j'})}{Y(X_{k'i'j'})} \right\} \frac{Y_{li}(X_{k'i'j'})}{Y(X_{k'i'j'})}.$$

Appendix C. Limiting distribution of the clustered log-rank statistic under H_1

For subunit $j(= 1, ..., m_{ki})$ in cluster $i(= 1, ..., n_k)$ that is randomized into arm $k(= 1, 2)$, let $M_{kij}(t) = N_{kij}(t) - \int_0^t Y_{kij}(s)d\Lambda_k(t)$ and $M_{ki}(t) = \sum_{j=1}^{m_{ki}} M_{kij}(t)$. By the definition of W for the log-rank statistic with $H(t) = n^{-1}Y_1(t)Y_2(t)/Y(t)$,

$$W = \frac{1}{\sqrt{n}} \left\{ \sum_{i=1}^{n_1} \int_0^\infty \frac{Y_2(t)}{Y(t)} dM_{1i}(t) - \sum_{i=1}^{n_2} \int_0^\infty \frac{Y_1(t)}{Y(t)} dM_{2i}(t) \right\}$$

$$+ \frac{1}{\sqrt{n}} \int_0^\infty \frac{Y_1(t)Y_2(t)}{Y(t)} \{d\Lambda_1(t) - d\Lambda_2(t)\}.$$

Let $\eta = \max\{t : S_1(t)S_2(t)G(t) > 0\}$, where $S_k(t) = \exp\{-\Lambda_k(t)\}$. Usually the upper limit of the support of survival distributions is longer than the study period, which is the upper limit of the censoring distribution so that η is the study period. As $n \to \infty$, $n^{-1}Y_k(t)$ uniformly converge to $y_k(t) = \bar{m}p_k S_k(t)G(t)$ so that we have

$$W = \frac{1}{\sqrt{n}} \left(\sum_{i=1}^{n_1} \epsilon_{1i} - \sum_{i=1}^{n_2} \epsilon_{2i} \right) + \omega\sqrt{n} + o_p(1),$$

where $\epsilon_{ki} = \sum_{j=1}^{m_{ki}} \epsilon_{kij}$,

$$\epsilon_{kij} = \int_0^\infty \frac{y_{3-k}(t)}{y_1(t) + y_2(t)} dM_{kij}(t)$$

and

$$\omega = \int_0^\infty \frac{y_1(t)y_2(t)}{y_1(t) + y_2(t)} \{d\Lambda_1(t) - d\Lambda_2(t)\}$$

$$= p_1 p_2 \bar{m} \int_0^\infty \frac{S_1(t)S_2(t)G(t)}{p_1 S_1(t) + p_2 S_2(t)} \{d\Lambda_1(t) - d\Lambda_2(t)\}. \quad (11.A5)$$

Since $\{\epsilon_{ki}, i = 1, ..., n_k, k = 1, 2\}$ are independent random variables with mean 0, by the central limit theorem, W is approximately normal with mean $\omega\sqrt{n}$ and variance

$$\sigma^2 = \sigma_1^2 + \sigma_2^2$$

with

$$\sigma_k^2 = p_k \text{var}(\epsilon_{ki}) = p_k\{\bar{m}\sigma_{k1}^2 + (\bar{\bar{m}} - \bar{m})\sigma_{k2}\}, \tag{11.A6}$$

where $\sigma_{k1}^2 = \text{var}(\epsilon_{kij})$ that is expressed as

$$\begin{aligned}\sigma_{k1}^2 =& \int_0^\infty \frac{y_{3-k}^2(t)}{\{y_1(t) + y_2(t)\}^2} S_k(t)G(t)d\Lambda_k(t) \\ =& p_{3-k}^2 \int_0^\infty \frac{S_k(t)S_{3-k}^2(t)G(t)}{\{p_1S_1(t) + p_2S_2(t)\}^2} d\Lambda_k(t)\end{aligned} \tag{11.A7}$$

since $M_{kij}(t)$ is marginally a 0-mean martingale. Further, by similar arguments to those in the lemma of Appendix C of Chapter 10, for $j \neq j'$, we have

$$\begin{aligned}E\{dM_{kij}(t_1)dM_{kij'}(t_2)\} =& E\{Y_{kij}(t_1)Y_{kij'}(t_2)\}dA_k(t_1, t_2) \\ =& S_k(t_1, t_2)G(t_1, t_2)dA_k(t_1, t_2),\end{aligned}$$

where

$$\begin{aligned}dA_k(t_1, t_2) =& \{\lambda_k(t_1, t_2) - \lambda_{k(1|2)}(t_1, t_2)\lambda_k(t_2) - \lambda_{k(2|1)}(t_1, t_2)\lambda_k(t_1) \\ &+ \lambda_k(t_1)\lambda_k(t_2)\}dt_1dt_2.\end{aligned}$$

So, $\sigma_{k2} = \text{cov}(\epsilon_{kij}, \epsilon_{kij'})$ is given as

$$\begin{aligned}\sigma_{k2} =& \int_0^\infty \int_0^\infty \frac{y_{3-k}(t_1)y_{3-k}(t_2)}{\{y_1(t_1) + y_2(t_1)\}\{y_1(t_2) + y_2(t_2)\}} E\{dM_{kij}(t_1)dM_{kij'}(t_2)\} \\ =& p_{3-k}^2 \int_0^\infty \int_0^\infty \frac{S_{3-k}(t_1)S_{3-k}(t_2)S_k(t_1, t_2)G(t_1, t_2)}{\{p_1S_1(t_1) + p_2S_2(t_1)\}\{p_1S_1(t_2) + p_2S_2(t_2)\}} dA_k(t_1, t_2).\end{aligned} \tag{11.A8}$$

On the other hand, by definition,

$$\begin{aligned}\hat{\sigma}^2 =& n \sum_{k=1}^{2} \sum_{i=1}^{n_k} \left[\int_0^\infty \frac{Y_{3-k}(t)}{Y_1(t) + Y_2(t)} dM_{ki}(t) \right. \\ &\left. + \int_0^\infty \frac{Y_{3-k}(t)}{Y_1(t) + Y_2(t)} Y_{ki}(t)\{d\Lambda_k(t) - d\hat{\Lambda}(t)\} \right]^2.\end{aligned}$$

By the uniform convergence of $n^{-1}Y_k(t)$ and $Y_k(t)^{-1}dN_k(t)$ to $y_k(t) = \bar{m}p_kS_k(t)G(t)$ and $d\Lambda_k(t)$, respectively, $d\hat{\Lambda}(t)$ uniformly converges to $\{y_1(t)+y_2(t)\}^{-1}\{y_1(t)d\Lambda_1(t)+y_2(t)d\Lambda_2(t)\}$ in $[0,\eta]$. Hence, we have

$$\hat{\sigma}^2 = \frac{1}{n}\sum_{k=1}^{2}\sum_{i=1}^{n_k}(\epsilon_{ki}+\xi_{ki})^2 + o_p(1).$$

Here,

$$\xi_{ki} = \int_0^\infty \frac{y_{3-k}(t)}{y_1(t)+y_2(t)}Y_{ki}(t)\{d\Lambda_1(t)-d\Lambda_2(t)\}$$

are negligible under the nearby alternative hypothesis, i.e., $H_1 : \Lambda_1(t) - \Lambda_2(t) = o_p(\sqrt{n})$. Therefore, $\hat{\sigma}^2 = n^{-1}\sum_{k=1}^{2}\sum_{i=1}^{n_k}\epsilon_{ki}^2 + o_p(1)$ converges to σ^2.

Note that, for the weighted rank tests, $H(t)$ converges to a square integrable process $h(t)$ which is a function of the survival and censoring distributions as in the log-rank test. Hence, the sample size formulas for different weighted rank tests can be similarly derived.

Appendix D. A simplified sample size formula for the clustered log-rank test under the nearby alternative hypothesis

Now, we consider the nearby alternative hypothesis, i.e., $S_1(t) \approx S_2(t)(= S(t))$ and $S_1(t_1,t_2) \approx S_2(t_1,t_2)(= S(t_1,t_2))$, and simplify ω and σ^2 that are derived in Appendix C.

Under this assumption, we have $\Lambda_1(t) - \Lambda_2(t) = (\Delta-1)\Lambda(t)$ and $y_k(t) = p_k\bar{m}S(t)G(t)$. So, from (11.A5), $\tilde{\omega} = \omega/(p_1p_2\bar{m})$ is expressed as

$$\tilde{\omega} = (\Delta-1)\int_0^\infty S(t)G(t)d\Lambda(t) \approx d\log\Delta,$$

where $d = -\int_0^\infty G(t)dS(t) = P(T_{kij} < C_{kij})$.

Furthermore, from (11.A7) and (11.A8), we have

$$\sigma_{k1}^2 = p_{3-k}^2\int_0^\infty S(t)G(t)d\Lambda(t) = p_{3-k}^2 d$$

since $S(t)d\Lambda(t) = -dS(t)$ and

$$\sigma_{k2} = p_{3-k}^2\int_0^\infty\int_0^\infty S(t_1,t_2)G(t_1,t_2)dA(t_1,t_2),$$

where $dA(t_1,t_2) = \{\lambda(t_1,t_2) - \lambda_{(1|2)}(t_1,t_2)\lambda(t_2) - \lambda_{(2|1)}(t_2,t_1)\lambda(t_1) + \lambda(t_1)\lambda(t_2)\}dt_1dt_2$ that is defined with respect to the common survival distribution.

Let $\rho = \sigma_{k2}/\sigma_{k1}^2 = \int_0^\infty \int_0^\infty S(t_1,t_2)G(t_1,t_2)dA(t_1,t_2)/d$ denote the ICC. Then, from (11.A6),

$$\sigma_k^2 = \bar{m}p_k\sigma_{k1}^2\{1+(\bar{\bar{m}}/\bar{m}-1)\rho\} = p_1p_2^2\bar{m}d\{1+(\bar{\bar{m}}/\bar{m}-1)\rho\}$$

so that $\sigma^2 = \sigma_1^2 + \sigma_2^2$ is expressed as

$$\sigma^2 = p_1p_2\bar{m}d\{1+(\bar{\bar{m}}/\bar{m}-1)\rho\}.$$

We propose to calculate $\rho = (p_1c_1+p_2c_2)/(p_1d_1+p_2d_2)$, where

$$c_k = \sigma_{k2}/p_{3-k}^2 = \int_0^\infty \int_0^\infty S_k(t_1,t_2)G(t_1,t_2)dA_k(t_1,t_2)$$

and

$$d_k = \sigma_{k2}/p_{3-k}^2 = -\int_0^\infty G(t)dS_k(t)$$

is the probability that a subunit in arm k experiences an event during the study.

Hence, under the nearby alternative hypothesis, (11.6) is expressed as

$$n = \frac{(z_{1-\alpha/2}+z_{1-\beta})^2}{\bar{m}dp_1p_2(\log\Delta)^2}\mathrm{IF},$$

where $\mathrm{IF} = 1+(\bar{\bar{m}}/\bar{m}-1)\rho$ is the inflation factor due to ICC.

Appendix E. Design parameters under bivariate exponential survival with Clayton and Cuzick's frailty and (i) common censoring or (ii) independent censoring case

For a marginal exponential survival distribution, we have $S_k(t) = e^{-\lambda_k t}$. Using Clayton and Cuzick's copula, the bivariate exponential distribution has

$$\lambda_k(t_1,t_2) = \frac{f_k(t_1,t_2)}{S_k(t_1,t_2)} = \lambda_k^2(1+\theta^{-1})e^{(t_1+t_2)\lambda_k/\theta}\left(e^{\lambda_k t_1/\theta}+e^{\lambda_k t_2/\theta}-1\right)^{-2}$$

$$\lambda_{k(1|2)}(t_1,t_2) = \frac{\partial S_k(t_1,t_2)/\partial t_1}{S_k(t_1,t_2)} = \lambda_k e^{\lambda_k t_1/\theta}\left(e^{\lambda_k t_1/\theta}+e^{\lambda_k t_2/\theta}-1\right)^{-1}$$

$$\lambda_{k(2|1)}(t_1,t_2) = \frac{\partial S_k(t_1,t_2)/\partial t_2}{S_k(t_1,t_2)} = \lambda_k e^{\lambda_k t_2/\theta}\left(e^{\lambda_k t_1/\theta}+e^{\lambda_k t_2/\theta}-1\right)^{-1}$$

and

$$dA_k(t_1,t_2) = \lambda_k^2\left\{\frac{(1+\theta^{-1})e^{(t_1+t_2)\lambda_k/\theta}}{(e^{\lambda_k t_1/\theta}+e^{\lambda_k t_2/\theta}-1)^2} - \frac{e^{\lambda_k t_1/\theta}+e^{\lambda_k t_2/\theta}}{e^{\lambda_k t_1/\theta}+e^{\lambda_k t_2/\theta}-1}+1\right\}dt_1dt_2.$$

With an accrual period of a and a follow-up period of b, the marginal censoring distribution is $U(b, a+b)$ in both common and independent censoring cases. So, the marginal survival function of the censoring distribution is given as

$$G(t) = I(t < a+b) - \frac{t-b}{a} I(b \le t < a+b).$$

Hence, using the formulas for the log-rank test, we have

$$\begin{aligned}\tilde{\omega} =& (\lambda_1 - \lambda_2)\left\{\int_0^{a+b} \frac{e^{-(\lambda_1-\lambda_2)t}}{(p_1e^{-\lambda_1 t} + p_2 e^{-\lambda_2 t})^2} dt\right.\\ &\left. - \frac{1}{a}\int_0^{a+b} \frac{(t-b)e^{-(\lambda_1-\lambda_2)t}}{(p_1e^{-\lambda_1 t} + p_2 e^{-\lambda_2 t})^2} dt\right\}\\ \sigma_{k1}^2 =& p_{3-k}^2 \lambda_k \left\{\int_0^{a+b} \frac{e^{-(\lambda_k+2\lambda_{3-k})t}}{(p_1e^{-\lambda_1 t} + p_2 e^{-\lambda_2 t})^2} dt\right.\\ &\left. - \frac{1}{a}\int_0^{a+b} \frac{(t-b)e^{-(\lambda_k+2\lambda_{3-k})t}}{(p_1e^{-\lambda_1 t} + p_2 e^{-\lambda_2 t})^2} dt\right\}.\end{aligned}$$

While $\tilde{\omega}$ and σ_{k1}^2 depend on the marginal censoring distribution, σ_{k1}^2 depends on the bivariate censoring distribution, which differs between the two censoring cases. In the common censoring case, we have $G(t_1, t_2) = G(t_1 \vee t_2)$ so that

$$\begin{aligned}\sigma_{k2} =& p_{3-k}^2 \int_0^{a+b}\int_0^{a+b} \frac{e^{-\lambda_{3-k}(t_1+t_2)}(e^{\lambda_k t_1/\theta} + e^{\lambda_k t_2/\theta} - 1)^{-\theta} G(t_1, t_2)}{(p_1 e^{-\lambda_1 t_1} + p_2 e^{-\lambda_2 t_1})(p_1 e^{-\lambda_1 t_2} + p_2 e^{-\lambda_2 t_2})}\\ & dA(t_1, t_2),\end{aligned}$$

where $G(t_1, t_2) = 1 - a^{-1}[t_1 \vee t_2 - b]_+$ and $[t]_+ = t \times I(t \ge 0)$.

On the other hand, in the independent censoring case, we have $G(t_1, t_2) = G(t_1)G(t_2)$ so that

$$\begin{aligned}\sigma_{k2} =& p_{3-k}^2 \int_0^{a+b}\int_0^{a+b} \frac{e^{-\lambda_{3-k}(t_1+t_2)}(e^{\lambda_k t_1/\theta} + e^{\lambda_k t_2/\theta} - 1)^{-\theta} G(t_1, t_2)}{(p_1 e^{-\lambda_1 t_1} + p_2 e^{-\lambda_2 t_1})(p_1 e^{-\lambda_1 t_2} + p_2 e^{-\lambda_2 t_2})}\\ & dA_k(t_1, t_2),\end{aligned}$$

where $G(t_1, t_2) = (1 - a^{-1}[t_1 - b]_+)(1 - a^{-1}[t_2 - b]_+)$.

References

Aalen O. Nonparametric inference for a family of counting processes. Annals of Statistics 1978;6(1): 701–726.

Andersen PK, Borgan O, Gill R, Keiding N. Linear nonparametric tests for comparison of counting processes, with applications to censored survival data, correspondent paper. International Statistical Review / Revue Internationale de Statistique 1982;50: 219–244.

Clayton D, Cuzick J. Multivariate generalizations of the proportional Hazards model. Journal of the Royal Statistical Society, Series A (General) 1985;148(2): 82–108.

Fleming TR, Harrington DP. Counting Processes and Survival Analysis. Hoboken, NJ: John Wiley & Sons; 2011.

Freedman LS. Tables of the number of patients required in clinical trials using the logrank test. Statistics in Medicine 1982;1(2):121–129.

Gangnon RE, Kosorok MR. Sample-size formula for clustered survival data using weighted log-rank statistics. Biometrika 2004;91(2):263–275.

Gehan EA. A generalized Wilcoxon test for comparing arbitrarily singly-censored samples. Biometrika 1965; 52(1–2): 203–224.

George SL, Desu MM. Planning the size and duration of a clinical trial studying the time to some critical event. Journal of Chronic Diseases 1974;27(1–2):15–24.

Gill RD. *Censoring and Stochastic Integrals.* Mathematical Centre Tracts 124, Mathematisch Centrum: Amsterdam, 1980.

Harper CC, Rocca CH, Thompson KM, et al. Reductions in pregnancy rates in the USA with long-acting reversible contraception: a cluster randomised trial. Lancet 2015;386(9993):562–568.

Harrington DP, Fleming TR. A class of rank test procedures for censored survival data. Biometrika 1982;69(3):553–566.

Hayes RJ, Bennett S. Simple sample size calculation for cluster-randomized trials. International Journal of Epidemiology 1999;28(2):319–326.

Howie VM, Schwartz RH. Acute otitis media: one year in general pediatric practice. American Journal of Diseases in Children 1983; 137: 155–158.

Jahn-Eimermacher A, Ingel K, Schneider A. Sample size in cluster-randomized trials with time-to-event as the primary endpoint. Statistics in Medicine 2013; 32(5): 739–751.

Jung SH. Sample size calculation for weighted rank tests comparing survival distributions under cluster randomization: a simulation method. Journal of Biopharmaceutical Statistics 2007; 17(5): 839–849.

Jung SH, Jeong JH. Rank tests for clustered survival data. Lifetime Data Analysis 2003; 9(1): 21–33.

Kaplan EL, Meier P. Nonparametric estimator from incomplete observations. Journal of the American Statistical Association 1958; 53: 457–481.

Lakatos E. Sample sizes based on the log-rank statistic in complex clinical trials. Biometrics 1988; 44(1): 229–241.

Lakatos E, Lan KKG. A comparison of sample size methods for the logrank statistic. Statistics in Medicine 1992; 11(2): 179–191.

Le CT. Counting Processes and Survival Analysis. Wiley: New York, 1997.

Le CT, Lindgren BR. Duration of ventilating tubes: a test for comparing two clustered samples of censored data. Biometrics 1996; 52: 328–334.

Lee EW, Wei LJ, Ying Z. Linear Regression Analysis for Highly Stratified Failure Time Data. Journal of American Statistical Association 1993; 88(422): 557–565.

Lee EW, Wei LJ, Amato DA, Leurgans S. Cox-Type Regression Analysis for Large Numbers of Small Groups of Correlated Failure Time Observations. Survival Analysis: State of the Art, edited by Klein JP and Goel PK, Springer New York, NY, 1992: 237–247.

Lee EW, Wei LJ, Ying Z. Linear Regression Analysis for Highly Stratified Failure Time Data. Journal of the American Statistical Association 1993; 88(422) ; 557–565.

Li J, Jung SH. Sample size calculation for cluster randomization trials with a time-to-event endpoint. Statistics in Medicine 2020; 39(25): 3608–3623.

Lin DY, Ying Z. A Simple Nonparametric Estimator of the Bivariate Survival function under univariate censoring. Biometrika 1993; 80: 573–581.

Manatunga AK, Chen S. Sample size estimation for survival outcomes in cluster-randomized studies with small cluster sizes. Biometrics 2000; 56(2): 616–621.

Moran PAP. Testing for correlation between non-negative variates. Biometrika 1967; 54: 385–394.

Nelson W. Hazard plotting for incomplete failure data. Journal of Quality Technology 1969; 1(1): 27–52.

Peto R, Peto J. Asymptotically efficient rank invariant test procedures (with discussion. Journal of the Royal Statistical Society, Series A 1972; 135: 185–206.

Prentice RL. Linear rank tests with right censored data. Biometrika 1978; 65: 167–179.

Schoenfeld DA. Sample-size formula for the proportional-hazards regression model. Biometrics 1983; 39(2): 499–503.

Stedman MR, Gagnon DR, Lew RA, Jung SH, Losina E, Brookhart MA. A SAS macro for a clustered logrank Test. Computer Methods and Programs in Biomedicine 2011; 104: 266–270.

Tarone RE, Ware J. On distribution-free tests for equality of survival distributions. Biometrika 1977; 64(1): 156–160.

Teele DW, Klein JO, Rosner B, et al. Epidemiology of otitis media during the first seven years of life in children in greater Boston. Journal of Infectious Diseases 1989; 160: 89–94.

Thernaeu TH, Grambsch PM. Modeling Survival Data: Extending the Cox Model Springer: New York, 2000.

Xie T, Waksman J. Design and sample size estimation in clinical trials with clustered survival times as the primary endpoint. Statistics in Medicine 2003; 22(18): 2835–2846.

Ying Z, Wei LJ. The Kaplan-Meier estimate for dependent failure time observations. Journal of Multivariate Analysis 1994; 50: 17–29.

12

Rank Tests for Clustered Survival Data and Sample Size Calculation under Subunit Randomization

In a clinical trial, more than one sites (such as teeth or ears) from each subject may be randomized into different treatment groups. In this case, the sites, called subunits, of each subject, called cluster, share common genetic, physiological, or environmental characteristics so that their observations tend to be positively correlated. Clinical trials involving clusters either randomize clusters or subunits within each cluster between treatment arms. Trials with the former randomization scheme, called cluster randomization trials (CRTs), are investigated in Chapter 11. In this chapter, we consider those with the latter randomization, called subunit randomization trials (SRTs).

Batchelor and Hackett (1970) conducted an SRT to evaluate the influence of HL-A match between donors and donees on the survival of allogeneic grafts for severely burned patients. Patients were classified by HL-A antigen types. Selected skin-grafts (subunits) from at least two unrelated types of donors were applied to the burned sites of each patient (cluster) when grafting became necessary. For each patient, allogeneic skin-grafts were selected so that some of them involved only slight HL-A incompatibility and the others were HL-A incompatible. The primary endpoint of the trial was the survival time of each skin-graft. In this trial, the number of skin-grafts varies patient by patient.

Mimicking an SRT, a litter-matched tumorigenesis experiment (Mantel et al. 1977) was conducted to randomize three rats (subunits) in each of 50 female litters (clusters) to a drug treatment group or the control group. The major study objective was to assess whether the time to tumor appearance in the drug-treated group tends to be longer than that in the control group. In this case, rats in each litter share common frailties, and consequently their times to tumor appearance are correlated. Contrary to the previous SRT, the cluster sizes are fixed at 3 in this animal study.

Note that these studies have survival endpoints. For independent survival data, non-parametric tests, such as the weighted rank tests, have been widely used for comparing the distributions between treatment groups, e.g., Harrington and Fleming (1982); Gehan (1965); Kalbfleisch and Prentice

DOI: 10.1201/9781003221951-12

(2011); Tarone and Ware (1977); Fleming and Harrington (2011). Sample size calculation based on weighted rank tests has been studied in various literatures, including George and Desu (1974), Schoenfeld (1983), Freedman (1982), Lakatos (1988), and Lakatos and Lan (1992).

To evaluate a treatment effect between groups marginally under subunit randomization, the standard rank test statistics can be used, but their variances should be modified to account for the intracluster dependence. The paired survival data we have investigated in Chapters 9 and 10 are the simplest form of clustered survival data with subunit randomization. In Chapter 11, we have investigated clustered survival data from CRTs. In such data, intracluster dependency exists within each treatment group, but not between groups. In the data from SRTs, however, intracluster dependency exists between treatment groups as well as within each treatment group.

In this chapter, we consider clustered survival data from SRTs. At first, we investigate Jeong and Jung's (2006) method extending the weighted rank tests to the clustered survival data under subunit randomization. And then, we discuss the sample size method proposed by Li and Jung (2022) of these weighted rank tests to be used to design SRTs. For large sample approximations, we assume that the number of clusters is large.

Two-Sample Weighted Rank Tests for Subunit Randomization Trials

Suppose that cluster $i(=1,...,n)$ has m_i subunits, of which m_{ki} are assigned to treatment $k(=1,2)$, i.e., $m_{1i}+m_{2i}=m_i$. Let $(T_{ki1},...,T_{kim_{ki}})$ be survival times of the subunits randomized into treatment k. Since subunits within a cluster share common characteristics, their survival times $T_{1i1},...,T_{1i,m_{1i}},T_{2i1},...,T_{2i,m_{2i}}$ tend to be positively correlated.

We assume that within treatment group k, $(T_{kij}, 1\le i\le n, 1\le j\le m_{ki})$ are marginally identically distributed with cumulative hazard function $\Lambda_k(t)$. We want to test the null hypothesis,

$$H_0:\Lambda_1(t)=\Lambda_2(t) \text{ for all } t\ge 0,$$

against the alternative hypothesis,

$$H_1:\Lambda_1(t)\neq\Lambda_2(t) \text{ for some } t\ge 0.$$

For subunits in cluster i, let $C_{1i1},...,C_{1i,m_{1i}},C_{2i1},...,C_{2i,m_{2i}}$ be the censoring times. We assume that censoring times are independent of survival times within each cluster. Note that the censoring times within each cluster may be correlated as in the case of common (or univariate) censoring, for which

$C_{kij} = C_i$ for $1 \le j \le m_{ki}$ and $k = 1, 2$. From an SRT, we observe clustered survival data

$$\{(X_{kij}, \delta_{kij}), i = 1, ..., n; j = 1, ..., m_{ki}; k = 1, 2\},$$

where $X_{kij} = \min(T_{kij}, C_{kij})$ and $\delta_{kij} = I(T_{kij} \le C_{kij})$.

Let $N_{kij}(t) = \delta_{kij} I(X_{kij} \le t)$ and $Y_{kij}(t) = I(X_{kij} \ge t)$ denote the event process and the at-risk process, respectively, for each subunit. Define $N_{ki}(t) = \sum_{j=1}^{m_{ki}} N_{kij}(t)$, $N_k(t) = \sum_{i=1}^{n} N_{ki}(t)$, $N(t) = N_1(t) + N_2(t)$, $Y_{ki}(t) = \sum_{j=1}^{m_{ki}} Y_{kij}(t)$, $Y_k(t) = \sum_{i=1}^{n} Y_{ki}(t)$, and $Y(t) = Y_1(t) + Y_2(t)$.

Suppose that $H(t)$ is a nonnegative bounded predictable process that uniformly converges in probability to a bounded left-continuous function $h(t)$ over $[0, \eta]$, where $\eta = \max\{t : \mathrm{P}[\min(X_{1ij}, X_{2ij'}) > t] > 0\}$. We consider the class of rank statistics

$$W = \sqrt{n} \int_0^\infty H(t)\{d\hat{\Lambda}_1(t) - d\hat{\Lambda}_2(t)\}, \tag{12.1}$$

where $\hat{\Lambda}_k(t) = \int_0^t Y_k^{-1}(s) dN_k(s)$ is the Nelson-Aalen (Nelson 1969, Aalen 1978) estimator of $\Lambda_k(t)$. The log-rank statistic (Peto and Peto 1972) uses $H(t) = n^{-1} Y_1(t) Y_2(t)/Y(t)$, the Gehan-Wilcoxon test uses $H(t) = n^{-2} Y_1(t) Y_2(t)$, and the Prentice-Wilcoxon test uses $H(t) = n^{-1} \hat{S}^-(t) Y_1(t) Y_2(t)/Y(t)$. Here, $\hat{S}^-(t)$ is the left-continuous version of the Kaplan-Meier estimate (1958) obtained from the pooled data $\{(X_{kij}, \delta_{kij}), 1 \le i \le n; k = 1, 2; 1 \le j \le m_{ki}\}$.

In Appendix A, we show that, under H_0, W is asymptotically (i.e., as $n \to \infty$) normal with mean 0 and variance σ^2 that can be consistently estimated by

$$\hat{\sigma}^2 = \frac{1}{n} \sum_{i=1}^n \hat{\varepsilon}_i^2, \tag{12.2}$$

where

$$n^{-1}\hat{\varepsilon}_i = \sum_{j=1}^{m_{1i}} \frac{\delta_{1ij} H(X_{1ij})}{Y_1(X_{1ij})} - \sum_{k'=1}^{2} \sum_{i'=1}^{n} \sum_{j'=1}^{m_{k'i'}} \frac{\delta_{k'i'j'} Y_{1i}(X_{k'i'j'}) H(X_{k'i'j'})}{Y_1(X_{k'i'j'}) Y(X_{k'i'j'})}$$

$$- \sum_{j=1}^{m_{2i}} \frac{\delta_{2ij} H(X_{2ij})}{Y_2(X_{2ij})} + \sum_{k'=1}^{2} \sum_{i'=1}^{n} \sum_{j'=1}^{m_{k'i'}} \frac{\delta_{k'i'j'} Y_{2i}(X_{k'i'j'}) H(X_{k'i'j'})}{Y_2(X_{k'i'j'}) Y(X_{k'i'j'})}.$$

Hence, we reject H_0 when the absolute value of $W/\hat{\sigma}$ is larger than $z_{1-\alpha/2}$, the $100(1 - \alpha/2)$ percentile of the standard normal distribution.

Shared Gamma Frailty Model

A popular approach to formulating correlations among subunits will be to introduce a frailty term (Batchelor and Hackett 1970) in the Cox's (1972, 1975) proportional hazards model. Under the shared frailty model, the hazard function for subunit j in cluster i specifies

$$\lambda_{ij}(t; v, z) = v_i \exp(\beta z_{ij})\lambda_0(t), \quad i = 1, ..., n; \quad j = 1, \ldots, m_i, \tag{12.3}$$

where $\lambda_0(t)$ is an unknown baseline hazard function and v_i is a frailty factor shared by the subunits in cluster i. In a two-sample test setting, the covariate z_{ij} is a treatment indicator for subunit j of cluster i. This model is called a gamma-exponential frailty model when the baseline hazard is a constant or a gamma-Weibull frailty model when the baseline survival follows a Weibull distribution with the cumulative hazard function $\Lambda_0(t) = (\zeta t)^{\xi}$, where ζ and ξ are scale and shape parameters, respectively. In Appendix B, the intracluster correlation coefficients (ICCs) are derived under the gamma-exponential and gamma-Weibull frailty models and it is noticed that the ICCs between and within treatment groups are the same under the gamma frailty model. These analytic formulas of the ICC will be used to generate the clustered survival data in our simulation studies.

A number of semiparametric inference methods have been proposed for testing a difference in survival distributions between two groups under model (12.3). For computational convenience, the frailties $v_1, ..., v_n$ are usually assumed to have a gamma distribution (Klein 1992; Nielsen et al. 1992) with shape parameter κ and scale parameter $1/\kappa$ with the probability density function

$$f_V(v; \kappa) = \frac{\kappa^\kappa}{\Gamma(\kappa)} v^{\kappa - 1} \exp(-\kappa v),$$

denoted as $V \sim \Gamma(\kappa, 1/\kappa)$. Therneau and Grambsch (2000) (Lemma, p. 254) proved that the EM approaches proposed by Klein (1992) and Nielsen et al. (1992) provided the same solutions as the penalized partial likelihood (PPL) approach, where the PPL is simply subtracting a penalty term $(1/\kappa)\sum_{i=1}^{n}\{v_i - \exp(v_i)\}$ from the usual partial likelihood function under model (12.3). To test the equality of marginal survival distributions under the gamma frailty model for our simulations, we use a Wald-type test statistic under the PPL procedure implemented in *coxph* in R, mainly because of availability of the procedure.

Simulation Studies

The weighted rank statistics are based on the asymptotic theory for a large number of clusters. Simulation studies are performed to assess their finite sample size performance. We also compare their performance with that of the standard test procedures ignoring intracluster dependency.

Two models are considered to generate clustered survival data, Moran's (1967) model and gamma frailty models (Vaupel 1979). For each survival distribution model, common censoring times C_i were generated from $U(0, c_1)$ for 30% censoring in the control group ($k = 1$). With the constant c_1 fixed at this value, censoring times with 10% censoring are generated from $U(c_0, c_0 + c_1)$ by choosing a proper constant c_0. Note that c_0 and c_1 would imply additional follow-up period and accrual period, respectively, in a clinical trial with uniform accrual. Cluster sizes m_i are generated from a discrete uniform distribution between 2 and 5, and these subunits are randomized into two treatment groups with an equal allocation probability, i.e., $m_{1i} \approx m_{2i}$.

Moran Model

For clustered survival random variables, we modify the Moran's (1967) algorithm. Suppose that $(A_{11}, ..., A_{1,m_1}, A_{21}, ..., A_{2,m_2})$ and $(B_{11}, ..., B_{1,m_1}, B_{21}, ..., B_{2,m_2})$ are mutually independent, but each vector has a multivariate normal distribution with marginal means of 0, variances of 1, and correlation coefficients, $\text{corr}(A_{kj}, A_{kj'}) = \text{corr}(B_{kj}, B_{kj'}) = \sqrt{\phi_w}$ for $j \neq j'$ and $\text{corr}(A_{1j}, A_{2j'}) = \text{corr}(B_{1j}, B_{2j'}) = \sqrt{\phi_b}$ for any j and j'. Then, for the new random vector $(T_{11}, ..., T_{1,m_1}, T_{21}, ..., T_{2,m_2})$ with $T_{kj} = 0.5(A_{kj}^2 + B_{kj}^2)/\lambda_k$, T_{kj} $(k = 1, 2)$ are marginally exponential random variables with hazard rate λ_k and correlation coefficients $\text{corr}(T_{kj}, T_{kj'}) = \phi_w$ for $j \neq j'$ and $\text{corr}(T_{1j}, T_{2j'}) = \phi_b$. Note that ϕ_w and ϕ_b are ICCs among subunits within each group and between different groups, respectively.

To evaluate the type I error probabilities under the null hypothesis $H_0 : \lambda_1 = \lambda_2 = 1$, 5,000 samples of $\{(X_{kij}, \delta_{kij}), 1 \leq i \leq n; k = 1, 2; 1 \leq j \leq m_{ki}\}$ are generated for $n = 10$, 30, or 50 with 10% or 30% censoring proportion. We assume that the ICCs are the same within and between treatment groups, i.e., $\phi_w = \phi_b (= \phi = 0, 0.3, 0.6, \text{ or } 0.9)$ for fair comparisons with the optimal semiparametric PPL procedure. The new (accounting for dependency) and standard (ignoring dependency) log-rank (LR), Prentice-Wilcoxon (PW), and Gehan-Wilcoxon (GW) tests, as well as the semiparametric PPL test from the gamma frailty model, are applied to each simulated data set. The two-sided nominal level of $\alpha = 0.05$ is used and an empirical type I error probability is obtained as the proportion of simulation samples rejecting H_0 among 5,000 samples.

Table 12.1 summarizes the empirical type I error probabilities. The clustered rank have empirical type I error probabilities that are very close to the nominal level for moderate sample sizes ($n = 30$ and 50) regardless of the dependence level. Note that the PW and GW tests tend to be slightly conservative for a small sample size ($n = 10$) and a high correlation ($\phi = 0.9$). The PPL test also has an empirical type I error probabilities close to the nominal level overall. However, the standard rank tests ignoring the intracluster correlation become more conservative as the ICC ϕ increases.

Power analyses have been performed under the same settings, but under a specific alternative hypothesis $H_1 : \lambda_1 = 1, \lambda_2 = 0.75$. Table 12.2 shows

TABLE 12.1

Empirical type I error probability of rank tests with nominal $\alpha = 0.05$ under $H_0 : \lambda_1 = \lambda_2 = 1$ when ICCs are the same within and between treatment groups, i.e., $\phi_w = \phi_b (= \phi)$ and common censoring

Censoring in group 1	n	PPL	New methods LR	New methods PW	New methods GW	Ignoring dependency LR	Ignoring dependency PW	Ignoring dependency GW
$\phi = 0$								
30%	10	0.059	0.064	0.049	0.044	0.042	0.046	0.047
	30	0.058	0.058	0.053	0.053	0.047	0.049	0.049
	50	0.052	0.052	0.053	0.051	0.047	0.049	0.051
10%	10	0.062	0.064	0.048	0.048	0.045	0.047	0.047
	30	0.052	0.055	0.049	0.049	0.043	0.046	0.046
	50	0.057	0.058	0.049	0.049	0.051	0.049	0.048
$\phi = 0.3$								
30%	10	0.054	0.066	0.047	0.043	0.028	0.027	0.029
	30	0.054	0.060	0.052	0.049	0.029	0.031	0.032
	50	0.048	0.054	0.047	0.044	0.025	0.028	0.029
10%	10	0.053	0.054	0.038	0.037	0.021	0.021	0.022
	30	0.047	0.049	0.045	0.046	0.018	0.023	0.024
	50	0.049	0.049	0.051	0.051	0.022	0.026	0.027
$\phi = 0.6$								
30%	10	0.044	0.050	0.032	0.029	0.009	0.010	0.010
	30	0.049	0.058	0.048	0.046	0.009	0.009	0.009
	50	0.054	0.055	0.045	0.045	0.007	0.007	0.009
10%	10	0.050	0.044	0.032	0.032	0.008	0.008	0.009
	30	0.052	0.051	0.047	0.047	0.005	0.006	0.006
	50	0.050	0.048	0.043	0.043	0.003	0.004	0.004
$\phi = 0.9$								
30%	10	0.037	0.044	0.026	0.022	0.000	0.001	0.000
	30	0.043	0.056	0.045	0.043	0.000	0.000	0.000
	50	0.055	0.051	0.045	0.045	0.000	0.000	0.000
10%	10	0.044	0.033	0.017	0.016	0.000	0.000	0.000
	30	0.053	0.043	0.036	0.035	0.000	0.000	0.000
	50	0.055	0.049	0.048	0.045	0.000	0.000	0.000

empirical powers for the clustered rank tests under subunit randomization and the PPL test. Note that the clustered log-rank test has comparable empirical powers with the PPL test when $\phi \leq 0.6$, but the latter has higher powers than the former when $\phi = 0.9$. Under the multivariate exponential simulation model, the two groups have marginally proportional hazards so that the log-rank test has a higher power than the two types of Wilcoxon tests.

Gamma Frailty Models

The comparisons using the Moran's model may be considered unfair to the PPL test since it does not have a gamma frailty. Our clustered log-rank test and the PPL test are compared by generating data from the gamma-exponential (GE) and gamma-Weibull (GW) frailty models. For example,

TABLE 12.2

Empirical power for the PPL test and the new rank tests with two-sided $\alpha = 0.05$ under $H_1 : \lambda_2/\lambda_1 = 0.75$ with $\phi_w = \phi_b (= \phi)$

		30% censoring in group 1				10% censoring in group 1			
ϕ	n	PPL	LR	PW	GW	PPL	LR	PW	GW
0	10	0.098	0.108	0.082	0.076	0.125	0.121	0.093	0.091
	30	0.218	0.213	0.185	0.171	0.257	0.251	0.216	0.211
	50	0.327	0.322	0.281	0.259	0.393	0.386	0.332	0.322
0.3	10	0.107	0.105	0.083	0.074	0.134	0.128	0.096	0.091
	30	0.248	0.248	0.213	0.197	0.304	0.302	0.253	0.249
	50	0.386	0.385	0.332	0.305	0.482	0.494	0.419	0.406
0.6	10	0.127	0.123	0.093	0.085	0.177	0.154	0.111	0.104
	30	0.348	0.324	0.273	0.248	0.436	0.422	0.352	0.342
	50	0.533	0.500	0.447	0.406	0.642	0.643	0.559	0.542
0.9	10	0.247	0.176	0.145	0.125	0.378	0.236	0.215	0.198
	30	0.683	0.520	0.548	0.512	0.827	0.772	0.778	0.763
	50	0.856	0.716	0.750	0.727	0.959	0.933	0.942	0.937

for the gamma-Weibull frailty model, frailty values $V_1, \ldots, V_n$ are first generated from $\Gamma(\kappa, 1/\kappa)$ with $\kappa = 2.7$ and Weibull baseline hazard function with shape parameter $\xi = 2.7$ and scale parameter $\zeta = 1$, corresponding to $\phi_w = \phi_b = \phi = 0.3$ (see Appendix B). Conditional on frailty value $V_i = v_i$ $(i = 1, \ldots, n)$, correlated survival times $(T_{kij}, k = 1, 2, 1 \leq j \leq m_{kij})$ are generated for each cluster by using the probability integral transformation,

$$T_{kij} = \left\{ \frac{-\log U_{kij}}{v_i \exp(\beta z_{ij})} \right\}^{1/2.7},$$

where U_{kij} are IID $U(0, 1)$ random variables and $z_{ij} = 0$ if $k = 1$ and $z_{ij} = 1$ if $k = 2$. We set the hazard ratio $\Delta = \exp(\beta)$ at 1, 0.75, or 0.5 with 10% or 30% censoring proportion, cluster size distribution of discrete $U(2, 5)$, and a number of clusters $n = 50$. The simulation results are summarized in Table 12.3. Note that both PPL and the clustered log-rank test have empirical type I error rates close to the nominal 5%. With a hazard ratio of 0.75 or 0.5, the clustered log-rank test has comparable powers to the optimal PPL procedure. We observe similar results under gamma-exponential model with $\kappa = 1.33$ that corresponds to $\phi_w = \phi_b = \phi = 0.3$.

Examples

The weighted rank tests for clustered survival data were applied to the data from the litter-matched tumorigenesis experiment, where three rats $(m_i = 3)$ were taken from each of $n = 50$ female litters, and one was randomized into a drug treatment group $(m_{1i} = 1)$ and the other two to the control

TABLE 12.3

Comparison of the clustered log-rank test and the PPL test with nominal two-sided $\alpha = 0.05$ under the gamma-exponential (GE) and gamma-Weibull (GW) models with a hazard ratio of 1, 0.75, or 0.5; $\phi_w = \phi_b = 0.3$. We considered $n = 50$ and 10% or 30% common censoring in group 1

Censoring in group 1	Hazard ratio	Under GE		Under GW	
		LR	PPL	LR	PPL
30%	1	0.053	0.050	0.057	0.047
	0.75	0.228	0.248	0.262	0.275
	0.5	0.771	0.800	0.848	0.858
10%	1	0.051	0.051	0.055	0.047
	0.75	0.272	0.305	0.356	0.370
	0.5	0.843	0.871	0.925	0.937

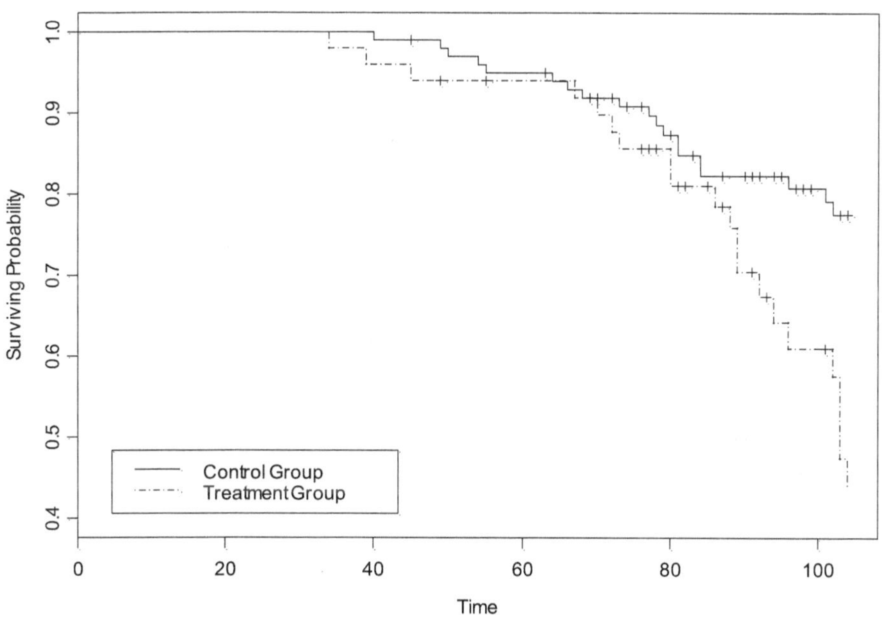

FIGURE 12.1
Kaplan-Meier estimates of time to tumor appearance for litter-matched rats assigned to either drug-treatment or control groups.

group ($m_{2i} = 2$). The times to tumor appearance are reported in Mantel, Bohidar, and Ciminera (1977) and Michalek and Mihalko (1983), and the Kaplan-Meier (1958) estimates for the two groups are shown in Figure 12.1. For testing equality of the two marginal survival distributions, the clustered test statistics using the adjusted variance estimators give the standardized test statistics (and two-sided p-values) of 2.766 (0.006) by the log-rank test, 2.590 (0.010) by the Prentice-Wilcoxon test, and 2.276 (0.023) by the Gehan-Wilcoxon test. All of the three rank tests give similarly significant results. Using the standard (unadjusted) variance formulas for independent observations, the corresponding test statistics (and p-values) are 2.453 (0.014), 2.272 (0.023), and 1.995 (0.046), respectively. We find that the amount of significance is slightly lowered by ignoring intracluster correlation, as expected. The PPL test under the gamma frailty model gives the most significant value of 2.830 (0.005).

Another example of clustered survival data is taken from a clinical trial conducted to evaluate the influence of HL-A antigens on the survival of allogeneic grafts in severely burned patients (Batchelor and Hackett 1970). Each patient received multiple grafts, some from donors with close HL-A antigen match and the others from donors with poor HL-A antigen match. The survival time for each allogeneic graft is defined as the time (days) to rejection of graft. Each donor contributed only one graft (subunit) to the trial so that the survival times are independent between patients (clusters). However, the survival times within each patient (donee) may be correlated because the grafts share the same condition of the patient. The data taken from Bachelor and Hackett (1970) are shown in Table 12.4. Kaplan-Meier estimates for the marginal survival functions of the two match types are shown in Figure 12.2. For testing equality of the two marginal survival distributions, clustered rank tests give standardized statistics (and two-sided p-values) of 2.299 (0.022) by the log-rank test, 2.193 (0.028) by the Prentice-Wilcoxon test, and 2.169 (0.030) by the Gehan-Wilcoxon test. All the three rank tests give similarly significant results again. The PPL test under the gamma frailty model gives a slightly more significant value of 2.619 (0.009) for this data set.

TABLE 12.4

Days of skin-graft survival on each burned patient

Patient	**1**	**2**	**3**	**4**	**5**	**6**	**7**	**8**
Close match	–	24	–	37	19	–	$57^+, 57^+$	93
Poor match	19	–	18,18	29	13	19,19	15	26
Patient	**9**	**10**	**11**	**12**	**13**	**14**	**15**	**16**
Close match	16	22	20	18	77,63,29	–	29	60^+
Poor match	11	17	26	21	43	$28^+, 28^+$	15,18	40

+ indicates censored observations and – indicates no observations.

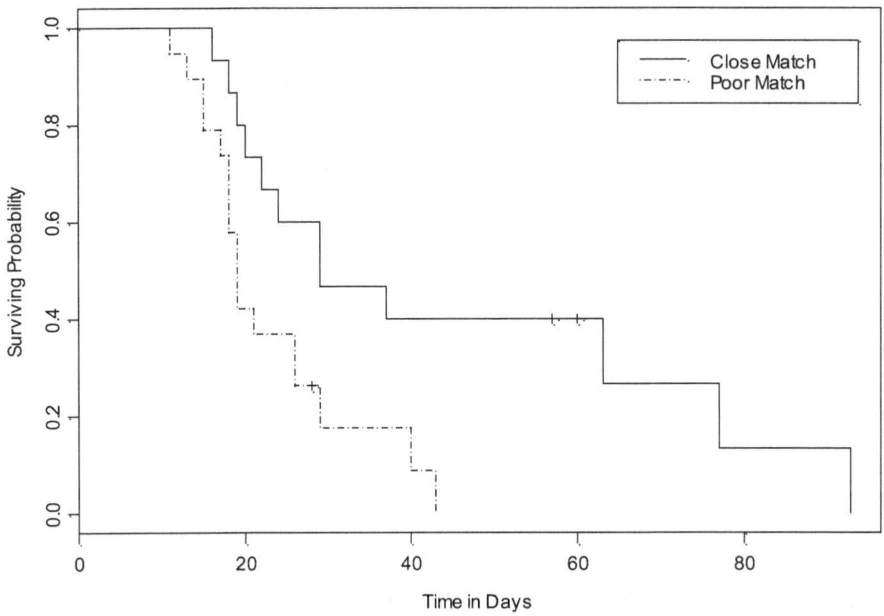

FIGURE 12.2
Kaplan-Meier estimates of survival of skin-grafts for burned patients that are closely matched and poorly matched.

Sample Size Calculation of the Log-Rank Test for SRTs

Usually in SRTs, (i) the number of subunits for each cluster is fixed and clusters are recruited over an accrual period or (ii) the number of clusters is pre-determined and subunits are recruited to each cluster over an accrual period. In this section, we derive a sample size formula for the former case first, and then modify it for the latter case.

When the number of subunits is fixed (i.e., not increasing over an accrual period) for each cluster, let $\bar{m} = E(m_i)$ and $\bar{\bar{m}} = E(m_i^2)$ denote the first and second moments, respectively, of the cluster size distribution. For a constant cluster size case with $m_i = m$, we have $\bar{m} = m$ and $\bar{\bar{m}} = m^2$. Let $p_k = m_{ki}/m_i$ denote the allocation proportion for arm k within each cluster $(p_1 + p_2 = 1)$.

The survival times of subunits within each cluster may be correlated, while those from different clusters are independent. There are two types of ICC in an SRT. One is the correlation between subunits assigned to the same treatment arm, called within-arm correlation, and the other is that between subunits assigned to different treatment arm, called between-arm correlation. For clustered data under subunit randomization, the survival times of subunits randomized into the same treatment arm from each cluster have an exchangeable dependency with a bivariate survival function

$$S_k(t_1,t_2) = P(T_{kij} \geq t_1, T_{kij'} \geq t_2)$$

for $1 \leq j \neq j' \leq m_{ki}$ and a bivariate probability density function

$$f_k(t_1,t_2) = \frac{\partial^2 S_k(t_1,t_2)}{\partial t_1 \partial t_2}.$$

We define the bivariate hazard function

$$\lambda_k(t_1,t_2) = f_k(t_1,t_2)/S_k(t_1,t_2)$$

and the conditional hazard function

$$\lambda_{k(1|2)}(t_1,t_2) = \lim_{\epsilon\to 0}\frac{P(t_1 \leq T_{kij} < t_1+\epsilon, T_{kij'} \geq t_2)}{P(T_{kij} \geq t_1, T_{kij'} \geq t_2)} = -\frac{\partial \log S_k(t_1,t_2)}{\partial t_1}$$

for $j \neq j'$. We define $\lambda_{k(2|1)}(t_1,t_2)$ similarly.

For two subunits randomized into different arms from the same cluster, the bivariate survival function is denoted as

$$S_b(t_1,t_2) = P(T_{1ij} \geq t_1, T_{2ij'} \geq t_2).$$

Like the within-arm distribution functions, we define between-arm distribution functions

$$f_b(t_1,t_2) = \frac{\partial S_b(t_1,t_2)}{\partial t_1 \partial t_2},$$

$$\lambda_b(t_1,t_2) = f_b(t_1,t_2)/S_b(t_1,t_2),$$

$$\lambda_{b(1|2)}(t_1,t_2) = \lim_{\epsilon\to 0}\frac{P(t_1 \leq T_{1ij} < t_1+\epsilon, T_{2ij'} \geq t_2)}{P(T_{1ij} \geq t_1, T_{2ij'} \geq t_2)} = -\frac{\partial \log S_b(t_1,t_2)}{\partial t_1},$$

and

$$\lambda_{b(2|1)}(t_1,t_2) = \lim_{\epsilon\to 0}\frac{P(T_{1ij} \geq t_1, t_2 \leq T_{2ij'} < t_2+\epsilon)}{P(T_{1ij} \geq t_1, T_{2ij'} \geq t_2)} = -\frac{\partial \log S_b(t_1,t_2)}{\partial t_2}.$$

We also need to specify censoring distribution for sample size calculation. While censoring time C_{kij} and survival time T_{kij} are assumed to be independent for each subunit, censoring times of subunits within each cluster may be dependent. Let $G(t) = P(C_{kij} \geq t)$ and $G(t_1,t_2) = P(C_{kij} \geq t_1, C_{kij'} \geq t_2)$ denote the marginal and bivariate survival functions, respectively, of the censoring distribution. The censoring distribution depends on both accrual and loss to follow-up patterns of clusters and subunits.

By Appendix C, under H_1, the clustered log-rank test statistic W in (12.1) is asymptotically normal with mean $\bar{m}p_1p_2\omega\sqrt{n}$ and variance

$$\sigma^2 = p_1^2p_2^2\left[\bar{m}\sigma_1^2\{1/p_1 + (\bar{\bar{m}}/\bar{m} - 1/p_1)\rho_1\} + \bar{m}\sigma_2^2\{1/p_2 + (\bar{\bar{m}}/\bar{m} - 1/p_2)\rho_2\} - 2\bar{\bar{m}}c_b\right],$$

where

$$\omega = \int_0^\infty \frac{S_1(t)S_2(t)G(t)}{p_1S_1(t)+p_2S_2(t)}\{d\Lambda_1(t)-d\Lambda_2(t)\},$$

$\rho_k = c_k/\sigma_k^2$, $\rho_b = c_b/(\sigma_1\sigma_2)$

$$\sigma_k^2 = \int_0^\infty \frac{S_k(t)S_{3-k}^2(t)G(t)}{\{p_1S_1(t)+p_2S_2(t)\}^2}d\Lambda_k(t),$$

$$c_k = \int_0^\infty\int_0^\infty \frac{S_{3-k}(t_1)S_{3-k}(t_2)S_k(t_1,t_2)G(t_1,t_2)}{\{p_1S_1(t_1)+p_2S_2(t_1)\}\{p_1S_1(t_2)+p_2S_2(t_2)\}}dA_k(t_1,t_2),$$

$$c_b = \int_0^\infty\int_0^\infty \frac{S_2(t_1)S_1(t_2)S_b(t_1,t_2)G(t_1,t_2)}{(p_1S_1(t_1)+p_2S_2(t_1))(p_1S_1(t_2)+p_2S_2(t_2))}dA_b(t_1,t_2),$$

$$\begin{aligned} dA_k(t_1,t_2) =& \{\lambda_k(t_1,t_2) - \lambda_{k(1|2)}(t_1,t_2)\lambda_k(t_2) - \lambda_{k(2|1)}(t_1,t_2)\lambda_k(t_1) \\ &+ \lambda_k(t_1)\lambda_k(t_2)\}dt_1dt_2 \end{aligned}$$

and

$$\begin{aligned} dA_b(t_1,t_2) =& \{\lambda_b(t_1,t_2) - \lambda_{b(1|2)}(t_1,t_2)\lambda_2(t_2) - \lambda_{b(2|1)}(t_1,t_2)\lambda_1(t_1) \\ &+ \lambda_1(t_1)\lambda_2(t_2)\}dt_1dt_2. \end{aligned}$$

We call $\rho_k = c_k/\sigma_k^2$ within-arm ICC and $\rho_b = c_b/(\sigma_1\sigma_2)$ between-arm ICC. Both within-arm and between-arm ICCs range between 0 and 1. In sample size calculations, we often assume that within-arm ICC and between-arm ICC are identical. However, within-arm ICC may be larger than between-arm ICC if there is an additional layer of common frailty by treatment. If correlation exists only within each treatment arm, then between-arm ICC will be 0. In this case, the data from an SRT has the same dependency structure as one from a CRT so that all statistical methods for the CRT that are investigated in Chapter 11 can be used for the SRT. Furthermore, if all subunits are independent, the within-arm ICC will become 0 as well, and the standard statistical methods for independent data can be used for such a trial.

In Appendix C, we show that $\hat{\sigma}^2$ in (12.2) converges to σ^2 under the nearby alternative hypothesis, i.e., $\Lambda_1(t) \approx \Lambda_2(t)$ for all $t \geq 0$. Hence, given sample size n, the power of the clustered log-rank test is given as

$$\begin{aligned} 1-\beta =& P\left(|\frac{W}{\hat{\sigma}}| > z_{1-\alpha/2}|H_1\right) \\ \approx& P\left(\frac{W-\bar{m}p_1p_2\omega\sqrt{n}}{\sigma} > z_{1-\alpha/2} - \frac{\bar{m}p_1p_2\omega\sqrt{n}}{\sigma}|H_1\right). \end{aligned} \tag{12.4}$$

As $(W-\bar{m}p_1p_2\omega\sqrt{n})/\sigma$ is asymptotically $N(0,1)$ under H_1, we derive the required sample size by solving the equation (12.3) with respect to n,

$$n = \frac{\sigma^2(z_{1-\alpha/2}+z_{1-\beta})^2}{(\bar{m}p_1p_2\omega)^2}. \tag{12.5}$$

Note that the components ω and σ^2 in (12.4) require specification of only the marginal and bivariate distribution functions for survival and censoring times even when cluster size is larger than 2.

Let's consider a proportional hazards assumption with hazard ratio $\Delta = \lambda_1(t)/\lambda_2(t)$. Under the nearby alternative hypothesis, we have $\Delta - 1 \approx \log\Delta$ by the Taylor expansion. In this case, by Appendix C, sample size formula (12.4) is simplified to

$$n = \frac{(z_{1-\alpha/2} + z_{1-\beta})^2}{\bar{m}dp_1p_2(\log\Delta)^2}\text{DE}, \tag{12.6}$$

where

$$\text{DE} = 1 - \rho_w + 2p_1p_2(\rho_w - \rho_b)\bar{\bar{m}}/\bar{m}$$

$\rho_w = c_w/d$, $\rho_b = c_b/d$,

$$c_w = \int_0^\infty \int_0^\infty S(t_1, t_2)G(t_1, t_2)dA(t_1, t_2)$$

$$c_b = \int_0^\infty \int_0^\infty S_b(t_1, t_2)G(t_1, t_2)dA_b(t_1, t_2)$$

and $d = -p_1 \int_0^\infty G(t)dS_1(t) - p_2 \int_0^\infty G(t)dS_2(t)$ is the probability that a subunit has an event. Since $M = n\bar{m}$ is the total number of subunits, $D = dM$ is the expected number of events from M subunits. Furthermore, by Schoenfeld (1983),

$$D_0 = \frac{(z_{1-\alpha/2} + z_{1-\beta})^2}{p_1p_2(\log\Delta)^2}$$

is the required number of events when subunits are independent so that (12.5) is expressed as $D = D_0 \times \text{DE}$. Hence, DE is the design effect modifying the Schoenfeld's (1983) formula accounting for intracluster dependencies. Recall that ρ_w and ρ_b are within-arm and between-arm ICCs. From this simplified formula, we observe that, with cluster sizes m_i larger than two, the required sample size increases in ρ_w (since $\bar{\bar{m}}/\bar{m} > 1$ in DE) and decreases in ρ_b.

If two subunits in each cluster have the same ICC whether they are assigned to the same arm or different arms, i.e., $\rho_w = \rho_b (= \rho)$, then $\text{DE} = 1 - \rho$ so that equation (12.5) is simplified to

$$n = \frac{(z_{1-\alpha/2} + z_{1-\beta})^2}{\bar{m}dp_1p_2(\log\Delta)^2}(1 - \rho). \tag{12.7}$$

Equation (12.6) implies that, when $\rho_b = \rho_w$, the variance of cluster size distribution, $\text{var}(m_i) = \bar{\bar{m}} - \bar{m}^2$, has no impact on the required number of clusters, and the required sample size decreases in ICC ρ. Gangnon and Kosorok (2004) implicitly assume that $\rho_b = \rho_w (= \rho)$ and propose a sample size formula that has the same form as equation (12.6). In their formula, however, ρ is specified as an input parameter without presenting its explicit form. Note that it is impossible to specify $\rho_w = \rho_b$ in the design stage of a trial without specifying the bivariate survival and censoring distributions. In the method discussed here, ρ_w and ρ_b are not specified, but are calculated from the specified bivariate survival and censoring distributions.

Some methods have been proposed for estimation of bivariate survival distribution (e.g., Lin and Ying 1993) that can be used when pilot data are available. In the following subsections, some practical models are presented for censoring and survival distributions to be used in sample size calculations.

Specification of Survival Distribution

Recall that the power or sample size for the clustered rank tests depend on the marginal and bivariate distributions for clustered survival times. Exponential distributions have been widely used in designing clinical trials collecting independent survival data for the following reasons. An exponential distribution is uniquely identified by hazard rate, median, or survival probability at a time point so that it is convenient to specify an exponential distribution by an estimate of any of these parameters from previous studies. Moreover, survival data in real clinical trials usually fit well by exponential models. For these reasons, we use exponential distributions to specify the marginal distributions of clustered survival too.

To account for the dependency among subunits within each cluster, we may use nested Archimedean copulas as a joint survival distribution model. For sample size calculation, we need to specify both within-arm bivariate survival function $S_k(t_1, t_2)$ and between-arm bivariate survival function $S_b(t_1, t_2)$. The outcomes of subunits within the same treatment arm are possibly more correlated than those of subunits assigned to different treatment arms. For example, in a hospital-based surgical study, outcomes of patients (subunits) in each hospital (cluster) can be correlated. In this case, if the surgeon teams are different between two surgical methods, then, among the patients in each hospital, those in the same surgical method share the common frailties of surgeon team as well as hospital, while those in different surgical methods share the common frailties of hospital only. Consequently, the within-arm dependency can be higher than the between-arm dependency (Pals et al. 2008). Nested Archimedean copula provides a convenient method to model bivariate survival distributions with different within-arm and between-arm dependencies at the same time.

One of the most popular Archimedean copulas is the Gumbel (1960) copula model. Using marginal exponential distributions with hazard rates λ_k for arms $k(= 1, 2)$, it is shown in Appendix D that the bivariate and conditional hazard functions are expressed as

$$\lambda_k(t_1,t_2) = \lambda_1\lambda_2(\lambda_k t_1)^{1/\theta_w-1}(\lambda_k t_2)^{1/\theta_w-1}\left\{(\lambda_k t_1)^{1/\theta_w}+(\lambda_k t_2)^{1/\theta_w}\right\}^{2\theta_w-2}$$
$$\times\left[1+(1/\theta_w-1)\left\{(\lambda_k t_1)^{1/\theta_w}+(\lambda_k t_2)^{1/\theta_w}\right\}^{-\theta_w}\right]$$
$$\lambda_{k(1|2)}(t_1,t_2) = \lambda_k(\lambda_k t_1)^{1/\theta_w-1}\left\{(\lambda_k t_1)^{1/\theta_w}+(\lambda_k t_2)^{1/\theta_w}\right\}^{\theta_w-1}$$
$$\lambda_b(t_1,t_2) = \lambda_1\lambda_2 e^{(\lambda_1 t_1+\lambda_2 t_2)/\theta_b}(1+1/\theta_b)\left\{e^{\lambda_1 t_1/\theta_b}+e^{\lambda_2 t_2/\theta_b}-1\right\}^{-2}$$
$$\lambda_{b(1|2)}(t_1,t_2) = \lambda_1 e^{\lambda_1 t_1/\theta_b}\left\{e^{\lambda_1 t_1/\theta_b}+e^{\lambda_2 t_2/\theta_b}-1\right\}^{-1},$$

where $\theta_l = 1-\tau_l$ characterizes the degree of correlation (within-arm for $l = w$ and between-arm for $l = b$) and τ_l is the Kendall's tau.

Specification of Censoring Distribution

The power and sample size of clustered rank tests depend on the marginal and bivariate censoring distributions of subunits as well as survival distributions. In an SRT, the joint censoring distribution of subunits is determined by the accrual pattern of clusters and subunits. In the study by Batchelor and Hackett (1970), for each patient (cluster), the number of skin-grafts (subunits) from different donors is determined by the size of burned area requiring skin-graft, and all of the skin-grafts of each patient are recruited at the time when the patient is recruited. In this case, if censoring occurs only by ending the study (administrative censoring), then all subunits in each cluster have identical censoring time. We call this a 'common censoring'.

On the other hand, in the Harper's trial (Harper et al. 2015), all clinics (clusters) participating in the study are selected by the time of study open and subjects (subunits) enter the study from each clinic independently over an accrual period. So, the censoring times of subunits within each cluster are independent in this case. We call this an 'independent censoring'. Our sample size formula allows any type of censoring patterns by modeling the appropriate bivariate censoring distribution, but we consider these two popular types in this chapter.

(i) Common Censoring Case

Suppose that each clusters are accrued at a constant rate r during a period of a, and followed for an additional period of b as in the Batchelor's trial. Furthermore, we assume that subunits of each cluster are recruited at the same time when the cluster is recruited, and consider administrative censoring only. In this case, subunits of each cluster have identical censoring times, i.e., $C_{kij} = C_i$ for $k = 1,2$ and $j = 1,...,m_{ki}$. The marginal distribution for censoring time C_{kij} is $U(b, a+b)$ with survival function

$$G(t) = I(t < a+b) - \frac{t-b}{a}I(b \le t < a+b).$$

The bivariate survival function of censoring times of subunits of each cluster is expressed by the marginal function as

$$G(t_1, t_2) = P(C_{kij} > t_1, C_{ki'j'} > t_2) = P(C_i > t_1 \vee t_2) = G(t_1 \vee t_2),$$

where $t_1 \vee t_2$ denotes the maximum of t_1 and t_2.

(ii) Independent Censoring Case
Suppose that all clusters are recruited before study opens and subunits of each cluster are independently accrued during an accrual period as in the Harper's trial. In this case, the censoring times are independent among subunits so that we have $G(t_1, t_2) = G(t_1)G(t_2)$. As in the common censoring case, the bivariate joint censoring distribution is expressed by the marginal distribution. If subunits are accrued at a constant rate for period of a and followed for an additional period of b after the completion of accrual, then, with administrative censoring only, censoring times C_{kij} are IID $U(b, a+b)$. Note that the marginal censoring distribution of subunits is identical to that of common censoring case although the meaning of a is different between the two censoring cases, i.e., accrual period for clusters vs. that for subunits.

Sample Size Calculation under Some Practical Design Settings

To calculate a sample size using formula (12.4), we have to calculate $\bar{m}$, $\bar{\bar{m}}$, ω, σ_k^2, c_k, and c_b for given survival and censoring distributions. Assuming marginal exponential distributions with hazard rate λ_k for survival and $U(b, a+b)$ distribution for censoring, we have

$$\omega = (\lambda_1 - \lambda_2) \int_0^{a+b} (1 - a^{-1}[t-b]_+) \frac{e^{-(\lambda_1 - \lambda_2)t}}{(p_1 e^{-\lambda_1 t} + p_2 e^{-\lambda_2 t})^2} dt$$

$$\sigma_k^2 = \lambda_k \int_0^{a+b} (1 - a^{-1}[t-b]_+) \frac{e^{-(\lambda_k + 2\lambda_{3-k})t}}{(p_1 e^{-\lambda_1 t} + p_2 e^{-\lambda_2 t})^2} dt,$$

where $[t]_+ = t \times I(t > 0)$.

While ω and σ_k^2 depend on the marginal survival and censoring distributions only, c_k and c_b depend on the bivariate survival and censoring distributions. In the following calculations, we use

$$dA_k(t_1, t_2) = \{\lambda_k(t_1, t_2) - \lambda_k \lambda_{k(1|2)}(t_1, t_2) - \lambda_k \lambda_{k(2|1)}(t_1, t_2) + \lambda_k^2\} dt_1 dt_2$$

and

$$dA_b(t_1, t_2) = \{\lambda_b(t_1, t_2) - \lambda_2 \lambda_{b(1|2)}(t_1, t_2) - \lambda_1 \lambda_{b(2|1)}(t_1, t_2) + \lambda_1 \lambda_2\} dt_1 dt_2$$

with $\lambda_k(t_1, t_2)$, $\lambda_{k(1|2)}(t_1, t_2)$, $\lambda_b(t_1, t_2)$, and $\lambda_{b(1|2)}(t_1, t_2)$ calculated based on the Gumbel copula as shown above.

(i) Common Censoring Case

In a common censoring case, we usually estimate the cluster size distribution from historical data. Let $q(m)$ denote the estimated probability mass function for cluster size distribution. Then, we have $\bar{m} = \sum_m mq(m)$ and $\bar{\bar{m}} = \sum_m m^2 q(m)$. In addition, Appendix D shows that

$$c_k = \int_0^{a+b} \int_0^{a+b} (1 - a^{-1}[t_1 \vee t_2 - b]_+)$$

$$\times \frac{e^{-\lambda_{3-k}(t_1+t_2)} \exp[-\{(\lambda_k t_1)^{1/\theta_w} + (\lambda_k t_2)^{1/\theta_w}\}^{\theta_w}]}{(p_1 e^{-\lambda_1 t_1} + p_2 e^{-\lambda_2 t_1})(p_1 e^{-\lambda_1 t_2} + p_2 e^{-\lambda_2 t_2})} dA_k(t_1, t_2)$$

and

$$c_b = \int_0^{a+b} \int_0^{a+b} (1 - a^{-1}[t_1 \vee t_2 - b]_+)$$

$$\times \frac{e^{-\lambda_1 t_1 + \lambda_2 t_2} \exp[-\{(\lambda_1 t_1)^{1/\theta_b} + (\lambda_2 t_2)^{1/\theta_b}\}^{\theta_b}]}{(p_1 e^{-\lambda_1 t_1} + p_2 e^{-\lambda_2 t_1})(p_1 e^{-\lambda_1 t_2} + p_2 e^{-\lambda_2 t_2})} dA_b(t_1, t_2).$$

(ii) Independent Censoring Case

In an independent censoring case, cluster size is estimated by the accrual period and the accrual rate of subunits for each cluster. If r_i denotes the accrual rate of subunits for cluster i, then, given accrual period a, the expected cluster size for cluster i is $m_i = a \times r_i$. Let $q(r)$ denote the probability mass function of accrual rate r_i among clusters, and $\bar{r} = \sum_r rq(r)$ and $\bar{\bar{r}} = \sum_r r^2 q(r)$ denote its first and second moments, respectively. Then, we have $\bar{m} = a\bar{r}$ and $\bar{\bar{m}} = a^2 \bar{\bar{r}}$. In Appendix D, we show that

$$c_k = \int_0^{a+b} \int_0^{a+b} (1 - a^{-1}[t_1 - b]_+)(1 - a^{-1}[t_2 - b]_+)$$

$$\times \frac{e^{-\lambda_{3-k}(t_1+t_2)} \exp[-\{(\lambda_k t_1)^{1/\theta_w} + (\lambda_k t_2)^{1/\theta_w}\}^{\theta_w}]}{(p_1 e^{-\lambda_1 t_1} + p_2 e^{-\lambda_2 t_1})(p_1 e^{-\lambda_1 t_2} + p_2 e^{-\lambda_2 t_2})} dA_k(t_1, t_2)$$

and

$$c_b = \int_0^{a+b} \int_0^{a+b} (1 - a^{-1}[t_1 - b]_+)(1 - a^{-1}[t_2 - b]_+)$$

$$\times \frac{e^{-\lambda_1 t_1 + \lambda_2 t_2} \exp[-\{(\lambda_1 t_1)^{1/\theta_b} + (\lambda_2 t_2)^{1/\theta_b}\}^{\theta_b}]}{(p_1 e^{-\lambda_1 t_1} + p_2 e^{-\lambda_2 t_1})(p_1 e^{-\lambda_1 t_2} + p_2 e^{-\lambda_2 t_2})} dA_b(t_1, t_2).$$

When Accrual Rate Is Specified Instead of Accrual Period

So far, we have calculated sample sizes by specifying accrual period a. In practice, however, it is easier to specify the accrual rate based on the number of clusters or subunits who have recently visited the clinics participating in the study. From the previous section, we observe that $\omega = \omega(a)$, $\sigma_k^2 = \sigma_k^2(a)$, $c_k = c_k(a)$, and $c_b = c_b(a)$ are functions of accrual period a. For the two censoring cases presented above, calculation of sample size is slightly different as follows.

(i) Common Censoring Case
The variance of the test statistic σ^2 is a function of accrual period a,

$$\sigma_C^2 = p_1^2 p_2^2 \left[\bar{m}\sigma_1^2(a)\{1/p_1 + (\bar{\bar{m}}/\bar{m} - 1/p_1)\rho_1(a)\} \right.$$

$$\left. + \bar{m}\sigma_2^2(a)\{1/p_2 + (\bar{\bar{m}}/\bar{m} - 1/p_2)\rho_2(a)\} - 2\bar{\bar{m}}c_b(a) \right].$$

Furthermore, if clusters are accrued at a constant rate r, the total sample size n is approximated by $a \times r$. Hence, equation (12.4) is expressed as

$$a \times r = \frac{\sigma_C^2(a)(z_{1-\alpha/2} + z_{1-\beta})^2}{\{\bar{m}p_1 p_2 \omega(a)\}^2}. \tag{12.8}$$

Let a^* denote the solution to equation (12.7), then the required sample size is $n = a^* \times r$. Similarly, we can solve the simplified sample size formula (12.5) with respect to accrual period a too.

(ii) Independent Censoring Case
In this case, we can calculate the number of clusters n for a given accrual period a, or the required accrual period a given a number of clusters n. Based on the equations in the previous section, the variance of W, σ^2, is a function of accrual period a with

$$\sigma_I^2 = p_1^2 p_2^2 \left[a\bar{r}\sigma_1^2(a)\{1/p_1 + (a\bar{\bar{r}}/\bar{r} - 1/p_1)\rho_1(a)\} \right.$$

$$\left. + a\bar{r}\sigma_2^2(a)\{1/p_2 + (a\bar{\bar{r}}/\bar{r} - 1/p_2)\rho_2(a)\} - 2a^2\bar{\bar{r}}c_b(a) \right]$$

by replacing $\bar{m}$ with $a\bar{r}$ and $\bar{\bar{m}}$ with $a^2\bar{\bar{r}}$. Hence, given accrual period a, the required number of clusters n is obtained by

$$n = \frac{\sigma_I^2(a)(z_{1-\alpha/2} + z_{1-\beta})^2}{\{a\bar{r}p_1 p_2 \omega(a)\}^2}. \tag{12.9}$$

On the other hand, for a given number of clusters n, the required accrual period a^* is obtained by solving equation (12.9) with respect to a.

Subunit Randomization versus Cluster Randomization

Recall that, when there is no intracluster dependency, the required number of clusters is

$$n_0 = \frac{(z_{1-\alpha/2} + z_{1-\beta})^2}{\bar{m}dp_1^c p_2^c (\log \Delta)^2},$$

where p_k^c is the proportion of clusters randomized into arm k. From Chapter 11, the required number of clusters for a CRT with a within-arm ICC ρ_w increases to $n_c = n_0 \times \text{IF}$, where $\text{IF} = 1+(\bar{\bar{m}}/\bar{m}-1)\rho_w$. On the other hand, from (12.5) above, the required number of clusters for an SRT with a within-arm ICC ρ_w and a between-arm ICC ρ_b is given as $n_s = n_0 \times \text{DE}$, where

$$\text{DE} = 1 - \rho_w + 2p_1p_2(\rho_w - \rho_b)\bar{\bar{m}}/\bar{m}.$$

Since ICC is non-negative, we always have $n_s/n_c = \text{DE}/\text{IF} \leq 1$. The difference between n_s and n_c increases in $\text{var}(m)$ and ρ_b. Therefore, when designing a trial with clusters, we always can save the sample size by using an SRT, rather than a CRT. But, due to some reasons, SRT may not be a feasible option sometimes.

Numerical Studies

Simulations

Simulations are conducted to evaluate the finite sample properties of the sample size formulas that are derived using large sample approximations. We use the algorithm proposed by McNeil (2008) to generate correlated survival times from nested Gumbel copula model. More specifically, we generate the correlated survival times of a cluster as follows.

1. Generate a random variable V_0 from stable distribution $S(\theta_b, 1, cos(\pi\theta_b/2), 0)$ using the method described by Nolan (2003).
2. Generate two IID random variables V_1 and V_2 from stable distribution $S(\theta_w/\theta_b, 1, cos(\pi\theta_w/2\theta_b), 0)$.
3. Generate $m_1 + m_2$ independent random variables $Z_{11}, ...Z_{1m_1}, Z_{21}, ...,$ Z_{2m_2} from $U(0,1)$ distribution.
4. Calculate $U_{kj} = \exp[-\{-\log(Z_{kj})/V_k\}^{\theta_w/\theta_b}], k = 1, 2, j = 1, 2, ..., m_k$.
5. Finally, generate correlated failure times $T_{kj} = \lambda_k^{-1}\{-\log(U_{kj})/V_0\}^{\theta_b}$ for $j = 1, ..., m_k$ and $k = 1, 2$.

We set $\alpha = 0.05$; $1 - \beta = 0.8, 0.85$, or 0.9; hazard ratio $\Delta = \lambda_1/\lambda_2 = 1.2$ or 1.4; 2 years of median survival for arm 1, i.e., $\lambda_1 = 2^{-1}\log 2$; $b = 1$ year of additional follow-up; $p_1 = p_2 = 1/2$ for a balanced randomization. We assume Kendall's $\tau_w = 0.1, 0.3$, or 0.5 for within-arm correlation, and Kendall's τ_b for between-arm correlation is set to be either $\tau_b = \tau_w$ or $\tau_b = \tau_w/2$.

At first, we consider the case where clusters are accrued over an accrual period and all the subunits of each cluster enter the study at the same time, i.e., common censoring case. We assume an accrual rate of $r = 100$ clusters per year, and three cluster size distributions: fixed at $m = 10$, random with a discrete uniform distribution $U(8, 12)$, or a discrete uniform distribution

TABLE 12.5

Common censoring case: Required number of clusters (empirical type I error rate and power in the parenthesis) with $\lambda_1 = 2^{-1} \log 2$

$1-\beta$	τ_w	τ_b	λ_1/λ_2	$m = 10$		$m \sim U(8,12)$		$m \sim U(2,18)$	
				by (12.4)	by (12.5)	by (12.4)	by (12.5)	by (12.4)	by (12.5)
0.9	0.1	0.05	1.2	288 (0.047, 0.910)	287 (0.045, 0.900)	289 (0.048,0.900)	288 (0.047,0.903)	301 (0.045,0.896)	299 (0.052,0.895)
			1.4	121 (0.048, 0.903)	119 (0.047, 0.894)	121 (0.053,0.903)	119 (0.051,0.894)	127 (0.050,0.898)	125 (0.051,0.894)
		0.1	1.2	232 (0.055, 0.900)	230 (0.049, 0.898)	232 (0.050,0.898)	230 (0.047,0.895)	232 (0.046,0.895)	231 (0.054,0.902)
			1.4	96 (0.048, 0.902)	94 (0.046, 0.878)	96 (0.051,0.899)	94 (0.048,0.891)	96 (0.057,0.895)	94 (0.049,0.892)
	0.3	0.15	1.2	350 (0.048, 0.895)	347 (0.044, 0.893)	353 (0.046,0.893)	350 (0.046,0.901)	385 (0.050,0.908)	382 (0.051,0.890)
			1.4	148 (0.052, 0.902)	145 (0.056, 0.893)	149 (0.049,0.909)	146 (0.048,0.890)	164 (0.051,0.903)	160 (0.055,0.888)
		0.3	1.2	186 (0.048, 0.910)	183 (0.051, 0.901)	186 (0.046,0.902)	183 (0.051,0.895)	187 (0.046,0.901)	183 (0.046,0.883)
			1.4	78 (0.049, 0.921)	75 (0.053, 0.898)	78 (0.052,0.909)	75 (0.048,0.893)	79 (0.048,0.901)	75 (0.049,0.885)
	0.5	0.25	1.2	404 (0.057, 0.892)	400 (0.051, 0.899)	408 (0.054,0.906)	405 (0.052,0.902)	459 (0.054,0.901)	455 (0.049,0.894)
			1.4	170 (0.047, 0.911)	166 (0.048, 0.898)	172 (0.051,0.907)	168 (0.050,0.894)	194 (0.047,0.906)	189 (0.049,0.892)
		0.5	1.3	139 (0.051, 0.915)	135 (0.046, 0.910)	140 (0.046,0.901)	135 (0.051,0.892)	141 (0.049,0.901)	136 (0.049,0.891)
			1.4	62 (0.047, 0.928)	58 (0.045, 0.909)	62 (0.047,0.928)	58 (0.049,0.907)	65 (0.044,0.925)	59 (0.046,0.891)
0.85	0.1	0.05	1.2	257 (0.053, 0.850)	255 (0.050, 0.846)	258 (0.047,0.851)	256 (0.050,0.842)	268 (0.047,0.896)	267 (0.046,0.850)
			1.4	107 (0.051, 0.852)	105 (0.049, 0.852)	107 (0.050,0.843)	105 (0.047,0.846)	112 (0.046,0.898)	110 (0.051,0.831)
		0.1	1.2	206 (0.046, 0.855)	205 (0.052, 0.846)	206 (0.046,0.841)	205 (0.048,0.847)	206 (0.050,0.895)	205 (0.053,0.848)
			1.4	84 (0.054, 0.847)	83 (0.051, 0.847)	84 (0.054,0.850)	83 (0.050,0.831)	85 (0.048,0.895)	83 (0.050,0.831)
	0.3	0.15	1.2	311 (0.050, 0.840)	309 (0.051, 0.856)	314 (0.053,0.852)	312 (0.055,0.851)	343 (0.049,0.908)	340 (0.051,0.849)
			1.4	131 (0.048, 0.846)	128 (0.051, 0.836)	132 (0.048,0.850)	129 (0.050,0.841)	145 (0.047,0.903)	142 (0.052,0.849)
		0.3	1.2	165 (0.049, 0.849)	162 (0.054, 0.839)	165 (0.051,0.842)	162 (0.045,0.850)	165 (0.050,0.901)	163 (0.049,0.839)
			1.4	68 (0.049, 0.859)	66 (0.051, 0.847)	68 (0.047,0.859)	66 (0.045,0.843)	69 (0.049,0.901)	66 (0.045,0.826)
	0.5	0.25	1.2	359 (0.052, 0.857)	355 (0.051, 0.840)	363 (0.049,0.844)	359 (0.050,0.848)	408 (0.051,0.901)	404 (0.056,0.854)
			1.4	151 (0.047, 0.863)	147 (0.047, 0.841)	153 (0.046,0.855)	149 (0.051,0.851)	172 (0.052,0.906)	168 (0.049,0.848)
		0.5	1.2	123 (0.048, 0.862)	120 (0.048, 0.853)	123 (0.053,0.846)	120 (0.053,0.829)	125 (0.049,0.901)	121 (0.046,0.831)
			1.4	54 (0.047, 0.886)	50 (0.051, 0.862)	55 (0.044,0.883)	51 (0.044,0.841)	57 (0.051,0.925)	52 (0.050,0.825)

(Continued)

TABLE 12.5 (Continued)

Common censoring case: Required number of clusters (empirical type I error rate and power in the parenthesis) with $\lambda_1 = 2^{-1}\log 2$

				$m = 10$		$m \sim U(8, 12)$		$m \sim U(2, 18)$	
$1-\beta$	τ_w	τ_b	λ_1/λ_2	by (12.4)	by (12.5)	by (12.4)	by (12.5)	by (12.4)	by (12.5)
0.8	0.1	0.05	1.2	232 (0.048, 0.804)	231 (0.046, 0.792)	233 (0.053,0.795)	232 (0.045,0.800)	243 (0.052,0.791)	241 (0.052,0.781)
			1.4	96 (0.048, 0.793)	94 (0.053, 0.785)	96 (0.048,0.802)	95 (0.049,0.787)	101 (0.047,0.787)	99 (0.049,0.792)
		0.1	1.2	186 (0.051, 0.805)	185 (0.047, 0.794)	186 (0.045,0.800)	185 (0.052,0.798)	187 (0.051,0.794)	185 (0.049,0.795)
			1.4	76 (0.052, 0.809)	74 (0.045, 0.791)	76 (0.051,0.797)	74 (0.046,0.788)	76 (0.052,0.798)	74 (0.048,0.788)
	0.3	0.15	1.2	282 (0.048, 0.801)	280 (0.057, 0.784)	284 (0.053,0.800)	282 (0.049,0.787)	310 (0.054,0.799)	308 (0.052,0.782)
			1.4	118 (0.051, 0.802)	116 (0.043, 0.786)	119 (0.051,0.812)	117 (0.046,0.782)	131 (0.044,0.802)	128 (0.046,0.794)
		0.3	1.2	148 (0.049, 0.802)	146 (0.044, 0.800)	148 (0.047,0.791)	146 (0.048,0.799)	149 (0.047,0.784)	147 (0.049,0.786)
			1.4	61 (0.046, 0.819)	59 (0.045, 0.812)	61 (0.049,0.797)	59 (0.048,0.788)	62 (0.048,0.805)	59 (0.046,0.779)
	0.5	0.25	1.2	324 (0.052, 0.800)	321 (0.047, 0.796)	328 (0.047,0.798)	325 (0.054,0.792)	368 (0.050,0.795)	365 (0.052,0.794)
			1.4	136 (0.048, 0.805)	133 (0.050, 0.794)	137 (0.045,0.809)	134 (0.051,0.792)	155 (0.052,0.797)	151 (0.047,0.785)
		0.5	1.2	111 (0.049, 0.816)	108 (0.046, 0.804)	111 (0.047,0.804)	108 (0.050,0.788)	112 (0.046,0.791)	109 (0.049,0.787)
			1.4	48 (0.050, 0.834)	45 (0.046, 0.798)	49 (0.044,0.831)	45 (0.046,0.783)	50 (0.050,0.813)	46 (0.051,0.778)

$U(2,18)$. These three cluster size distributions have the same mean $\bar{m} = 10$, but different variances $\bar{\bar{m}} - \bar{m}^2 = 0, 2$, and 24, respectively. Under each design setting, we calculate the required accrual period of the clustered log-rank test by solving equations (12.4) and (12.5) with respect to a, generate simulation data sets of size $n = a \times r$ under the design setting, and apply the clustered log-rank test to the generated data. We repeat this procedure 5,000 times for each simulation setting, and estimate an empirical power $1 - \hat{\beta}$ as the proportion of simulation data sets rejecting the null hypothesis among the 5,000 data sets. Empirical type I error $\hat{\alpha}$ is also calculated to evaluate the finite sample property of the clustered log-rank test under subunit randomization by generating simulation data of size n under $H_0 : \lambda_1 = \lambda_2 = 2^{-1} \log 2$. Table 12.5 reports the calculated sample size n, and empirical type I error rate $\hat{\alpha}$ and power $1 - \hat{\beta}$ under the various design settings.

In the second set of simulations, we calculate the number of required clusters when clusters are determined before the study opens, and subunits are recruited independently from each cluster during accrual period a at a constant rate, i.e., independent censoring case. The follow-up period b is fixed at 1 year, and the accrual period is fixed at 0.5 year. Accrual rate of subunits is either fixed at $r_i = 20$ per year for all clusters or randomly selected from 10, 20, or 30 with an equal probability of $1/3$ assuming that small, medium, and large size clinics (clusters) are equally distributed among the participating clinics. The mean subunit accrual rate is $\bar{r} = 20$ for the both cases, but the variances are $\bar{\bar{r}} - \bar{r}^2 = 0$ and $200/3$, respectively. Table 12.6 reports sample size, and empirical type I error rate and power from 5,000 simulation samples for each of the various design settings with independent censoring.

In the both censoring cases, the required number of clusters decreases in α and hazard ratio Δ, and increases in $1 - \beta$. For a fixed within-arm correlation τ_w, a larger between-arm correlation τ_b leads to a smaller sample size. When $\tau_b = \tau_w$, the variance of cluster size distribution or subunit accrual rate distribution has limited effect on the sample size. However, when $\tau_b = \tau_w/2$, a larger variance in cluster size distribution leads to a larger sample size. Formula (12.5) gives a slightly smaller sample size than (12.4), but both formulas have empirical powers close to the nominal level. Since the empirical type I error rates $\hat{\alpha}$ are close to the nominal level of $\alpha = 0.05$, we find that the clustered log-rank test controls the type I error rate quite accurately for SRTs.

Examples

Example 1: Suppose that we are designing the Batchelor-Hackett trial as an example with common censoring pattern. The hazard rate estimated from the trial data is $\lambda_1 = 0.043$ per day for the poorly matched arm and $\lambda_2 = 0.025$ per day for the closely matched arm. Since the donors are independent, the dependency between the skin-grafts on each patient results only from sharing the body of the patient (donee). We use the Gumbel's copula to model the joint survival distribution with marginal exponential distributions, with

TABLE 12.6

Independent censoring case: Required number of clusters (empirical type I error rate and power in the parenthesis) with $\lambda_1 = 2^{-1}\log 2$

				$r_i = 20$		$r_i \sim U(10, 20, 30)$	
$1-\beta$	τ_w	τ_b	λ_1/λ_2	$n(\hat{\alpha}, 1-\hat{\beta})$ by (12.4)	$n(\hat{\alpha}, 1-\hat{\beta})$ by (12.5)	$n(\hat{\alpha}, 1-\hat{\beta})$ by (12.4)	$n(\hat{\alpha}, 1-\hat{\beta})$ by (12.5)
0.9	0.1	0.05	1.2	463 (0.052, 0.901)	460 (0.048, 0.890)	483 (0.050,0.901)	480 (0.051,0.893)
			1.4	147 (0.055, 0.904)	143 (0.054, 0.887)	153 (0.045,0.902)	150 (0.049,0.887)
		0.1	1.2	342 (0.053, 0.896)	339 (0.042, 0.902)	342 (0.050,0.896)	340 (0.049,0.900)
			1.4	109 (0.046, 0.901)	106 (0.044, 0.894)	109 (0.050,0.892)	107 (0.049,0.897)
	0.3	0.15	1.2	595 (0.052, 0.896)	590 (0.050, 0.901)	653 (0.042,0.895)	648 (0.047,0.900)
			1.4	189 (0.045, 0.893)	185 (0.049, 0.892)	208 (0.050,0.901)	203 (0.045,0.906)
		0.3	1.2	254 (0.051, 0.896)	250 (0.048, 0.904)	255 (0.055,0.898)	251 (0.047,0.888)
			1.4	84 (0.050, 0.909)	81 (0.050, 0.900)	85 (0.044,0.903)	81 (0.051,0.888)
	0.5	0.25	1.2	703 (0.046, 0.898)	697 (0.051, 0.904)	792 (0.048,0.897)	786 (0.047,0.899)
			1.4	225 (0.046, 0.904)	219 (0.048, 0.902)	254 (0.049,0.902)	247 (0.047,0.905)
		0.5	1.3	176 (0.052, 0.913)	171 (0.047, 0.902)	178 (0.053,0.893)	172 (0.050,0.885)
			1.4	65 (0.046, 0.938)	59 (0.051, 0.906)	67 (0.044,0.923)	61 (0.037,0.898)
0.85	0.1	0.05	1.2	395 (0.056, 0.851)	393 (0.048, 0.854)	413 (0.048,0.849)	410 (0.048,0.850)
			1.4	125 (0.047, 0.847)	123 (0.048, 0.849)	131 (0.051,0.856)	128 (0.047,0.839)
		0.1	1.2	292 (0.043, 0.848)	290 (0.050, 0.842)	293 (0.048,0.846)	290 (0.049,0.840)
			1.4	93 (0.048, 0.856)	91 (0.043, 0.839)	94 (0.047,0.844)	91 (0.054,0.838)
	0.3	0.15	1.2	508 (0.052, 0.855)	504 (0.049, 0.847)	558 (0.047,0.848)	553 (0.053,0.835)
			1.4	162 (0.046, 0.851)	158 (0.057, 0.851)	178 (0.050,0.850)	173 (0.048,0.840)
		0.3	1.2	217 (0.049, 0.852)	214 (0.047, 0.846)	218 (0.047,0.846)	214 (0.050,0.837)
			1.4	72 (0.051, 0.867)	69 (0.047, 0.855)	73 (0.048,0.850)	69 (0.048,0.823)
	0.5	0.25	1.2	600 (0.050, 0.848)	595 (0.053, 0.855)	677 (0.053,0.850)	672 (0.051,0.847)
			1.4	192 (0.053, 0.861)	187 (0.045, 0.853)	217 (0.048,0.856)	211 (0.047,0.842)
		0.5	1.2	150 (0.049, 0.858)	146 (0.046, 0.852)	152 (0.045,0.846)	147 (0.048,0.834)
			1.4	55 (0.043, 0.883)	51 (0.046, 0.854)	57 (0.043,0.878)	52 (0.050,0.842)

0.8	0.1	0.05	1.2	346 (0.050, 0.803)	343 (0.049, 0.802)	361 (0.051,0.788)	358 (0.048,0.786)
			1.4	109 (0.047, 0.801)	107 (0.049, 0.790)	114 (0.050,0.791)	112 (0.048,0.777)
		0.1	1.2	256 (0.050, 0.799)	254 (0.051, 0.791)	256 (0.044,0.794)	254 (0.052,0.797)
			1.4	82 (0.052, 0.808)	79 (0.047, 0.795)	82 (0.050,0.791)	80 (0.052,0.787)
	0.3	0.15	1.2	444 (0.045, 0.794)	441 (0.059, 0.795)	487 (0.054,0.798)	484 (0.046,0.792)
			1.4	141 (0.050, 0.805)	138 (0.051, 0.791)	155 (0.047,0.795)	152 (0.051,0.784)
		0.3	1.2	190 (0.052, 0.796)	187 (0.049, 0.795)	190 (0.054,0.799)	187 (0.047,0.789)
			1.4	63 (0.046, 0.810)	60 (0.048, 0.792)	64 (0.051,0.799)	61 (0.049,0.777)
	0.5	0.25	1.2	525 (0.052, 0.806)	521 (0.048, 0.808)	592 (0.051,0.782)	587 (0.055,0.800)
			1.4	168 (0.048, 0.801)	163 (0.052, 0.800)	190 (0.043,0.797)	184 (0.044,0.800)
		0.5	1.2	131 (0.049, 0.813)	127 (0.051, 0.801)	133 (0.050,0.796)	129 (0.050,0.781)
			1.4	48 (0.050, 0.832)	44 (0.045, 0.803)	50 (0.047,0.818)	45 (0.049,0.770)

identical within-arm and between arm correlations, $\tau_w = \tau_b$. We further assume two-sided $\alpha = 0.05$, $1-\beta = 0.9$, a balanced allocation ($p_1 = p_2 = 1/2$), cluster sizes to be 2, 3, or 4 with probability $1/3$ each, a follow-up period of $b = 2$ months, and an accrual rate of $r = 50$ patients per month. For these input parameters, the required sample size for the clustered log-rank test is $n = 242, 198$, and 165 for $\tau_w = 0.3, 0.5$, and 0.7, respectively.

Example 2: The original Harper's study described above was conducted as a CRT. Suppose that it is newly conducted as an SRT assuming that both control and experimental interventions are available from each clinic. This trial has an independent censoring pattern. We want to calculate the sample size (i.e., the required number of clinics) of this study as a balanced ($p_1 = p_2 = 1/2$) SRT. From Harper et al. (2015), the 1-year pregnancy rate is approximately 0.2 ($\lambda_1 = -\log 0.2$ per year) for the control arm and the hazard ratio is about $\lambda_1/\lambda_2 = 1/0.6$. Suppose that the yearly accrual rate for each clinic is $r_i = 100$, 150, or 200 women with an equal probability of $1/3$ for each value so that we have $\bar{r} = 150$ and $\bar{\bar{r}} = 5000/3$. We consider an accrual period of $a = 0.2$ years and an additional follow-up period of $b = 1$ year as in the original study. We use the Gumbel's copula to model the joint survival distribution with marginal exponential distributions. If within-arm and between-arm ICCs are identical with Kendall's $\tau_w = \tau_b = 0.05$, then the required sample size (i.e., number of clinics) is $n = 31$ for the clustered log-rank test with $(\alpha, 1-\beta) = (0.05, 0.9)$. If the between-arm correlation is half of the within-arm correlation with $\tau_b = \tau_w/2 = 0.025$, then the required sample size is $n = 47$.

On the other hand, suppose that we design this study as a CRT like the original study using the same design parameter values. If the intracluster correlation is Kendall's $\tau_w = 0.05$, then using the sample size formula (11.7) of Chapter 11, the required sample size is $n = 96$. Note that this sample size is much larger than that for an SRT.

Appendix A. Asymptotic Normality of W under H_0

By the definition of W and $\hat{\Lambda}_k$, under H_0, we have

$$\begin{aligned} W =& \sqrt{n}\int_0^\infty H(t)\left\{\frac{dN_1(t)}{Y_1(t)} - \frac{dN_2(t)}{Y_2(t)}\right\} \\ =& \sqrt{n}\int_0^\infty \frac{H(t)}{Y_1(t)}\{dN_1(t) - Y_1(t)d\Lambda_1(t)\} \\ &- \sqrt{n}\int_0^\infty \frac{H(t)}{Y_2(t)}\{dN_2(t) - Y_2(t)d\Lambda_2(t)\} + \sqrt{n}\omega. \end{aligned}$$

Let $M_{kij}(t) = N_{kij}(t) - \int_0^t Y_{kij}(s)d\Lambda_k(s)$, $M_{ki}(t) = \sum_{j=1}^{m_{ki}} M_{kij}(t)$. Then,

$$W = \frac{1}{\sqrt{n}}\sum_{i=1}^n \int_0^\infty H(t)\left\{\frac{dM_{1i}(t)}{n^{-1}Y_1(t)} - \frac{dM_{2i}(t)}{n^{-1}Y_2(t)}\right\}.$$

Let $h(t)$ and $y_k(t)$ be the limit of $H(t)$ and $n^{-1}Y_k(t)$ $(k = 1, 2)$. Because of possible intracluster dependence, M_{ki} may not be martingales. By Ying and Wei (1994), $n^{1/2}\sum_{i=1}^{n} M_{ki}$ converges weakly and uniformly to a Gaussian process $U_k(t)$. Since $nH(t)/Y_k(t)$ is of bounded variation that is convergent to $h(t)/y_k(t)$, as in Lee, Wei and Ying (1993), we can show that

$$W_k = \frac{1}{\sqrt{n}}\sum_{i=1}^{n_k}\int_0^{\infty}\frac{H(t)}{n^{-1}Y_k(t)}dM_{ki}(t)$$

and

$$W_k^* = \frac{1}{\sqrt{n}}\sum_{i=1}^{n_k}\int_0^{\infty}\frac{h(t)}{y_k(t)}dM_{ki}(t)$$

converge a.s. to the same limit

$$\int_0^{\infty} h(t)/y_k(t)dU_k(t).$$

Hence, W is asymptotically equivalent to

$$W^* = \frac{1}{\sqrt{n}}\sum_{i=1}^{n}(\varepsilon_{1i} - \varepsilon_{2i}),$$

where

$$\varepsilon_{ki} = \int_0^{\infty}\frac{h(t)}{y_k(t)}dM_{ki}(t).$$

By the standard central limit theorem for sum of independent random variables, W^* converges to a normal distribution with mean 0 and variance

$$\sigma^2 = \lim_{n\to\infty}\frac{1}{n}\sum_{i=1}^{n}(\varepsilon_{1i} - \varepsilon_{2i})^2.$$

A consistent estimate of σ^2 is given as

$$\hat{\sigma}^2 = \frac{1}{n}\sum_{i=1}^{n}(\hat{\varepsilon}_{1i} - \hat{\varepsilon}_{2i})^2,$$

where $\hat{\varepsilon}_{ki}$ are obtained from ε_{ki} by replacing $h(t)$, $y_k(t)$ and $\Lambda_k(t)$ with $H(t)$, $Y_k(t)/n$, and $\hat{\Lambda}_k(t)$ respectively.

Appendix B. ICC under Gamma Frailty Model

Since correlation coefficient is invariant to a scale transformation, we set the scale parameter ζ at 1 in the Weibull baseline hazard function under the model (12.3). Let V be a gamma frailty term with the probability density function

$$f_V(v) = \frac{\kappa^\kappa}{\Gamma(\kappa)} v^{\kappa-1} \exp(-\kappa v).$$

Let's consider two subunits $j = 1, 2$ in a cluster. Given $V = v$, $(T_j, j = 1, 2)$ are independent Weibull random variables with the survival functions

$$S_j(t|v) = \exp(-v\theta_j t^\xi),$$

where $\theta_j = 1$ and $= e^\beta$ if subunit j belongs to group 1 and group 2, respectively). We can show that

$$E(T_j^l|V = v) = \frac{\Gamma(l/\xi + 1)}{(v\theta_j)^{l/\xi}} \qquad (12.A1)$$

for $l = 1, 2$. It is also easy to show that

$$E(V^{-l/\xi}) = \frac{\kappa^{l/\xi}\Gamma(\kappa - l/\xi)}{\Gamma(\kappa)} \qquad (12.A2)$$

for $l = 1, 2$ when $\kappa > 2/\xi$. From (12.A1) and (12.A2), we obtain

$$E(T_j^l) = E_V E(T_j^l|V) = \frac{\kappa^{l/\xi}\Gamma(l/\xi + 1)\Gamma(\kappa - l/\xi)}{\theta_j^{l/\xi}\Gamma(\kappa)}$$

for $l = 1, 2$. Hence,

$$\text{var}(T_j) = \frac{\kappa^{2/\xi}}{\theta_j^{2/\xi}\Gamma(\kappa)} \left\{ \Gamma(2/\xi + 1)\Gamma(\kappa - 2/\xi) - \frac{\Gamma(1/\xi + 1)^2\Gamma(\kappa - 1/\xi)^2}{\Gamma(\kappa)} \right\}.$$

Since, given V, T_1 and T_2 are independent, $E(T_1T_2|V) = E(T_1|V)E(T_2|V)$. So, from (12.A1), we have

$$E(T_1T_2|V = v) = \frac{\Gamma(1/\xi + 1)^2}{(\theta_1\theta_2)^{1/\xi}} v^{-2/\xi}.$$

Combining this with (12.A2), we obtain

$$E(T_1T_2) = E_V E(T_1T_2|V) = \frac{\kappa^{2/\xi}\Gamma(1/\xi + 1)^2\Gamma(\kappa - 2/\xi)}{(\theta_1\theta_2)^{1/\xi}\Gamma(\kappa)}.$$

Hence,

$$\text{cov}(T_1, T_2) = \frac{\kappa^{2/\xi}\Gamma(1/\xi + 1)^2}{(\theta_1\theta_2)^{1/\xi}\Gamma(\kappa)} \left\{ \Gamma(\kappa - 2/\xi) - \frac{\Gamma(\kappa - 1/\xi)^2}{\Gamma(\kappa)} \right\}.$$

Finally, we obtain the ICC, $\phi_{1,2} = \text{cov}(T_1, T_2)/\sqrt{\text{var}(T_1)\text{var}(T_2)}$, by

$$\phi_{1,2} = \frac{\Gamma(1/\xi+1)^2\{\Gamma(\kappa)\Gamma(\kappa-2/\xi) - \Gamma(\kappa-1/\xi)^2\}}{\Gamma(\kappa)\Gamma(2/\xi+1)\Gamma(\kappa-2/\xi) - \Gamma(1/\xi+1)^2\Gamma(\kappa-1/\xi)^2}. \quad (12.A3)$$

Note that the gamma-Weibull frailty distribution has a marginal ICC only for $\kappa > 2/\xi$. Also, the marginal intracluster correlation is free of θ_j so that it is the same whether two subunits are assigned to the same group or different groups. The ICC (12.A3) reduces to $1/\kappa$ ($\kappa > 2$) for the gamma-exponential model when $\xi = 1$.

Appendix C. Sample Size Formula of the Log-Rank Statistic for SRTs

We derive the limiting distribution of the clustered log-rank test W with $H(t) = n^{-1}Y_1(t)Y_2(t)/Y(t)$. For subunit j in cluster i that is randomized into arm k, let $M_{kij}(t) = N_{kij}(t) - \int_0^t Y_{kij}(s)d\Lambda_k(t)$ and $M_{ki}(t) = \sum_{j=1}^{m_{ki}} M_{kij}(t)$. By the definition of W,

$$W = \frac{1}{\sqrt{n}}\{\sum_{i=1}^{n_1}\int_0^\infty \frac{Y_2(t)}{Y(t)}dM_{1i}(t) - \sum_{i=1}^{n_2}\int_0^\infty \frac{Y_1(t)}{Y(t)}dM_{2i}(t)\}$$
$$+\frac{1}{\sqrt{n}}\int_0^\infty \frac{Y_1(t)Y_2(t)}{Y(t)}\{d\Lambda_1(t) - d\Lambda_2(t)\}.$$

Let $\eta = \max\{t : S_1(t)S_2(t)G(t) > 0\}$. Usually the upper limit of the support of survival distributions is longer than the study period which is the upper limit of the support of censoring distribution so that η denotes the study period. For the log-rank statistic, as $n \to \infty$, $n^{-1}Y_k(t)$ uniformly converges to $y_k(t) = \bar{m}p_kS_k(t)G(t)$ in $[0, \eta]$, respectively so that we have

$$W = \frac{1}{\sqrt{n}}\sum_{i=1}^{n}(\epsilon_{1i} - \epsilon_{2i}) + \sqrt{n}\int_0^\infty \frac{y_1(t)y_2(t)}{y(t)}\{d\Lambda_1(t) - d\Lambda_2(t)\} + o_p(1),$$

where $y(t) = y_1(t)+y_2(t)$, $\epsilon_{ki} = \sum_{j=1}^{m_{ki}}\epsilon_{kij}$, and $\epsilon_{kij} = \int_0^\infty y_{3-k}(t)/y(t)dM_{kij}(t)$.

Since $\{\epsilon_{1i} - \epsilon_{2i}, i = 1, ..., n\}$ are independent random variables with mean 0, by the central limit theorem, W is approximately normal with mean $p_1p_2\bar{m}\omega\sqrt{n}$, where

$$\omega = (p_1p_2\bar{m})^{-1}\int_0^\infty \frac{y_1(t)y_2(t)}{y(t)}\{d\Lambda_1(t) - d\Lambda_2(t)\}$$
$$= \int_0^\infty \frac{S_1(t)S_2(t)G(t)}{p_1S_1(t) + p_2S_2(t)}\{d\Lambda_1(t) - d\Lambda_2(t)\}.$$

Now, we derive $\sigma^2 = \text{var}(W)$,

$$\sigma^2 = \frac{1}{n}\sum_{i=1}^{n}\text{var}\left(\sum_{j=1}^{m_{1i}}\epsilon_{1ij} - \sum_{j=1}^{m_{2i}}\epsilon_{2ij}\right)$$

$$= \frac{1}{n}\sum_{i=1}^{n}\left\{\text{var}(\sum_{j=1}^{m_{1i}}\epsilon_{1ij}) + \text{var}(\sum_{j=1}^{m_{2i}}\epsilon_{2ij}) - 2\text{cov}(\sum_{j=1}^{m_{1i}}\epsilon_{1ij}, \sum_{j=1}^{m_{2i}}\epsilon_{2ij})\right\}$$

$$\equiv v_1 + v_2 - 2\sigma_b. \qquad (12.A4)$$

Here,

$$v_k = \frac{1}{n}\sum_{i=1}^{n}\left\{\sum_{j=1}^{m_{ki}}\text{var}(\epsilon_{kij}) + 2\sum_{j=1}^{m_{ki}-1}\sum_{j'=j+1}^{m_{ki}}\text{cov}(\epsilon_{kij}, \epsilon_{kij'})\right\}. \qquad (12.A5)$$

Since $M_{kij}(t)$ are marginally 0-mean martingales, the first term of (12.A5) is

$$\frac{1}{n}\sum_{i=1}^{n}\sum_{j=1}^{m_{ki}}\text{var}(\epsilon_{kij}) = \frac{1}{n}\int_0^\infty \frac{y_{3-k}^2(t)}{y(t)^2}Y_k(t)d\Lambda_k(t)$$

$$= \int_0^\infty \frac{y_k(t)y_{3-k}^2(t)}{y(t)^2}d\Lambda_k(t) + o_p(1)$$

$$= p_k p_{3-k}^2 \bar{m}\int_0^\infty \frac{S_k(t)S_{3-k}^2(t)G(t)}{\{p_1 S_(t) + p_2 S_2(t)\}^2}d\Lambda_k(t) + o_p(1). \qquad (12.A6)$$

Further, by similar arguments to those in the lemma of Appendix C of Chapter 10, for $j \neq j'$,

$$E\{dM_{kij}(t_1)dM_{kij'}(t_2)\} - Y_{kij}(t_1)Y_{kij'}(t_2)dA_k(t_1, t_2)\} = 0$$

and $n^{-1}\sum_{i=1}^{n}\sum_{j=1}^{m_{ki}-1}\sum_{j'=j+1}^{m_{ki}}\{M_{kij}(t_1)M_{kij'}(t_2) - dA_b(t_1, t_2)\}$ converges to a 0-mean two-dimensional Gaussian process with

$$dA_k(t_1, t_2) = \{\lambda_k(t_1, t_2) - \lambda_{k(1|2)}(t_1, t_2)\lambda_k(t_2) - \lambda_{k(2|1)}(t_1, t_2)\lambda_k(t_1) + \lambda_k(t_1)\lambda_k(t_2)\}dt_1 dt_2$$

so that the second term of (12.A5) is

$$\frac{2}{n}\sum_{i=1}^{n}\sum_{j=1}^{m_{ki}-1}\sum_{j'=j+1}^{m_{ki}}\text{cov}(\epsilon_{kij}, \epsilon_{kij'})$$

$$= (p_k^2\bar{\bar{m}} - p_k\bar{m})\int_0^\infty\int_0^\infty \frac{y_{3-k}(t_1)y_{3-k}(t_2)}{y(t_1)y(t_2)}y_k(t_1, t_2)dA_k(t_1, t_2) + o_p(1)$$

$$= p_1^2 p_2^2 \bar{m}(\bar{\bar{m}}/\bar{m} - 1/p_k)$$
$$\times \int_0^\infty \int_0^\infty \frac{S_{3-k}(t_1)S_{3-k}(t_2)S_k(t_1,t_2)G(t_1,t_2)}{\{p_1S_1(t_1)+p_2S_2(t_1)\}\{p_1S_1(t_2)+p_2S_2(t_2)\}} dA_k(t_1,t_2) \tag{12.A7}$$

since $m_{ki} = p_k m_i$, where $y_k(t_1,t_2) = E\{Y_{kij}(t)Y_{kij'}(t)\} = P(X_{kij} \geq t_1, X_{kij'} \geq t_2) = S_k(t_1,t_2)G(t_1,t_2)$. By plugging (12.A6) and (12.A7) in (12.A5), we have

$$v_k = p_1^2 p_2^2 \bar{m}\sigma_k^2\{1/p_k + (\bar{\bar{m}}/\bar{m} - 1/p_k)\rho_k\}, \tag{12.A8}$$

where $\rho_k = c_k/\sigma_k^2$,

$$\sigma_k^2 = \int_0^\infty \frac{S_k(t)S_{3-k}^2(t)G(t)}{\{p_1S_(t)+p_2S_2(t)\}^2} d\Lambda_k(t)$$

and

$$c_k = \int_0^\infty \int_0^\infty \frac{S_{3-k}(t_1)S_{3-k}(t_2)S_k(t_1,t_2)G(t_1,t_2)}{\{p_1S_1(t_1)+p_2S_2(t_1)\}\{p_1S_1(t_2)+p_2S_2(t_2)\}} dA_k(t_1,t_2).$$

Also, by similar arguments to those in the lemma of Appendix C of Chapter 10,

$$E\{dM_{1ij}(t_1)dM_{2ij'}(t_2)\} - Y_{1ij}(t_1)Y_{2ij'}(t_2)dA_b(t_1,t_2)\} = 0$$

and $n^{-1}\sum_{i=1}^n \sum_{j=1}^{m_{1i}} \sum_{j'=1}^{m_{2i}} \{M_{1ij}(t_1)M_{2ij'}(t_2) - dA_b(t_1,t_2)\}$ converges to a 0-mean two-dimensional Gaussian process with

$$\begin{aligned} dA_b(t_1,t_2) =& \{\lambda_b(t_1,t_2) - \lambda_{b(1|2)}(t_1,t_2)\lambda_2(t_2) - \lambda_{b(2|1)}(t_1,t_2)\lambda_1(t_1) \\ &+ \lambda_1(t_1)\lambda_2(t_2)\}dt_1dt_2 \end{aligned}$$

so that, from (12.A4), σ_b is

$$\begin{aligned} \sigma_b =& \frac{1}{n}\sum_{j=1}^{m_{1i}}\sum_{j'=1}^{m_{2i}} \text{cov}(\epsilon_{1ij}, \epsilon_{2ij'}) \\ =& p_1p_2\bar{\bar{m}} \int_0^\infty \int_0^\infty \frac{y_2(t_1)y_1(t_2)}{y(t_1)y(t_2)} y_b(t_1,t_2)dA_b(t_1,t_2) + o_p(1) \\ =& p_1^2p_2^2\bar{\bar{m}} \int_0^\infty \int_0^\infty \frac{S_2(t_1)S_1(t_2)S_b(t_1,t_2)G(t_1,t_2)}{\{p_1S_1(t_1)+p_2S_2(t_1)\}\{p_1S_1(t_2)+p_2S_2(t_2)\}} dA_b(t_1,t_2) \\ &+ o_p(1), \end{aligned}$$

where $y_b(t_1,t_2) = E\{Y_{1ij}(t)Y_{2ij'}(t)\} = P(X_{1ij} \geq t_1, X_{2ij'} \geq t_2) = S_b(t_1,t_2)G(t_1,t_2)$. Hence,

$$\sigma_b = p_1^2p_2^2\bar{\bar{m}}c_b, \tag{12.A9}$$

where

$$c_b = \int_0^\infty \int_0^\infty \frac{S_2(t_1)S_1(t_2)S_b(t_1,t_2)G(t_1,t_2)}{\{p_1S_1(t_1)+p_2S_2(t_1)\}\{p_1S_1(t_2)+p_2S_2(t_2)\}} dA_b(t_1,t_2).$$

From (12.A4), (12.A8), and (12.A9), we have

$$\sigma^2 = p_1^2 p_2^2 \left[\bar{m}\sigma_1^2\{1/p_1 + (\bar{\bar{m}}/\bar{m} - 1/p_1)\rho_1\} + \bar{m}\sigma_2^2\{1/p_2 + (\bar{\bar{m}}/\bar{m} - 1/p_2)\rho_2\} \right.$$
$$\left. -2\bar{\bar{m}}c_b \right].$$

Under the nearby alternative hypothesis, $\sigma_1^2 = \sigma_2^2 = d$ and $\rho_1 = \rho_2 = \rho_w$, where $d = -\int_0^\infty G(t)dS(t) = P(T_{ij} < C_{ij})$ denotes the probability that a subunit experiences an event. Hence,

$$\sigma^2 = p_1 p_2 \bar{m} d\{1 - \rho_w + 2p_1p_2(\rho_w - \rho_b)\bar{\bar{m}}/\bar{m}\}$$

under the nearby alternative hypothesis. Further, under the nearby alternative hypothesis, $\hat{\sigma}^2$ converges to σ^2.

We consider a proportional hazards model, $\Delta = \lambda_1(t)/\lambda_2(t)$. Under the nearby assumption, we have $\log \Delta \approx \Delta - 1$ by the Taylor expansion and

$$\omega = (\Delta - 1)\int_0^\infty S(t)G(t)d\Lambda(t) = -(\Delta - 1)\int_0^\infty G(t)dS(t) \approx (\log \Delta)d.$$

Hence, under the nearby alternative hypothesis, (12.5) is expressed as

$$n = \frac{(z_{1-\alpha/2} + z_{1-\beta})^2}{\bar{m} d p_1 p_2 (\log \Delta)^2}\text{DE},$$

where $\text{DE} = 1 - \rho_w + 2p_1p_2(\rho_w - \rho_b)\bar{\bar{m}}/\bar{m}$.

Appendix D. Calculation of parameters under practical settings

Assuming uniform accrual during accrual period a and with additional follow-up period b, we have

$$G(t) = I(t < a + b) - \frac{t - b}{a} I(b \le t < a + b).$$

Further, we have $G(t_1, t_2) = G(t_1 \vee t_2)$ (i) under common censoring within each cluster, and $G(t_1, t_2) = G(t_1)G(t_2)$ (ii) under independent censoring.

We assume Gumbel's copula and the exponential marginal distribution with hazard rate λ_k. The within-treatment group joint distribution becomes,

$$S_k(t_1, t_2) = \exp\left[-\left\{ (\lambda_k t_1)^{1/\theta_w} + (\lambda_k t_2)^{1/\theta_w} \right\}^{\theta_w} \right]$$
$$f_k(t_1, t_2) = S_k(t_1, t_2)\lambda_k^2 (\lambda_k t_1)^{1/\theta_w - 1}(\lambda_k t_2)^{1/\theta_w - 1}$$
$$\times \left\{ (\lambda_k t_1)^{1/\theta_w} + (\lambda_k t_2)^{1/\theta_w} \right\}^{2\theta_w - 2}$$

$$\times \left[1 + (1/\theta_w - 1)\left\{(\lambda_k t_1)^{1/\theta_w} + (\lambda_k t_2)^{1/\theta_w}\right\}^{-\theta_w}\right]$$

$$\frac{\partial S_k(t_1, t_2)}{\partial t_1} = - S_k(t_1, t_2)\lambda_k(\lambda_k t_1)^{1/\theta_w - 1}\left\{(\lambda_k t_1)^{1/\theta_w} + (\lambda_k t_2)^{1/\theta_w}\right\}^{\theta_w - 1}.$$

Hence, we have

$$\lambda_k(t_1, t_2) = \lambda_k^2(\lambda_k t_1)^{1/\theta_w - 1}(\lambda_k t_2)^{1/\theta_w - 1}\left\{(\lambda_k t_1)^{1/\theta_w} + (\lambda_k t_2)^{1/\theta_w}\right\}^{2\theta_w - 2}$$
$$\times \left[1 + (1/\theta_w - 1)\left\{(\lambda_k t_1)^{1/\theta_w} + (\lambda_k t_2)^{1/\theta_w}\right\}^{-\theta_w}\right]$$

and

$$\lambda_{k(1|2)}(t_1, t_2) = \lambda_k(\lambda_k t_1)^{1/\theta_w - 1}\left\{(\lambda_k t_1)^{1/\theta_w} + (\lambda_k t_2)^{1/\theta_w}\right\}^{\theta_w - 1}.$$

Similarly for the between-arm distributions, we have

$$S_b(t_1, t_2) = \exp\left[-\left\{(\lambda_1 t_1)^{1/\theta_b} + (\lambda_2 t_2)^{1/\theta_b}\right\}^{\theta_b}\right]$$

$$\lambda_b(t_1, t_2) = \lambda_1\lambda_2(\lambda_1 t_1)^{1/\theta_b - 1}(\lambda_2 t_2)^{1/\theta_b - 1}\left\{(\lambda_1 t_1)^{1/\theta_b} + (\lambda_2 t_2)^{1/\theta_b}\right\}^{2\theta_b - 2}$$
$$\times \left[1 + (1/\theta_b - 1)\left\{(\lambda_1 t_1)^{1/\theta_b} + (\lambda_2 t_2)^{1/\theta_b}\right\}^{-\theta_b}\right]$$

and

$$\lambda_{b(1|2)}(t_1, t_2) = \lambda_1(\lambda_1 t_1)^{1/\theta_b - 1}\left\{(\lambda_1 t_1)^{1/\theta_b} + (\lambda_2 t_2)^{1/\theta_b}\right\}^{\theta_b - 1}.$$

Therefore, we have

$$\omega = (\lambda_1 - \lambda_2)\int_0^{a+b}(1 - a^{-1}[t - b]_+)\frac{e^{-(\lambda_1 - \lambda_2)t}}{(p_1 e^{-\lambda_1 t} + p_2 e^{-\lambda_2 t})^2}dt$$

$$\sigma_k^2 = \lambda_k\int_0^{a+b}(1 - a^{-1}[t - b]_+)\frac{e^{-(\lambda_k + 2\lambda_{3-k})t}}{(p_1 e^{-\lambda_1 t} + p_2 e^{-\lambda_2 t})^2}dt,$$

where $[t]_+ = t \times I(t > 0)$.

Furthermore, (i) in common censoring case, we have

$$c_k = \int_0^{a+b}\int_0^{a+b}(1 - a^{-1}[t_1 \vee t_2 - b]_+)$$
$$\times \frac{e^{-\lambda_{3-k}(t_1 + t_2)}\exp[-\{(\lambda_k t_1)^{1/\theta_w} + (\lambda_k t_2)^{1/\theta_w}\}^{\theta_w}]}{(p_1 e^{-\lambda_1 t_1} + p_2 e^{-\lambda_2 t_1})(p_1 e^{-\lambda_1 t_2} + p_2 e^{-\lambda_2 t_2})}dA_k(t_1, t_2)$$

and

$$c_b = \int_0^{a+b}\int_0^{a+b} (1 - a^{-1}[t_1 \vee t_2 - b]_+)$$

$$\times \frac{e^{-\lambda_1 t_1 + \lambda_2 t_2} \exp[-\{(\lambda_1 t_1)^{1/\theta_b} + (\lambda_2 t_2)^{1/\theta_b}\}^{\theta_b}]}{(p_1 e^{-\lambda_1 t_1} + p_2 e^{-\lambda_2 t_1})(p_1 e^{-\lambda_1 t_2} + p_2 e^{-\lambda_2 t_2})} dA_b(t_1, t_2),$$

And, (ii) in independent censoring case, we have

$$c_k = \int_0^{a+b}\int_0^{a+b} (1 - a^{-1}[t_1 - b]_+)(1 - a^{-1}[t_2 - b]_+)$$

$$\times \frac{e^{-\lambda_{3-k}(t_1+t_2)} \exp[-\{(\lambda_k t_1)^{1/\theta_w} + (\lambda_k t_2)^{1/\theta_w}\}^{\theta_w}]}{(p_1 e^{-\lambda_1 t_1} + p_2 e^{-\lambda_2 t_1})(p_1 e^{-\lambda_1 t_2} + p_2 e^{-\lambda_2 t_2})} dA_k(t_1, t_2)$$

and

$$c_b = \int_0^{a+b}\int_0^{a+b} (1 - a^{-1}[t_1 - b]_+)(1 - a^{-1}[t_2 - b]_+)$$

$$\times \frac{e^{-\lambda_1 t_1 + \lambda_2 t_2} \exp[-\{(\lambda_1 t_1)^{1/\theta_b} + (\lambda_2 t_2)^{1/\theta_b}\}^{\theta_b}]}{(p_1 e^{-\lambda_1 t_1} + p_2 e^{-\lambda_2 t_1})(p_1 e^{-\lambda_1 t_2} + p_2 e^{-\lambda_2 t_2})} dA_b(t_1, t_2).$$

References

Aalen O. Nonparametric inference for a family of counting processes. Annals of Statistics 1978;6(4):701–726.

Batchelor JR, Hackett M. HL-A matching in treatment of burned patients with skin allografts. The Lancet 1970; 296(7673): 581–583.

Cox DR. Regression models and life-tables (with discussion). Journal of the Royal Statistical Society, Series B 1972; 34: 187–220.

Cox DR. Partial likelihood. Biometrika 1975; 62: 269–276.

Fleming TR, Harrington DP. Counting Processes and Survival Analysis. Hoboken, NJ: John Wiley & Sons; 2011.

Freedman LS. Tables of the number of patients required in clinical trials using the logrank test. Statistics in Medicine 1982;1(2):121–129.

Gangnon RE, Kosorok MR. Sample-size formula for clustered survival data using weighted log-rank statistics. Biometrika 2004; 91(2): 263–275.

Gehan EA. A generalized Wilcoxon test for comparing arbitrarily singly-censored samples. Biometrika 1965; 52(1–2): 203–224.

George SL, Desu MM. Planning the size and duration of a clinical trial studying the time to some critical event. Journal of Chronical Disease 1974; 27(1–2): 15–24.

Gumbel EJ. Bivariate exponential distributions. Journal of the American Statistical Association 1960; 55(292): 698–707.

Harper CC, Rocca CH, Thompson KM, et al. Reductions in pregnancy rates in the USA with long-acting reversible contraception: a cluster randomised trial. Lancet 2015; 386(9993): 562–568.

Harrington DP, Fleming TR. A class of rank test procedures for censored survival data. Biometrika 1982; 69(3): 553–566.

Jeong JH, Jung SH. Rank tests for clustered survival data when dependent subunits are randomized. Statistics in Medicine 2006; 25(3): 361–373.

Kalbfleisch JD, Prentice RL. The statistical analysis of failure time data. John Wiley & Sons: New Jersey, 2011.
Kaplan EL, Meier P. Nonparametric estimator from incomplete observations. Journal of the American Statistical Association 1958; 53: 457–481.
Klein JP. Semiparametric estimation of random effects using the Cox model based on the EM algorithm. Biometrics 1992; 48: 795–806.
Lakatos E. Sample sizes based on the log-rank statistic in complex clinical trials. Biometrics 1988; 44(1): 229–241.
Lakatos E, Lan KKG. A comparison of sample size methods for the logrank statistic. Statistics in Medicine 1992; 11(2): 179–191.
Lee EW, Wei LJ, Ying Z. Linear regression analysis for highly stratified failure time data. Journal of American Statistical Association 1993; 88(422): 557–565.
Li J, Jung SH. Sample size calculation for clustered survival data under subunit randomization. Lifetime Data Analysis 2022; 28: 40–67.
Lin DY, Ying Z. A simple nonparametric estimator of the bivariate survival function under univariate censoring. Biometrika 1993; 80: 573–581.
Mantel N, Bohidar NR, Ciminera JL. Mantel-Haenszel analyses of litter-matched time-to-response data, with modifications for recovery of interlitter information. Cancer Research 1977; 37; 3863–3868.
McNeil AJ. Sampling nested Archimedean copulas. Journal of Statistical Computation and Simulation 2008; 78(6): 567–581.
Michalek JE, Mihalko D. On the use of logrank scores in the analysis of litter-matched data on time to tumour appearance. Statistics in Medicine 1983; 2: 315–321.
Moran PAP. Testing for correlation between non-negative variates. Biometrika 1967; 54: 385–394.
Nelson W. Hazard plotting for incomplete failure data. Journal of Quality Technology 1969; 1(1): 27–52.
Nielsen G, Gill RD, Andersen PK, Sorensen TIA. A counting process approach to maximum likelihood estimation of frailty models. Scandinavian Journal of Statistics 1992; 19: 25–43.
Nolan J. Stable distributions: models for heavy-tailed data. Birkhauser 2003, New York.
Pals SL, Murray DM, Alfano CM, Shadish WR, Hannan PJ, Baker WL. Individually randomized group treatment trials: a critical appraisal of frequently used design and analytic approaches. American Journal of Public Health 2008; 98(8): 1418–1424.
Peto R, Peto J. Asymptotically efficient rank invariant test procedures (with discussion. Journal of the Royal Statistical Society, Series A 1972; 135: 185–206.
Schoenfeld DA. Sample-size formula for the proportional-hazards regression model. Biometrics 1983; 39(2): 499–503.
Tarone RE, Ware J. On distribution-free tests for equality of survival distributions. Biometrika 1977; 64(1): 156–160.
Thernaeu TH, Grambsch PM. Modeling Survival Data: Extending the Cox Model. Springer: New York, 2000.
Vaupel JW, Manton KG, Stallard E. The impact of heterogeneity in individual frailty on the dynamics of mortality. Demography 1979; 16: 439–454.
Ying Z, Wei LJ. The Kaplan-Meier estimate for dependent failure time observations. Journal of Multivariate Analysis 1994; 50: 17–29.

13

Group Sequential Testing for Cluster Randomized Trials with Time-to-Event Endpoint

Due to ethical and economical reasons, clinical trials are usually monitored using a group sequential testing method during the study period. We consider cluster randomized trials (CRT) with a survival endpoint. In a CRT. clusters are randomization between treatment arms, and the outcome variable is observed from each subunit. In this case, the outcome data of subunits within each cluster tend to be positively correlated due to the common frailties shared by the subunits, while those from different clusters are independent. For example, in an otology study (Howie and Schwartz 1983; Teele et al. 1989), 78 children suffering from otitis media in the ears received ventilating tubes as a surgical intervention and were randomized into either no treatment or a post-surgery treatment of the ventilating tubes. Children were regularly followed to check whether the tubes were functioning properly or not. One of the study objectives was to determine whether the post-surgery treatment extended the functioning of tubes or not. In this study, children are clusters and ears are subunits.

In another example study, Harper et al. (2015) studied interventions for reducing unintended pregnancy. In this trial, 20 clinics were randomized into a specialized training on intrauterine devices or progestin implants, while another 20 clinics were randomized into standard care. Each clinic recruited women who were attending family planning or abortion care and had no intention of pregnancy in the following 12 months. One of the study endpoints was the time to unintended pregnancy during the follow-up. The outcomes of women in each clinic tend to be correlated, while those in different clinics are independent. In this study, clinics are clusters and women are subunits.

For comparing survival distributions between treatment arms, weighted rank tests, such as the log-rank test (Peto and Peto 1972), have been widely used for both independent and clustered survival data. Sample size calculation for weighted rank tests has been studied by many researchers including Schoenfeld (1983) and Freedman (1982) for independent survival data. For clustered survival data, Jung and Jeong (2003) proposed the clustered weighted rank test adjusting the original weighted rank tests accounting for

DOI: 10.1201/9781003221951-13

possible dependency among subunits of each cluster, as reviewed in Chapter 11. Li and Jung (2020) derived power and sample size formulas for these clustered rank tests.

Numerous methods have been proposed to maintain the overall type I error rate in group sequential testing. Pocock (1977) and O'Brien and Fleming (1979) proposed group sequential procedures that require the total number of interim analyses be prespecified in the design stage and equal number of patients be accumulated in each monitoring stage. Later, Lan and DeMets (1983) developed the alpha spending function approach that allows unspecified frequencies and timing of interim looks during the study. The key to this approach is to estimate the fraction of maximal information of a study, called the information time, at each interim analysis. Early development of the alpha spending function is based on the independent increment assumption, meaning that the information accumulated between disjoint time intervals is statistically independent. However, DeMets and Lan (1994) later claimed that the alpha spending approach was also applicable to sequential studies with more complicated correlation structure of test statistics.

For group sequential tests with independent survival data, Tsiatis (1982) proved the independent increment property for the log-rank test. Lan and Lachin (1990) proposed to define the information time of the log-rank test with total time of exposure, while Kim et al. (1995) proposed to estimate the information time with the number events observed by the time of interim analysis divided by the expected number of events at the end of the trial.

For CRT, however, only limited literatures have discussed group sequential testing methods. Hasan et al. (2011) generalized the clustered log-rank test to group sequential design in the context of genetic association family studies. In their derivation, they assumed that the independent increment condition was still valid for clustered log-rank test. However, the information accumulated between interim analyses is not independent, due to the intracluster dependency, as shown by Li and Jung (2022). In this chapter, we investigate the group sequential testing method based on the log-rank test for clustered survival endpoint that was proposed by Li and Jung (2022).

Single-Stage Clustered Log-Rank Tests

We briefly review the log-rank test for CRTs, as investigated in Chapter 12. Suppose that arm 1 is a control arm and arm 2 is an experimental arm, and n_k clusters are randomized into arm $k(=1,2)$, $n = n_1 + n_2$. Cluster $i(=1,...,n_k)$ in arm k consists of m_{ki} subunits, called cluster size. For subunit $j(=1,...,m_{ki})$ of cluster i in arm k, T_{kij} denotes the survival time with marginal survival function $S_k(t) = P(T_{kij} \geq t)$ and cumulative hazard function $\Lambda_k(t) = -\log S_k(t)$. We want to test the superiority of the experimental arm, that is $H_0 : \Lambda_1(t) = \Lambda_2(t)$ against $H_1 : \Lambda_1(t) > \Lambda_2(t)$.

Let C_{kij} denote the censoring time associated with T_{kij}. From the CRT, we observe $X_{kij} = T_{kij} \wedge C_{kij}$ together with the event indicator $\delta_{kij} = I(T_{kij} \le C_{kij})$, where $a \wedge b = \min(a, b)$. Censoring times may be dependent within each cluster, but should be independent of survival times. Let $N_k(t) = \sum_{i=1}^{n_k} \sum_{j=1}^{m_{ki}} N_{kij}(t)$ and $Y_k(t) = \sum_{i=1}^{n_k} \sum_{j=1}^{m_{ki}} Y_{kij}(t)$ denote the event process and the at-risk process for arm k, respectively, where $N_{kij}(t) = \delta_{kij} I(X_{kij} \le t)$ and $Y_{kij}(t) = I(X_{kij} \ge t)$. Define $N(t) = N_1(t) + N_2(t)$ and $Y(t) = Y_1(t) + Y_2(t)$. The log-rank statistic is defined as:

$$
\begin{aligned}
W &= \int_0^\infty \frac{Y_1(t)Y_2(t)}{Y(t)} \left\{ d\hat{\Lambda}_1(t) - d\hat{\Lambda}_2(t) \right\} \\
&= \int_0^\infty \frac{Y_2(t)}{Y(t)} dN_1(t) - \int_0^\infty \frac{Y_1(t)}{Y(t)} dN_2(t), \qquad (13.1)
\end{aligned}
$$

where $\hat{\Lambda}_k(t) = \int_0^t Y_k^{-1}(s) dN_k(s)$ is the Nelson-Aalen (Nelson 1969; Aalen 1978) estimator for the marginal cumulative hazard function $\Lambda_k(t)$.

Jung and Jeong (2003) showed that, under H_0, W is approximately normal with mean 0, and its variance can be consistently estimated by

$$
\hat{\sigma}^2 = \sum_{i=1}^{n_1} \hat{\epsilon}_{1i}^2 + \sum_{i=1}^{n_2} \hat{\epsilon}_{2i}^2, \qquad (13.2)
$$

where

$$
\hat{\epsilon}_{ki} = \sum_{j=1}^{m_{ki}} \int_0^\infty \frac{Y_{3-k}(t)}{Y(t)} d\hat{M}_{kij}(t).
$$

$\hat{M}_{kij}(t) = N_{kij}(t) - \int_0^t Y_{kij}(s) d\hat{\Lambda}(s)$, and $\hat{\Lambda}(t) = \int_0^t Y^{-1}(s) dN(s)$ is the Nelson-Aalen estimator of the common cumulative hazard function under H_0 estimated from the pooled data. With a one-sided type I error rate α, we reject H_0 when $W/\hat{\sigma} > z_{1-\alpha}$, where $z_{1-\alpha}$ is the $100(1-\alpha)$ percentile of the standard normal distribution.

Li and Jung (2020) proposed a sample size formula for the clustered log-rank test as investigated in Chapter 11. Although the test statistic is completely non-parametric, its sample size sample size formula requires specification of the marginal and bivariate survival distributions and the projected accrual pattern of subunits and clusters. For arm k, suppose that subunits have marginal hazard function $\lambda_k(t) = \partial \Lambda_k(t)/\partial t$. Any two subunits in each cluster have bivariate joint survival function

$$
S_k(t, s) = P(T_{kij} \ge t, T_{kij'} \ge s)
$$

and joint probability density function $f_k(t, s) = \partial^2 S_k(t, s)/\partial t \partial s$. We also define the joint hazard function

$$
\lambda_k(t, s) = f_k(t, s)/S_k(t, s)
$$

and conditional hazard function

$$\lambda_{k(1|2)}(t,s) = \lim_{\epsilon \to 0} P(t \le T_{kij} < t+\epsilon | T_{kij} \ge t, T_{kij'} \ge s) = -\frac{\partial S_k(t,s)/\partial t}{S_k(t,s)}$$

for $j \neq j'$. Due to the exchangeable dependency property of clustered data, we have $\lambda_{k(2|1)}(t,s) = \lambda_{k(1|2)}(s,t)$.

In addition, let e_{kij} denote the entry time of subunit j of cluster i in arm k, $Q(t) = P(e_{kij} \le t)$ the marginal cumulative density function (CDF) of the entry time of a subunit, and $Q(t,s) = P(e_{kij} \le t, e_{kij'} \le s)$ the bivariate CDF of entry times of two subunits in the same cluster. If censoring occurs only due to early termination of study (i.e., assuming administrative censoring only), $Q(t)$ and $Q(t,s)$ are sufficient to capture the censoring distribution. In more general cases, suppose $\tilde{G}(t)$ and $\tilde{G}(t,s)$ denote the marginal and bivariate survival functions, respectively, of the non-administrative censoring (e.g., loss to follow-up) times $(\tilde{C}_{kij}, j = 1, ..., m_{kij})$, which is independent of administrative censoring and survival times. If the total study period is τ_0, then the administrative censoring time of each patient is $\tau_0 - e_{kij}$. Further, let $\tilde{C}_{kij}$ denote the non-administrative censoring time. Then, the censoring time for each patient is $C_{kij} = \min(\tau_0 - e_{kij}, \tilde{C}_{kij})$ so that we have $G(t) \equiv P(C_{kij} \ge t) \equiv Q(\tau_0 - t)\tilde{G}(t)$ and $G(t,s) \equiv P(C_{kij} \ge t, C_{kij'} \ge s) = Q(\tau_0 - t, \tau_0 - s)\tilde{G}(t,s)$. With administrative censoring only, we have $\tilde{C}_{kij} = \infty$, $\tilde{G}(t) = 1$, and $\tilde{G}(t,s) = 1$ for $t, s \ge 0$.

Let $p_k = n_k/n$ denote the allocation proportion for arm k $(p_1 + p_2 = 1)$, and $\bar{m} = E(m_{ki})$ and $\bar{\bar{m}} = E(m_{ki}^2)$ denote the first and second moments, respectively, of the distribution of cluster sizes among clusters. If the cluster sizes are constant $m_{ki} = m$, then we have $\bar{m} = m$ and $\bar{\bar{m}} = m^2$.

Li and Jung (2020) show that, under $H_1 : \Lambda_1(t) \neq \Lambda_2(t)$, the log-rank statistic W in (13.1) is approximately normal with mean

$$E(W) = n\bar{m}p_1p_2 d \log \Delta$$

and variance

$$\sigma^2 = np_1p_2\{\bar{m}d + (\bar{\bar{m}} - \bar{m})c\},$$

where $\Delta = \lambda_1(t)/\lambda_2(t)$ is the hazard ratio under H_1, $c = p_1c_1 + p_2c_2$, $d = p_1d_1 + p_2d_2$,

$$c_k = \int_0^\infty \int_0^\infty S_k(t,s)G(t,s)dA_k(t,s)$$

$$dA_k(t,s) = \{\lambda_k(t,s) - \lambda_{k(1|2)}(t,s)\lambda_k(s) - \lambda_{k(2|1)}(t,s)\lambda_k(t) + \lambda_k(t)\lambda_k(s)\}dtds$$

and

$$d_k = P(T_{kij} < C_{kij}) = -\int_0^\infty G(t)dS_k(t)$$

is the probability that a subunit in arm k has an event during the study period.

Based on this asymptotic result, the sample size (i.e., number of clusters) for the single-stage clustered log-rank test to have a power of $1-\beta$ under H_1 is

$$n = \frac{(z_{1-\alpha} + z_{1-\beta})^2}{\bar{m} d p_1 p_2 (\log \Delta)^2} \text{IF}, \tag{13.3}$$

where

$$\text{IF} = 1 + (\bar{\bar{m}}/\bar{m} - 1)\rho$$

denotes the inflation factor and $\rho = c/d$. This formula extends the Schoenfeld's (1983) sample size formula accounting for the intracluster dependency of clustered survival data by IF.

Group Sequential Testing for the Clustered Log-Rank Statistic

Suppose that we are conducting L interim analyses at calendar time $t_1, t_2, ..., t_L (= \tau_0)$. At the lth interim analysis, we observe $(X_{kij}^{(l)}, \delta_{kij}^{(l)})$, where $X_{kij}^{(l)} = T_{kij} \wedge C_{kij}^{(l)}$, $C_{kij}^{(l)} = \max\{\min(C_{kij}, t_l - e_{kij}), 0\}$ and $\delta_{kij}^{(l)} = I\{T_{kij} \le C_{kij}^{(l)}\}$. If cluster i or subunit j of cluster i has not been entered by the l-th interim analysis time t_l yet, then $C_{kij} = 0$ so that this subunit does not contribute any data to the interim analysis. With the data collected at t_l, we calculate the log-rank statistic $W^{(l)}$ and standard error estimator $\hat{\sigma}^{(l)}$ using the formulas (13.1) and (13.2), respectively.

To derive the asymptotic distribution of $(W^{(1)}, ..., W^{(L)})$, we introduce a few more notations. Let $Q^{(l)}(t) = P(e_{kij} \le t | e_{kij} \le t_l)$ denote the marginal CDF of the entry time of a subunit that has been recruited before t_l, and $Q^{(l_1 l_2)}(t, s) = P(e_{kij} \le t, e_{kij'} \le s | e_{kij} \le t_{l_1}, e_{kij'} \le t_{l_2})$ denote the bivariate CDF for entry times of two subunits that have been recruited from the same cluster before t_{l_1} and t_{l_2}. Using these notations, $G^{(l)}(t) = \tilde{G}(t) Q^{(l)}(t)$ denotes the marginal survival function of the censoring time for subunits who entered the study before t_l and $G^{(l_1 l_2)}(t, s) = \tilde{G}(t, s) Q^{(l_1 l_2)}(t, s)$ denotes the bivariate survival function of censoring times for two subunits who enter the study from the same cluster before t_l and t_2 each. We later show that the bivariate survival function of the entry times $Q^{(l_1 l_2)}(t, s)$ is expressed by the marginal survival function $Q^{(l)}(t)$ for some popular types of CRT designs.

The cluster sizes as well as the number of clusters at each interim analysis depend on the accrual pattern of clusters and subunits. Let $n_k^{(l)}$ and $m_{ki}^{(l)}$ denote the number of clusters and the number of subunits of cluster i in arm k, respectively, at the lth interim analysis $(n_1^{(l)} + n_2^{(l)} = n^{(l)})$. At the final analysis, we have $n_k^{(L)} = n_k$ and $m_{ki}^{(L)} = m_{ki}$. Since clusters and subunits are recruited during the course of the study, we have $n_k^{(1)} \le n_k^{(2)} \le ... \le n_k^{(L)}$ and $m_{ki}^{(1)} \le m_{ki}^{(2)} \le ... \le m_{ki}^{(L)}$.

Now we introduce our major result in the following theorem.

THEOREM 1: For interim analysis time t_l, let

$$d_k^{(l)} = \int_0^\infty S_k(t)G^{(l)}(t)d\Lambda_k(t) = -\int_0^\infty G^{(l)}(t)dS_k(t) \qquad (13.4)$$

denote the probability that a subunit in arm k has an event by t_l and $d^{(l)} = p_1 d_1^{(l)} + p_2 d_2^{(l)}$. For any two interim analysis times t_{l_1} and t_{l_2}, let

$$c_k^{(l_1 l_2)} = \int_0^\infty \int_0^\infty S_k(t,s)G^{(l_1 l_2)}(t,s)dA_k(t,s) \qquad (13.5)$$

and $c^{(l_1 l_2)} = p_1 c_1^{(l_1 l_2)} + p_2 c_2^{(l_1 l_2)}$. Then, under H_1, the random vector $(W^{(1)}, ..., W^{(L)})$ converges to a multivariate normal distribution with mean $\Omega = p_1 p_2 \log \Delta(\omega_1, ..., \omega_L)$ and covariance $\Sigma = \{\sigma_{l_1 l_2}\}_{L\times L}$, where

$$\omega_l = n^{(l)} \bar{m}_l d^{(l)} \qquad (13.6)$$

$$\sigma_{l_1 l_2} = n^{(l_1)} p_1 p_2 \left\{\bar{m}_{l_1} d^{(l_1)} + (\bar{m}_{l_1 l_2} - \bar{m}_{l_1})c^{(l_1 l_2)}\right\} \quad \text{for } 1 \le l_1 \le l_2 \le L \qquad (13.7)$$

$\bar{m}_l = E(m_{ki}^{(l)})$ is the mean cluster size at the interim analysis, and $\bar{m}_{l_1 l_2} = E(m_{ki}^{(l_1)} m_{ki}^{(l_2)})$.

Note that $\bar{m}_l$ and $\bar{m}_{l_1 l_2}$ are determined by the accrual pattern of clusters and subunits. We will elaborate their calculations under some specific accrual patterns in the next section. A proof of the theorem is given in Appendix A. Using Theorem 1, we derive following result in Appendix A.

THEOREM 2: For $1 \le l_1 < l_2 \le L$, we have

$$\text{cov}(W^{(l_1)}, W^{(l_2)}) \ge \text{var}(W^{(l_1)}).$$

The two sides are equal if and only if intracluster correlation is zero.

This result is consistent with the result shown by Tsiatis (1982) for independent survival data. When there exists a non-zero intracluster correlation, however, the independent increment assumption does not hold in group sequential tests with clustered survival data.

Asymptotic Distribution under Some Practical Design Settings

We consider some practical assumptions to specify the survival and censoring distributions for sample size calculation. To model the joint survival distribution of subunits within each cluster, we may use a copula. In this chapter, we demonstrate the methods using Clayton and Cuzick's (1985) copula model with marginally exponential distributions. More specifically, suppose that subunits in arm k have an exponential survival distribution with hazard rate λ_k. For any two subunits of a cluster in arm k, the bivariate survival function is given as

$$S_k(t,s) = \{\exp(\lambda_k t/\theta) + \exp(\lambda_k s/\theta) - 1\}^{-\theta},$$

where $\theta = 1/(2\tau) - 1/2$ and $\tau \in [0,1]$ is the Kendall's tau with value 0 meaning no association and 1 meaning a perfect association between the paired survival times. Under this correlation structure, we have (see Appendix B)

$$dA_k(t,s) = \lambda_k \left\{ \frac{\lambda_k(1+1/\theta)e^{(t+s)\lambda_k/\theta}}{(e^{\lambda_k t/\theta} + e^{\lambda_k s/\theta} - 1)^2} - \frac{e^{\lambda_k t/\theta} + e^{\lambda_k s/\theta}}{e^{\lambda_k t/\theta} + e^{\lambda_k s/\theta} - 1} + \lambda_k \right\} dtds.$$

To simplify our discussions, we consider administrative censoring only, but it is easy to incorporate other types of censoring, such as time to loss to follow-up which is independent of the administrative censoring time. With administrative censoring only, at each interim analysis, the censoring distribution, cluster sizes, and the number of clusters are determined by the accrual patterns. In the beginning of this chapter, we have reviewed two CRTs with different accrual patterns of clusters and subunits. In Howie's trial (Howie and Schwartz 1983), the patients (clusters) were recruited during an accrual period and both ears (subunits) of each patient were accrued at the time of cluster accrual. In this case, with administrative censoring only, all subunits in each cluster have the same censoring time. We call this case 'common entry'. On the other hand, in the Harper's trial (Harper et al. 2015), all clinics (clusters) were recruited at the beginning of the study and patients (subunits) were accrued independently to each clinic over an accrual period. In this case, the censoring times are independent among subunits whether they belong to the same cluster or not. We call this case 'independent entry'. We investigate the censoring distributions of these two types of censoring in detail.

(i) Common entry case

If all subunits of each cluster have a common entry time, i.e., $e_{kij} = e_{ki}$, then, for the cluster size distribution, $\bar{m}_l = \bar{m}$ and $\bar{m}_{l_1 l_2} = \bar{\bar{m}}$ are constants over the analysis times. Furthermore, if clusters are accrued at a constant rate r during an accrual period of a and followed for an additional period of b after the completion of accrual, then $n^{(l)} = r \times (t_l \wedge a)$ and the marginal CDF of entry time at the lth interim analysis is

$$Q^{(l)}(t_l - t) = \begin{cases} \frac{(t_l - t)\wedge a}{t_l \wedge a} & 0 \le t \le t_l \\ 0 & t > t_l. \end{cases}$$

And the bivariate CDF is

$$Q^{(l_1 l_2)}(t_{l_1} - t, t_{l_2} - s) = \begin{cases} \frac{(t_{l_1}-t)\wedge(t_{l_2}-s)\wedge a}{t_{l_1}\wedge t_{l_2}\wedge a} & 0 \le t \le t_{l_1}, 0 \le s \le t_{l_2} \\ 0 & t > t_{l_1} \text{ or } s > t_{l_2}. \end{cases}$$

(ii) Independent entry case
As in Harper's trial, suppose that all the clusters are recruited before study opens, and the subunits of cluster i are independently accrued at constant rate r_{ki} during accrual period a and followed for an additional period of b. Then, the number of clusters is fixed throughout the study period with $n^{(l)} = n$ and $Q^{(l)}(t)$ is exactly the same as the common entry case. However, the entry times are independent among subunits so that we have $Q^{(l_1 l_2)}(t_{l_1} - t, t_{l_2} - s) = Q^{(l_1)}(t_{l_1} - t)Q^{(l_2)}(t_{l_2} - s)$ and

$$Q^{(l_1 l_2)}(t_{l_1} - t, t_{l_2} - s) = \begin{cases} \frac{(t_{l_1}-t)\wedge a}{t_{l_1}\wedge a} \times \frac{(t_{l_2}-t)\wedge a}{t_{l_2}\wedge a} & 0 \le t \le t_{l_1}, 0 \le s \le t_{l_2} \\ 0 & t > t_{l_1} \text{ or } s > t_{l_2}. \end{cases}$$

Suppose that the accrual rate of subunits is random among clusters with the first and second moment of $E(r_{ki}) = \bar{r}$ and $E(r_{ki}^2) = \bar{\bar{r}}$, respectively. Then, we have $\bar{m}_l = \bar{r} \times (t_l \wedge a)$ at time t_l and $\bar{m}_{l_1 l_2} = \bar{\bar{r}} \times (t_{l_1} \wedge a) \times (t_{l_2} \wedge a)$ at times t_{l_1} and t_{l_2}.

Under both common and independent entry cases, the design parameter of (13.4) is expressed as

$$d_k^{(l)} = \int_0^{t_l} e^{-\lambda_k t} \frac{(t_l - t) \wedge a}{t_l \wedge a} d\Lambda_k(t) = \lambda_k \int_0^{t_l} e^{-\lambda_k t} \frac{(t_l - t) \wedge a}{t_l \wedge a} dt. \quad (13.8)$$

In (13.5), $c_k^{(l_1 l_2)}$ under common entry is

$$c_k^{(l_1 l_2)} = \int_0^{t_{l_1}} \int_0^{t_{l_2}} \{\exp(\lambda_k t/\theta) + \exp(\lambda_k s/\theta) - 1\}^{-\theta} \times \frac{(t_{l_1} - t) \wedge (t_{l_2} - s) \wedge a}{t_{l_1} \wedge t_{l_2} \wedge a} dA_k(t, s) \quad (13.9)$$

and under independent entry is

$$c_k^{(l_1 l_2)} = \int_0^{t_{l_1}} \int_0^{t_{l_2}} \{\exp(\lambda_k t/\theta) + \exp(\lambda_k s/\theta) - 1\}^{-\theta} \frac{(t_{l_1} - t) \wedge a}{t_{l_1} \wedge a} \times \frac{(t_{l_2} - s) \wedge a}{t_{l_2} \wedge a} dA_k(t, s). \quad (13.10)$$

Estimation of Covariance Matrix and Information Times

Lan and DeMets (1983) proposed the alpha spending function method which enables flexible group sequential procedure that does not require prespecification of interim analysis times. They proposed to specify a monotonically increasing function $\alpha^*(\iota)$, such that $\alpha^*(0) = 0$ and $\alpha^*(1) = \alpha$. The argument ι of the function is called information time or information fraction, which is the fraction of the maximum statistical information available at the current analysis. The maximum information of a study is called information horizon. For group sequential monitoring with the log-rank test, information time ι_l is calculated as $\iota_l = \text{var}(W^{(l)})/\text{var}(W^{(L)})$.

At the lth analysis, critical value ξ_l is calculated with respect to significance level of $\alpha^*(\iota_l) - \alpha^*(\iota_{l-1})$ so that H_0 is rejected if $W^{(l)}/\sigma^{(l)} > \xi_l$. Using this approach, the overall type I error rate is maintained at α level no matter how many interim analyses are performed during study. When the independent increment assumption holds, calculation of $\{\xi_l\}$ is related to information time $\{\iota_l\}$ only, regardless of the survival and censoring distributions. However, we have shown in Theorem 2 that the independent increment property does not hold for sequentially calculated log-rank statistics in CRT. Therefore, in order to calculate $\{\xi_l\}$ during the course of the study, we also need to estimate the covariance matrix of the clustered log-rank statistics from observed data.

Appendix C shows that for any two interim analyses l_1 and $l_2 (l_1 < l_2)$, the covariance between $W^{(l_1)}$ and $W^{(l_2)}$ is consistently estimated by

$$\hat{\sigma}_{l_1 l_2} = \sum_{k=1}^{2} p_{3-k}^2 \sum_{i=1}^{n_k^{(l_1)}} \left\{ D_{ki}^{(l_1)} - \sum_{j=1}^{m_{ki}^{(l_1)}} \hat{\Lambda}_k(X_{kij}^{(l_1)}) \right\} \left\{ D_{ki}^{(l_2)} - \sum_{j=1}^{m_{ki}^{(l_2)}} \hat{\Lambda}_k(X_{kij}^{(l_2)}) \right\} \tag{13.11}$$

where $D_{ki}^{(l)}$ is the observed total number of events at interim analysis time t_l from cluster i in arm k. Let $\hat{\Sigma}^{(l)}$ denote the estimated covariance matrix of $(W^{(1)}, ..., W^{(l)})$, test statistics calculated up to the lth interim analysis. By (13.11), $\hat{\Sigma}^{(l)}$ is the leading principle submatrix of $\hat{\Sigma}^{(L)}$ and depends only on the amount of information available up to the lth interim analysis.

The information time ι_l can be estimated by the ratio of $\hat{\sigma}_{ll}$ to $\hat{\sigma}_{LL}$. However, $\hat{\sigma}_{LL}$ is not known until the end of study. Similarly to the approach proposed by Kim et al. (1995) for independent survival data, we can use the variance of $W^{(L)}$ as the information horizon. In the following sections, we use $\sigma_0^2 = \text{var}(W^{(L)}|H_0)$ to estimate the information time $\hat{\iota}_l$ as

$$\hat{\iota}_l = \begin{cases} \hat{\sigma}_{ll}/\sigma_0^2 & \text{if } l < L \\ 1 & \text{if } l = L. \end{cases} \tag{13.12}$$

Given an alpha spending function and the covariance matrix estimator $\hat{\Sigma}^{(l)}$, we obtain the critical value ξ_l sequentially by solving

$$P[\cup_{l'=1}^{l}\{W^{(l')}/\hat{\sigma}^{(l')} > \xi_{l'}\}|\hat{\Sigma}^{(l)}] = \alpha^*(\hat{\iota}_l) \tag{13.13}$$

starting from $\xi_1 = -\Phi^{-1}\{\alpha^*(\hat{\iota}_1)\}$, where $\Phi(t)$ is the CDF for the standard normal distribution.

In a CRT, the 'group sequential testing using the clustered log-rank test is conducted as follows:

- **Design stage**:
  Specify
  - Overall type I error probability α and alpha spending function $\alpha^*(\iota)$
  - Accrual pattern of clusters and subunits (to determine censoring and cluster size distributions)
  - Accrual period a and additional follow-up period b
  - Survival distribution under H_0

  And, calculate σ_0^2 using (13.6) with $l_1 = l_2 = L$.
- **At the lth interim analysis**:
  - Calculate $W^{(l)}$ and $\hat{\sigma}^{(l)}$.
  - Compute correlation matrix estimator $\hat{\Sigma}^{(l)}$ using (13.11).
  - Estimate information fraction $\hat{\iota}_l$ using (13.12).
  - Using $\hat{\iota}_l$ and $\hat{\Sigma}^{(l)}$, calculate the critical value ξ_l by solving equation (13.13).
  - If $W^{(l)}/\hat{\sigma}^{(l)} > \xi_l$, then reject H_0 and terminate the trial. Otherwise, proceed to the next stage if $l < L$.

Maximal Sample Size

If the interim analysis times are pre-determined, we can calculate the maximal sample size $n = n^L$ for a given power $1 - \beta$.

At first, a calculation method of maximal sample size for the common entry case is investigated. We consider a group sequential study with L interim analyses, an accrual rate for clusters of r, and a follow-up period of b. Suppose that, for an unknown accrual period a, the interim looks are evenly scheduled throughout the whole study period $a + b$, i.e., the time for the lth analysis is $t_l = l(a+b)/L$. Then, given an accrual rate r, the number of clusters at interim analysis l is $n^{(l)} = r\{t_l \wedge a\}$. In addition, by 13.6–13.10, the mean and variance of $(W^{(1)}, ..., W^{(L)})$ under H_1 are functions of a with $\omega_l = n^{(l)}\bar{m}d^{(l)}$ and $\Sigma = \{\sigma_{l_1 l_2}\}_{L\times L}$, respectively. In the group sequential clustered log-rank testing, the covariance matrix estimator $\hat{\Sigma}^{(L)}$ converges to Σ. Therefore, the critical values solved with Σ and alpha spending function $\alpha^*(\iota)$ are also functions of a. The type II error rate constraint for the testing procedure can be written as

$$\beta = P\{\cap_{l=1}^{L}(W^{(l)}/\hat{\sigma}^{(l)} \leq \xi_l)|H_1\}$$

$$\approx P\left\{\bigcap_{l=1}^{L}\left(\frac{W^{(l)} - p_1 p_2 n^{(l)}\bar{m}d^{(l)}}{\hat{\sigma}^{(l)}} \leq \xi_l - \frac{p_1 p_2 n^{(l)}\bar{m}d^{(l)}}{\sqrt{\sigma_{ll}}}\right)|\Sigma, H_1\right\}. \quad (13.14)$$

Under H_1, $\{(W^{(l)} - p_1 p_2 n^{(l)}\bar{m}d^{(l)})/\hat{\sigma}^{(l)}, l = 1, ..., L\}$ asymptotically multivariate normal with means 0, variances 1, and correlation coefficients specified by Σ so that we can solve equation (13.14) with respect to accrual period a. If a^* denotes the solution to equation (13.14), then the required maximal sample size is given as $n = r \times a^*$ for a given accrual rate r.

For independent entry case, the mean and covariance of $(W^{(1)}, ...W^{(L)})$ become functions of the maximal sample size n. Therefore, we can calculate the required maximal sample size by directly solving equation (13.14) with respect to n.

Numerical Studies

Comparison of Stopping Boundaries

As we have shown so far, the critical values for group sequential clustered log-rank test statistics depend not only on the information times, but also on the survival and censoring distributions. We want to investigate how the different design parameters result in different stopping boundaries and how these different stopping boundaries are compared with the 'standard stopping boundaries' that are derived under independent increment assumption.

We compute the stopping boundaries for a few different design settings. In all of the calculations, we set $\alpha = 0.05$; $p_1 = p_2 = 1/2$ for balanced allocation; exponential survival with median for arm 1 at 7 months, i.e., $\lambda_1 = 7^{-1}\log 2$ per month; hazard ratio $\Delta = \lambda_1/\lambda_2 = 1.4$; an accrual period of $a = 2$ years; a follow-up period of $b = 1$ year. We consider a CRT with either common entry or independent entry.

For common entry case, we assume an annual accrual rate of $r = 100$ clusters so that the sample size is $n = 200$. The cluster sizes are constant with $m_{ki} = 11$. For independent entry case, we also assume a sample size of $n = 200$ clusters with an annual accrual rate of $r_{ki} = 10$ subunits per cluster so that the cluster sizes are $m_{ki} = 20$ per cluster over the accrual period of 2 years.

We also consider two types of alpha spending functions:

(a) O'Brien-Fleming (OBF) function, $\alpha^*(\iota) = 2\{1 - \Phi(Z_\alpha/\sqrt{\iota})\}$

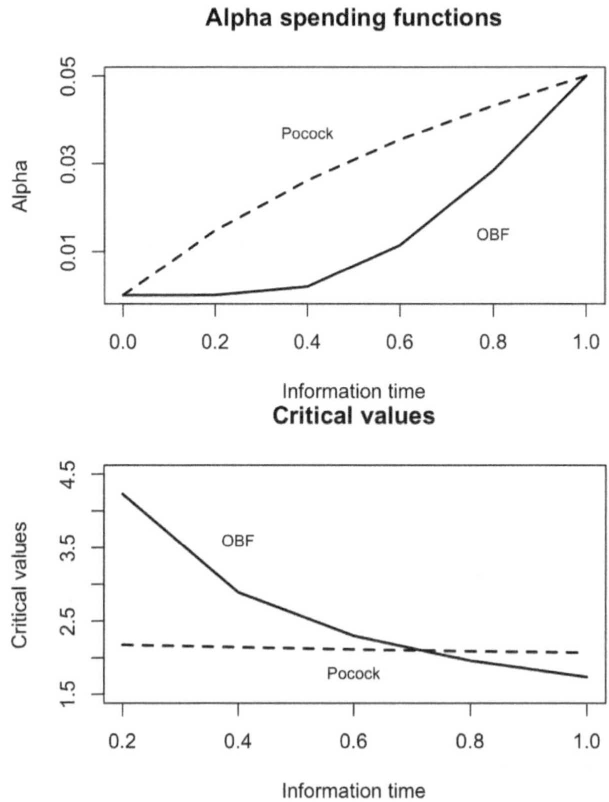

FIGURE 13.1
(a) Alpha spending functions and (b) stopping boundaries for Pocock's boundary and O'Brien-Fleming's (OBF) boundary when $\alpha = 0.05$.

(b) Pocock function, $\alpha^*(\iota) = \alpha \log\{1 + (e-1)\iota\}$

The shape of these two alpha spending functions and their corresponding 'standard boundaries' are shown in Figure 13.1. The OBF function is convex and has large critical values (or small alpha values) in early stages, and the critical value in the last stage is close to $z_{1-\alpha} = \Phi^{-1}(\alpha)$. In contrast, the Pocock function is concave and its stopping boundary is close to a horizontal line. We plan five interim analyses at $(t_1, t_2, t_3, t_4, t_5)$ with information times $(0.2, 0.4, 0.6, 0.8, 1)$, respectively. We use Clayton's (1985) copula to model the joint survival distribution for subunits in each cluster. We set Kendall's tau at $\tau = 0$, 0.05, 0.1, or 0.2. Note that when Kendall's $\tau = 0$, all the subunits are independent and the independent increment assumption holds. Therefore, we can investigate the impact of dependent increment, by comparing the boundary for Kendall's $\tau = 0$ against boundaries for positive Kendall's

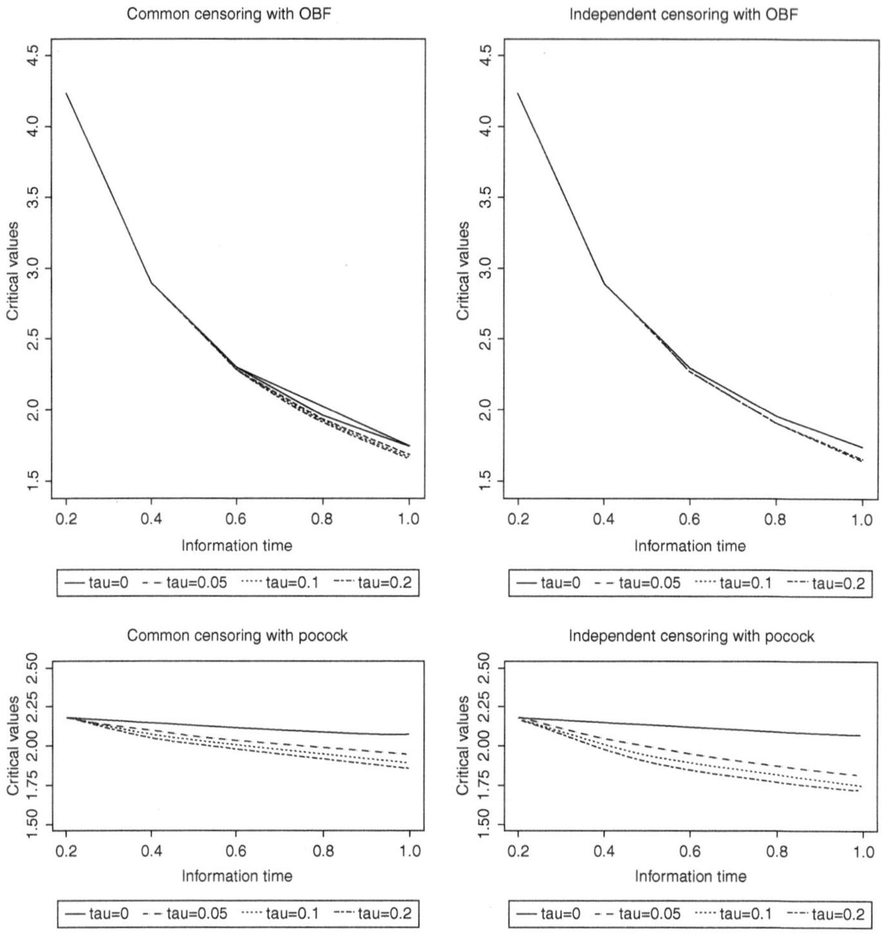

FIGURE 13.2
Pocock and O'Brien-Fleming's (OBF) boundaries for the clustered log-rank test under common entry and independent entry cases.

tau values. The curves with positive Kendall's tau values are called 'derived boundaries'.

From Figure 13.2, we find that the derived boundaries ($\tau > 0$) are all below the standard boundaries ($\tau = 0$). This implies that we will have a conservative testing result for CRT if we use a standard stopping boundary that is used for test statistics with independent increment. In addition, for the Pocock alpha spending function, the derived boundaries for $\tau > 0$ are noticeably different from the standard boundary for $\tau = 0$, even when the correlation is relatively small, and the stopping boundaries are well separated from the second interim analysis. On the other hand, for the OBF alpha spending function, the stopping boundaries look less dependent on the Kendall's τ value. Later, however, we will show an example that this small difference among the stopping boundaries actually makes a significant impact on the testing result. In conclusion, we recommend not to use the standard boundaries for the group sequential testing of CRT with positive intracluster dependency.

Simulations

The proposed group sequential testing and sample size calculation methods are based on asymptotic theories so that simulations are conducted to evaluate their finite sample performance. With superiority testing for early termination as in this chapter, the performance of a stopping boundary can be measured by the expected sample size under H_1, which can be calculated by the expected accrual period under H_1

$$EA = t_1 \wedge a + \sum_{k=2}^{L} (t_l \wedge a - t_{l-1} \wedge a) P\left\{ \left(\cap_{l=1}^{k-1} W^{(l)}/\hat{\sigma}^{(l)} \leq \xi_l \right) | H_1 \right\}.$$

Another performance measure of a group sequential testing is expected study period under H_1 that is calculated by

$$ET = t_1 + \sum_{k=2}^{L} (t_l - t_{l-1}) P\left\{ \cap_{l=1}^{k-1} \left(W^{(l)}/\hat{\sigma}^{(l)} \leq \xi_l \right) | H_1 \right\}.$$

The expected sample size is calculated by multiplying EA with expected accrual rate, i.e., the expected number of clusters $EN = r \times EA$ in common entry case, and the expected number of subunits per cluster is calculated by $EM = \bar{r} \times EA$ in independent entry case.

We use the algorithm proposed by McNeil (2008) to generate clustered exponential survival data using the Clayton and Cuzick's (1985) copula. To generate survival times for a cluster of size m in arm k, at first we generate a variable X from Gamma distribution $\Gamma(\theta, 1)$. And then, we generate random variables $V_1, ..., V_m \sim$ IID $U(0, 1)$. Let $U_j = (1 - \log V_j/X)^{-\theta}$ $(j = 1, ..., m)$, then the joint distribution of $(T_1, ..., T_m)$ with $T_j = -\log U_j/\lambda_k$ has the Clayton's copula with Kendall's $\tau = 1/(2\theta + 1)$.

We consider both common entry and independent entry cases. For the both entry cases, we set $\alpha = 0.05$; $1 - \beta = 0.8$ or 0.9; $p_1 = p_2 = 1/2$; $\Delta = 1.4$ or 1.6; $\lambda_1 = 7^{-1} \log 2$ per month; Kendall's $\tau = 0.3$ or 0.6; follow up period $b = 1$ year. Five analyses ($L = 5$) are conducted during the course of study, and the interim analysis times are evenly distributed. Both O'Brien-Fleming type and Pocock type alpha spending functions are considered in the simulations.

(i) For common entry case, we assume an accrual rate of $r = 100$ clusters per year. The cluster sizes are either fixed at $m_{ki} = 11$, or randomly chosen from discrete uniform distribution between 2 to 20, denoted as $m_{ki} \sim$

$U(2,20)$. Note that the two cluster size distributions have the same mean $\bar{m} = 11$, but the variances are different, with $\text{var}(m_{ki}) = 0$ and 30, respectively. For each parameter setting, we calculate the required accrual period a by solving equation (13.14), and obtain the required sample size by $n = r \times a$.

(ii) For independent entry case, accrual period for subunits is fixed at $a = 2$ years, and the accrual rate for subunits per cluster is either fixed at $r_{ki} = 10$ per year among clusters, or randomly selected from 5, 10, or 15 per year with an equal probability of $1/3$ each. For the both cases, the mean cluster sizes in the final analysis is $\bar{m}_L = 20$, but the variances are $\bar{m}_{LL} - \bar{m}_L^2 = 0$ and $200/3$, respectively. Sample size n is calculated by solving equation (13.14).

For each design setting, we calculate the maximal sample size n, the expected accrual period EA, and expected study period ET. Next, we generate clustered survival data of size n under the design setting, and apply the group sequential testing using clustered log-rank test statistics. We repeat this 5,000 times under each design setting and estimate the empirical power $1 - \hat{\beta}$ by the proportion of simulation samples rejecting the null hypothesis at any analysis time among 5,000 simulation samples. In addition, we also calculate an empirical type I error rate $\hat{\alpha}$ by generating 5,000 simulation samples of size n under the same design setting except that λ_2 is set to be equal to λ_1.

Table 13.1 reports the simulation results. Under each design setting, we also calculate the sample size of the single-stage design (denoted as n_s) calculated using (13.3). We find that all the empirical type I error rates and empirical powers are close to the corresponding nominal levels, but for some design settings, the empirical type I error rates are a little higher the nominal $\alpha = 0.05$. The required sample size decreases in hazard ratio Δ, and increases in $1 - \beta$, τ, and the variance of cluster size distribution. While the maximal sample size for OBF alpha spending function is almost identical to the sample size of a single-stage design, Pocock alpha spending function requires a much larger maximal sample size under each design setting. However, reflected by EA and ET, Pocock alpha spending function has a smaller expected sample size and shorter study period under H_1 than OBF spending function by spending higher alpha levels in early interim looks.

Examples

We apply our methods to design the real studies that are discussed in the beginning of this chapter.

Example 1: Suppose that we want to design the Howie's trial (Howie and Schwartz 1983) using the group sequential testing using clustered log-rank tests as an example with common entry type. In this study, the cluster sizes are constant, $m = 2$. We use the Clayton and Cuzick's (1985) copula with marginal exponential distributions to model the survival times. We schedule $L = 5$ sequential tests with evenly distributed interim analysis

TABLE 13.1

Sample size for single-stage design n_s, and maximal sample size (empirical type I error rate $\hat{\alpha}$ and power $1-\hat{\beta}$ from 5,000 simulations), and expected accrual period EA and study period ET under H_1 for multi-stage designs using Pocock o O'Brien-Fleming (OBF) stopping boundary

					O'Brien-Fleming			Pocock		
$1-\beta$	τ	λ_1/λ_2	m_i	n_s	n	$(\hat{\alpha}, 1-\hat{\beta})$	(EA, ET)	n	$(\hat{\alpha}, 1-\hat{\beta})$	(EA, ET)
(i) Common entry										
0.8	0.3	1.4	11	143	143	(0.052, 0.808)	(1.43, 1.99)	152	(0.048, 0.799)	(1.33, 1.67)
			$U(2, 20)$	175	175	(0.055, 0.814)	(1.72, 2.25)	186	(0.057, 0.800)	(1.58, 1.91)
		1.6	11	76	76	(0.054, 0.812)	(0.76, 1.44)	79	(0.057, 0.801)	(0.74, 1.15)
			$U(2, 20)$	92	92	(0.056, 0.819)	(0.92, 1.58)	96	(0.058, 0.801)	(0.88, 1.27)
	0.6	1.4	11	223	224	(0.052, 0.808)	(2.15, 2.64)	249	(0.055, 0.806)	(2.03, 2.36)
			$U(2, 20)$	273	275	(0.057, 0.799)	(2.60, 3.05)	307	(0.056, 0.811)	(2.45, 2.76)
		1.6	11	123	123	(0.062, 0.804)	(1.22, 1.82)	132	(0.051, 0.806)	(1.18, 1.56)
			$U(2, 20)$	150	150	(0.054, 0.801)	(1.49, 2.05)	163	(0.055, 0.819)	(1.42, 1.78)
0.9	0.3	1.4	11	197	197	(0.050, 0.902)	(1.89, 2.27)	210	(0.054, 0.890)	(1.64, 1.84)
			$U(2, 20)$	240	241	(0.051, 0.906)	(2.26, 2.61)	259	(0.057, 0.902)	(1.94, 2.13)
		1.6	11	104	104	(0.058, 0.906)	(1.03, 1.56)	109	(0.050, 0.899)	(0.94, 1.20)
			$U(2, 20)$	126	126	(0.058, 0.910)	(1.26, 1.74)	132	(0.051, 0.905)	(1.12, 1.36)
	0.6	1.4	11	301	304	(0.055, 0.903)	(2.77, 3.06)	337	(0.055, 0.904)	(2.46, 2.64)
			$U(2, 20)$	370	373	(0.059, 0.898)	(3.34, 3.58)	417	(0.050, 0.908)	(2.95, 3.11)
		1.6	11	165	166	(0.052, 0.903)	(1.62, 2.04)	179	(0.053, 0.907)	(1.46, 1.69)
			$U(2, 20)$	202	202	(0.062, 0.891)	(1.94, 2.33)	220	(0.055, 0.908)	(1.73, 1.95)

TABLE 13.1 (Continued)

Sample size for single-stage design n_s, and maximal sample size (empirical type I error rate $\hat{\alpha}$ and power $1-\hat{\beta}$ from 5,000 simulations), and expected accrual period EA and study period ET under H_1 for multi-stage designs using Pocock o O'Brien-Fleming (OBF) stopping boundary

					O'Brien-Fleming			Pocock		
$1-\beta$	τ	λ_1/λ_2	m_i	n_s	n	$(\hat{\alpha}, 1-\hat{\beta})$	(EA, ET)	n	$(\hat{\alpha}, 1-\hat{\beta})$	(EA, ET)
(ii) Independent entry										
0.8	0.3	1.4	11	134	134	(0.057, 0.806)	(1.96, 2.50)	134	(0.054, 0.805)	(1.55, 1.84)
			$U(2,20)$	155	155	(0.053, 0.800)	(1.96, 2.50)	155	(0.061, 0.804)	(1.55, 1.83)
		1.6	11	69	69	(0.063, 0.812)	(1.96, 2.53)	70	(0.053, 0.809)	(1.57, 1.86)
			$U(2,20)$	80	80	(0.056, 0.806)	(1.97, 2.53)	81	(0.056, 0.803)	(1.56, 1.85)
	0.6	1.4	11	216	216	(0.055, 0.803)	(1.95, 2.48)	220	(0.053, 0.817)	(1.56, 1.86)
			$U(2,20)$	251	251	(0.056, 0.809)	(1.96, 2.48)	255	(0.052, 0.805)	(1.56, 1.86)
		1.6	11	112	112	(0.052, 0.815)	(1.96, 2.51)	114	(0.053, 0.812)	(1.58, 1.88)
			$U(2,20)$	131	131	(0.057, 0.811)	(1.96, 2.51)	133	(0.057, 0.820)	(1.57, 1.88)
0.9	0.3	1.4	11	185	185	(0.048, 0.907)	(1.93, 2.33)	186	(0.050, 0.900)	(1.39, 1.56)
			$U(2,20)$	214	214	(0.056, 0.907)	(1.93, 2.33)	215	(0.052, 0.907)	(1.38, 1.54)
		1.6	11	96	96	(0.060, 0.915)	(1.94, 2.36)	96	(0.054, 0.901)	(1.41, 1.58)
			$U(2,20)$	111	111	(0.053, 0.901)	(1.94, 2.37)	111	(0.055, 0.904)	(1.40, 1.57)
	0.6	1.4	11	298	299	(0.055, 0.904)	(1.93, 2.31)	304	(0.053, 0.906)	(1.41, 1.58)
			$U(2,20)$	347	348	(0.052, 0.899)	(1.93, 2.31)	353	(0.053, 0.905)	(1.42, 1.57)
		1.6	11	156	156	(0.058, 0.908)	(1.93, 2.34)	158	(0.056, 0.913)	(1.42, 1.60)
			$U(2,20)$	181	181	(0.051, 0.904)	(1.93, 2.34)	184	(0.058, 0.910)	(1.42, 1.59)

times. Input parameters of $(\alpha, 1-\beta, \lambda_1, \Delta,$ Kendall's $\tau, m, r, b, p_1)$ =(0.05, 0.9, $7^{-1}\log 2$ per month, 1/0.7, 0.56, 2, 50 per year, 1 year, 0.5) are considered. For OBF alpha spending function, the maximal sample size is $n = 268$ with $EA = 4.63$ years and $EN = 50 \times 4.63 = 232$ patients. From 5,000 simulations, we obtain an empirical type I error rate of 0.052 and an empirical power of 0.899. On the other hand, for Pocock alpha spending function, the maximal sample size is $n = 306$ with $EA = 4.18$ years and $EN = 50 \times 4.18 = 209$ patients. From 5,000 simulations, we obtain an empirical type I error rate of 0.056 and an empirical power of 0.901. For reference, the single-stage design under the design parameter values requires $n = 263$ with total study period of 6.25 years. We find that the maximal sample size of OBF alpha spending function is smaller than that of Pocock alpha spending function, whereas the latter has a smaller EN than the former under H_1. Further, the maximal sample size of group sequential testing using OBF alpha spending function is close to the sample size of the single stage design, but, if H_1 is true, the former requires much smaller EN compared to the sample size of the single stage design (232 vs. 263). In this sense, OBF spending function has a similar property of the minimax designs, while Pocock spending function has a similar property of the optimal designs for 2-stage phase II clinical trials proposed by Simon (1989).

Example 2: Suppose that we design the Harper's trial using a five-stage $(L = 5)$ group sequential testing design with evenly distributed interim analysis times in information. This trial has an independent entry pattern. By Harper et al. (2015), the 12-month pregnancy rate for the control arm is approximately 0.2, and the hazard ratio is about $\lambda_1/\lambda_2 = 1/0.6$. In addition, the patients (subunits) are recruited for an accrual period of $a = 0.2$ years, and then followed for another $b = 1$ year after completion of accrual. Clinics (clusters) potentially have different accrual rate based on their patient volumes. Suppose that the yearly accrual rate is 100, 150, or 200 per clinic with an equal probability of $1/3$ each among clinics so that we have $\bar{r} = 150$ for an average cluster size of $\bar{m} = a \times \bar{r} = 30$, $\bar{\bar{m}} = a^2\bar{\bar{r}} = 24{,}166.67$, and $\text{var}(m) = 66.67$ during the accrual period of $a = 0.2$ years. We use the Clayton and Cuzick's copula to model the joint survival distribution with Kendall's $\tau = 0.05$ which corresponds to a Pearson correlation coefficient of 0.067 in the control arm. For $(\alpha, 1-\beta) = (0.05, 0.9)$, a single-stage design requires $n = 40$ clinics, whereas the multi-stage designs require $(n, EA, ET) = (43, 0.20, 0.70)$ using Pocock boundary and $(n, EA, ET) = (40, 0.20, 0.96)$ using OBF boundary. Note that the maximal sample size of the group sequential testing using OBF alpha spending function is identical to the sample size of the single-stage design. From 5,000 simulations, the empirical type I error rate and power are $(\hat{\alpha}, 1-\hat{\beta}) = (0.049, 0.888)$ for the Pocock boundary and $(0.048, 0.879)$ for the OBF boundary.

Discussion

We have investigated a group sequential testing method for CRT with a survival endpoint in this chapter. The group sequential testing method can be combined with any alpha spending function. Unlike in independent survival data case, the sequentially computed log-rank statistics do not have independent increment property with clustered survival data.

We find that the critical values with dependent increments are less extreme than those with independent increments. Probably with a positive intracluster correlation, we spend less alpha values at the interim looks. So, if we ignore such correlation and use the 'standard boundaries', we will have overly conservative results. For instance, in Example 1, when using OBF alpha spending function, we can well maintain both type I error and power with the maximal sample size of $n = 268$. However, if we use the standard boundary with this sample size, the empirical type I error is 0.029 while the empirical power is only 0.845 compared to the nominal $1 - \beta = 0.9$. Similarly, when using Pocock alpha spending function, for a maximal sample size of $n = 306$, the power of the standard boundary is only 0.820 and the type I error is 0.040.

We have investigated Pocock and OBF alpha spending functions. While Pocock stopping boundaries for clustered survival data are very different from that for independent survival data, OBF stopping boundaries are less sensitive to the intracluster dependency of survival data. By saving alpha spending until data are mature, an OBF stopping boundary has a similar statistical property to that of a single-stage design and the its maximal sample size is very close to the sample size of the single-stage design. On the other hand, compared to OBF stopping boundary, Pocock stopping boundary has a probability to stop the trial early by using more aggressive alpha spending from the beginning so that it has a smaller expected sample size and a shorter expected study period in spite of its larger maximal sample size. We observed these properties from simulations and real study examples.

Appendix A. Asymptotic distribution of clustered log-rank test

For subunit j in cluster i that is randomized into arm k before interim analysis time t_l, we define the counting process and at risk process as $N_{kij}^{(l)}(t) = \delta_{kij}^{(l)} I(X_{kij}^{(l)} \leq t)$ and $Y_{kij}^{(l)}(t) = I(X_{kij}^{(l)} \geq t)$, respectively. Let $M_{kij}^{(l)}(t) = N_{kij}^{(l)}(t) - \int_0^t Y_{kij}^{(l)}(s) d\Lambda_k(t)$ and $M_{ki}^{(l)}(t) = \sum_{j=1}^{m_{ki}^{(l)}} M_{kij}^{(l)}(t)$.

By definition,

$$W^{(l)} = \left\{ \sum_{i=1}^{n_1^{(l)}} \int_0^\infty \frac{Y_2^{(l)}(t)}{Y^{(l)}(t)} dM_{1i}^{(l)}(t) - \sum_{i=1}^{n_2^{(l)}} \int_0^\infty \frac{Y_1^{(l)}(t)}{Y^{(l)}(t)} dM_{2i}^{(l)}(t) \right\}$$

$$+ \int_0^\infty \frac{Y_1^{(l)}(t) Y_2^{(l)}(t)}{Y^{(l)}(t)} \{d\Lambda_1(t) - d\Lambda_2(t)\}.$$

Let $\eta = \max\{t : S_1(t)S_2(t)G(t) > 0\}$. Usually the upper limit of the support of survival distributions is longer than the study period so that η denotes the study period. For the log-rank statistic, as $n \to \infty$, $Y_k^{(l)}(t)/n^{(l)}$ and $Y^{(l)}(t)/n^{(l)}$ uniformly converge to $y_k^{(l)}(t) = \bar{m}_l p_k S_k(t) G^{(l)}(t)$ and $y^{(l)}(t) = \bar{m}_l\{p_1 S_1(t) + p_2 S_2(t)\} G^{(l)}(t)$, respectively, in $[0, \eta]$ so that we have

$$W^{(l)} = \left(\sum_{i=1}^{n_1^{(l)}} \epsilon_{1i}^{(l)} - \sum_{i=1}^{n_2^{(l)}} \epsilon_{2i}^{(l)} \right) + n^{(l)} \int_0^\infty \frac{y_1^{(l)}(t) y_2^{(l)}(t)}{y^{(l)}(t)} \{d\Lambda_1(t) - d\Lambda_2(t)\} + o_p(1),$$

where $\epsilon_{ki}^{(l)} = \sum_{j=1}^{m_{ki}^{(l)}} \epsilon_{kij}^{(l)}$ and

$$\epsilon_{kij}^{(l)} = \int_0^\infty \frac{y_{3-k}^{(l)}(t)}{y^{(l)}(t)} dM_{kij}^{(l)}(t). \qquad (13.A1)$$

Since $\{\epsilon_{ki}^{(l)}, i = 1, ..., n_k^{(l)}, k = 1, 2\}$ are independent 0-mean random variables, by the central limit theorem, $W^{(l)}$ is approximately normal with mean $n^{(l)}\omega^{(l)}$, where

$$\omega^{(l)} = \int_0^\infty \frac{y_1^{(l)}(t) y_2^{(l)}(t)}{y^{(l)}(t)} \{d\Lambda_1(t) - d\Lambda_2(t)\}.$$

Next, we calculate the covariance of test statistics for any two interim looks l_1 and l_2 ($l_1 < l_2$). Note that $\{\epsilon_{ki}^{(l)}, i = 1, ..., n_l, l = 1, ..., L\}$ are independent variables, therefore for given cluster sizes, we have

$$\mathrm{cov}\left(\sum_{i=1}^{n_k^{(l_1)}} \epsilon_{ki}^{(l_1)}, \sum_{i=1}^{n_k^{(l_2)}} \epsilon_{ki}^{(l_2)} | m_{ki}^{(l_1)}, m_{ki}^{(l_2)} \right) = \sum_{i=1}^{n_k^{(l_1)}} \mathrm{cov}\left(\epsilon_{ki}^{(l_1)}, \epsilon_{ki}^{(l_2)} | m_{ki}^{(l_1)}, m_{ki}^{(l_2)} \right)$$

$$= \sum_{i=1}^{n_k^{(l_1)}} \sum_{j=1}^{m_{ki}^{(l_1)}} E\left(\epsilon_{kij}^{(l_1)} \epsilon_{kij}^{(l_2)} \right) + \sum_{i=1}^{n_k^{(l_1)}} \sum_{j \neq j'}^{m_{ki}^{(l_1)}} E\left(\epsilon_{kij}^{(l_1)} \epsilon_{kij'}^{(l_2)} \right)$$

$$= n_k^{(l_1)} m_{ki}^{(l_1)} E\left(\epsilon_{kij}^{(l_1)} \epsilon_{kij}^{(l_2)} \right) + n_k^{(l_1)} \left(m_{ki}^{(l_1)} m_{ki}^{(l_2)} - m_{ki}^{(l_1)} \right) E\left(\epsilon_{kij}^{(l_1)} \epsilon_{kij'}^{(l_2)} \right). \qquad (13.A2)$$

In the second term (13.A2). we have

$$E(\epsilon_{kij}^{(l_1)}\epsilon_{kij'}^{(l_2)}) = \int_0^\infty \int_0^\infty \frac{y_{3-k}^{(l_1)}(t)y_{3-k}^{(l_2)}(s)}{y^{(l_1)}(t)y^{(l_2)}(s)} E\left\{dM_{kij}^{(l_1)}(t)dM_{kij'}^{(l_2)}(s)\right\}$$

$$= \int_0^\infty \int_0^\infty \frac{y_{3-k}^{(l_1)}(t)y_{3-k}^{(l_2)}(s)}{y^{(l_1)}(t)y^{(l_2)}(s)} E\left\{dN_{kij}^{(l_1)}(t)dN_{kij'}^{(l_2)}(s) - Y_{kij}^{(l_1)}(t)\lambda_k(t)dtdN_{kij'}^{(l_2)}(s)\right.$$

$$\left. - Y_{kij'}^{(l_2)}(s)\lambda_k(s)dN_{kij}^{(l_1)}(t)ds + Y_{kij}^{(l_1)}(t)\lambda_k(t)Y_{kij'}^{(l_2)}(s)\lambda_k(s)dtds\right\}. \quad (13.A3)$$

We can simplify (13.A3) with a direct method. For the first term of (13.A3), since subunit j and j' have been recruited before interim looks l_1 and l_2, respectively, based on the independent entry assumption, we have

$$E\{dN_{kij}^{(l_1)}(t)dN_{kij'}^{(l_2)}(s)\} = P(t \le T_{kij} < t + dt, s \le T_{kij'} < s + ds)$$

$$\times P(C_{kij} \ge t, C_{kij'} \ge s, t_{l_1} - e_{kij} \ge t, t_{l_2} - e_{kij'} \ge s | e_{kij} \le t, e_{kij'} \le s)$$

$$= \lambda_k(t,s)S_k(t,s)G^{(l_1 l_2)}(t,s).$$

Similarly, other terms in (13.A3) can be derived as

$$E\{Y_{kij}^{(l_1)}(t)\lambda_k(t)dtdN_{kij'}^{(l_2)}(s)\} = \lambda_{k(2|1)}(t,s)\lambda_k(t)S_k(t,s)G^{(l_1 l_2)}(t,s)dtds$$

$$E\{Y_{kij'}^{(l_2)}(s)\lambda_k(s)dN_{kij}^{(l_1)}(t)ds\} = y_k(t,s)\lambda_{k(1|2)}(t,s)\lambda_k(s)S_k(t,s)G^{(l_1 l_2)}(t,s) - s)dtds$$

and

$$E\{Y_{kij}^{(l_1)}(t)\lambda_k(t)Y_{kij'}^{(l_2)}(s)\lambda_k(s)dtds\} = y_k(t,s)\lambda_k(t)\lambda_k(s)S_k(t,s)G^{(l_1 l_2)}(t,s) - s)dtds.$$

Therefore, we have

$$E(\epsilon_{kij}^{(l_1)}\epsilon_{kij'}^{(l_2)}) = \int_0^\infty \int_0^\infty \frac{y_{3-k}^{(l_1)}(t)y_{3-k}^{(l_2)}(s)}{y^{(l_1)}(t)y^{(l_2)}(s)} S_k(t,s)G^{(l_1 l_2)}(t,s)dA_k(t,s). \quad (13.A4)$$

For the log-rank test statistics under the nearby alternative hypothesis, (13.A4) and $\omega^{(l)}$ are further simplified to

$$E(\epsilon_{kij}^{(l_1)}\epsilon_{kij'}^{(l_2)}) = p_{3-k}^2 \int_0^\infty \int_0^\infty S_k(t,s)G^{(l_1 l_2)}(t,s)dA_k(t,s)$$

and

$$\omega^{(l)} = \log\Delta \int_0^\infty S_k(t)G^{(l)}(t)d\Lambda_k(t) = -\log\Delta \int_0^\infty G^{(l)}(t)dS_k(t)$$

respectively.

For the first term in (13.A2), Tsiatis (1982) has shown that

$$\begin{aligned} E(\epsilon_{kij}^{(l_1)}\epsilon_{kij}^{(l_2)}) =&\text{var}(\epsilon_{kij}^{(l_1)}) = p_{3-k}^2 \int_0^\infty S_k(t)G^{(l)}(t)d\Lambda_k(t) \\ =& - p_{3-k}^2 \int_0^\infty G^{(l)}(t)dS_k(t). \end{aligned}$$

Finally, since $\text{cov}(W^{(l_1)}, W^{(l_2)}) = E\{\text{cov}(W^{(l_1)}, W^{(l_2)}|m_{ki}^{(l_1)}, m_{ki}^{(l_2)})\}$, we have

$$\text{cov}(W^{(l_1)}, W^{(l_2)}) = n^{(l_1)}p_1p_2\{\bar{m}_{l_1}d^{(l_1)} + (\bar{m}_{l_1l_2} - \bar{m}_{l_1})c^{(l_1l_2)}\}.$$

Now, we want to show that independent increment assumption does not hold with a positive intracluster correlation. Recall that $\bar{m}_l$ is the mean cluster size for a cluster accrued before time t_l. So, if e_{ki}^c denotes the entry time of cluster i in arm k, $\bar{m}_l$ is expressed as

$$\bar{m}_l = E\{\sum_{j=1}^{m_{ki}} I(e_{kij} \le t_l | e_{ki}^c \le t_l)\} = \bar{m}\frac{P(e_{kij} \le t_l)}{P(e_{ki}^c \le t_l)}.$$

Similarly, we have

$$\begin{aligned} \bar{m}_{l_1l_2} =&E\left\{\sum_{j=1}^{m_{ki}}\sum_{j'=1}^{m_{ki}} I(e_{kij} \le t_{l_1}, e_{kij'} \le t_{l_2} | e_{ki}^c \le t_{l_1})\right\} \\ =&\bar{\bar{m}}\frac{P(e_{kij} \le t_{l_1}, e_{kij'} \le t_{l_2})}{P(e_{ki}^c \le t_{l_1})}. \end{aligned}$$

We have $(\bar{m}_{l_1l_2} - \bar{m}_{l_1})c^{(l_1l_2)} > (\bar{m}_{l_1l_1} - \bar{m}_{l_1})c^{(l_1l_1)}$ because:

- If $c^{(l_1l_2)} > c^{(l_1l_1)}$, then we have

  $$(\bar{m}_{l_1l_2} - \bar{m}_{l_1})c^{(l_1l_2)} > (\bar{m}_{l_1l_2} - \bar{m}_{l_1})c^{(l_1l_1)} \ge (\bar{m}_{l_1l_1} - \bar{m}_{l_1})c^{(l_1l_1)}$$

- If $c^{(l_1l_2)} \le c^{(l_1l_1)}$, then it suffices to show that $\bar{m}_{l_1l_2}c^{(l_1l_2)} > \bar{m}_{l_1l_1}c^{(l_1l_1)}$. Note that $Q^{(l_1l_2)}(t,s) = P(e_{kij} \le t, e_{kij'} \le s | e_{kij} \le t_{l_1}, e_{kij'} \le t_{l_2})$. For any $l_2 > l_1$, we have

$$\begin{aligned} \bar{m}_{l_1l_2}c_k^{(l_1l_2)} =& \bar{\bar{m}}\frac{P(e_{kij} \le t_{l_1}, e_{kij'} \le t_{l_2})}{P(e_{ki}^c \le t_{l_1})} \\ &\times \int_0^{t_{l_1}}\int_0^{t_{l_2}} S_k(t,s)G(t,s)\frac{P(e_{kij} \le t_{l_1} - t, e_{kij'} \le t_{l_2} - s)}{P(e_{kij} \le t_{l_1}, e_{kij'} \le t_{l_2})}dA_k(t,s) \\ =& \bar{\bar{m}}\frac{1}{P(e_{ki}^c \le t_{l_1})}\int_0^{t_{l_1}}\int_0^{t_{l_2}} S_k(t,s)G(t,s) \end{aligned}$$

$$\times P(e_{kij} \le t_{l_1} - t, e_{kij} \le t_{l_2} - s) dA_k(t,s)$$
$$> \bar{\bar{m}} \frac{1}{P(e_{ki}^c \le t_{l_1})} \int_0^{t_{l_1}} \int_0^{t_{l_1}} S_k(t,s) G(t,s)$$
$$\times P(e_{kij} \le t_{l_1} - t, e_{kij} \le t_{l_1} - s) dA_k(t,s)$$
$$= \bar{\bar{m}} \frac{P(e_{kij} \le t_{l_1}, e_{kij'} \le t_{l_1})}{P(e_{ki}^c \le t_{l_1})} \int_0^{t_{l_1}} \int_0^{t_{l_1}} S_k(t,s) G(t,s)$$
$$\times \frac{P(e_{kij} \le t_{l_1} - t, e_{kij'} \le t_{l_1} - s)}{P(e_{kij} \le t_{l_1}, e_{kij'} \le t_{l_1})} dA_k(t,s)$$
$$= \bar{m}_{l_1 l_1} c_k^{(l_1 l_1)}.$$

Therefore, we have

$$\text{cov}(W^{(l_1)}, W^{(l_2)}) > n^{(l_1)} p_1 p_2 \{\bar{m}_{l_1} d^{(l_1)} + (\bar{m}_{l_1 l_1} - \bar{m}_{l_1}) c^{(l_1 l_1)}\} = \text{var}(W^{(l_1)}, W^{(l_1)}).$$

Appendix B. Design parameters under bivariate exponential survival with Clayton and Cuzick's frailty

For a marginal exponential survival distribution, we have $S_k(t) = e^{-\lambda_k t}$. Using Clayton and Cuzick's copula, the bivariate exponential distribution has

$$\lambda_k(t,s) = \frac{f_k(t,s)}{S_k(t,s)} = \lambda_k^2 (1 + 1/\theta) e^{(t+s)\lambda_k/\theta} \{e^{\lambda_k t/\theta} + e^{\lambda_k s/\theta} - 1\}^{-2}$$

$$\lambda_{k(1|2)}(t,s) = \frac{\partial S_k(t,s)/\partial t}{S_k(t,s)} = \lambda_k e^{\lambda_k t/\theta} (e^{\lambda_k t/\theta} + e^{\lambda_k s/\theta} - 1)^{-1}$$

$$\lambda_{k(2|1)}(t,s) = \frac{\partial S_k(t,s)/\partial s}{S_k(t,s)} = \lambda_k e^{\lambda_k s/\theta} (e^{\lambda_k t/\theta} + e^{\lambda_k s/\theta} - 1)^{-1}$$

and

$$dA_k(t,s) = \lambda_k^2 \left\{ \frac{(1 + 1/\theta) e^{(t+s)\lambda_k/\theta}}{(e^{\lambda_k t/\theta} + e^{\lambda_k s/\theta} - 1)^2} - \frac{e^{\lambda_k t/\theta} + e^{\lambda_k s/\theta}}{e^{\lambda_k t/\theta} + e^{\lambda_k s/\theta} - 1} + 1 \right\} dtds.$$

With an accrual period of a, the marginal CDF for entry time is $U(0, a)$ in both common and independent entry cases. So, the marginal CDF of the entry time conditioning on the fact that the subunit enters before t_l is written as

$$Q^{(l)}(t) = \frac{P(e_{kij} \le t, e_{kij} \le t_l)}{P(e_{kij} \le t_l)} = \frac{t \wedge t_l \wedge a/a}{t_l \wedge a/a} = \frac{t \wedge t_l \wedge a}{t_l \wedge a}.$$

Similarly, $Q^{(l)}(t,s)$ can be derived for $0 \le t \le t_{l_1}, 0 \le s \le t_{l_2}$

$$Q^{(l_1 l_2)}(t,s) = \frac{P(e_{kij} \le t, e_{kij'} \le s, e_{kij} \le t_{l_1}, e_{kij'} \le t_{l_2})}{P(e_{kij} \le t_{l_1}, e_{kij'} \le t_{l_2})} = \frac{t \wedge s \wedge t_{l_1} \wedge t_{l_2} \wedge a}{t_{l_1} \wedge t_{l_2} \wedge a}$$

in (i) common entry case, and

$$Q^{(l_1 l_2)}(t_{l_1} - t, t_{l_2} - s) = \frac{\{(t_{l_1} - t) \wedge a\}\{(t_{l_2} - t) \wedge a\}}{(t_{l_1} \wedge a)(t_{l_2} \wedge a)}$$

in (ii) independent entry case. We have $Q^{(l)}(t,s) = 0$ for $t > t_{l_1}$ or $s > t_{l_2}$ for the both entry cases.

Appendix C. A consistent estimator of covariance matrix of $(W^{(1)}, \ldots W^{(L)})$

Based on the derivation in Appendix A and the law of large numbers, for $l_1 < l_2$, $\text{cov}(W^{(l_1)}, W^{(l_2)})/n^{(l_1)}$ is equivalent to

$$\lim_{n^{(l_1)} \to \infty} \frac{1}{n^{(l_1)}} \left(\sum_{i=1}^{n_1^{(l_1)}} \epsilon_{1i}^{(l_1)} - \sum_{i=1}^{n_2^{(l_1)}} \epsilon_{2i}^{(l_1)} \right) \left(\sum_{i=1}^{n_1^{(l_2)}} \epsilon_{1i}^{(l_2)} - \sum_{i=1}^{n_2^{(l_2)}} \epsilon_{2i}^{(l_2)} \right)$$

$$= \lim_{n^{(l_1)} \to \infty} \frac{1}{n^{(l_1)}} \sum_{k=1}^{2} \sum_{i=1}^{n_k^{(l_1)}} \epsilon_{ki}^{(l_1)} \epsilon_{ki}^{(l_2)}, \tag{13.A5}$$

where, as given in (13.A1),

$$\epsilon_{ki}^{(l)} = \sum_{j=1}^{m_{ki}^{(l)}} \int_0^\infty \frac{y_{3-k}^{(l)}(t)}{y^{(l)}(t)} dM_{kij}^{(l)}(t).$$

Here, $y_{3-k}^{(l)}(t)/y^{(l)}(t) = p_{3-k} + o_p(1)$ under nearby alternative hypothesis. Let

$$\hat{\epsilon}_{ki}^{(l)} = p_{3-k} \int_0^\infty \{dN_{ki}^{(l)}(t) - Y_{ki}^{(l)}(t) d\hat{\Lambda}_k(t).$$

which is obtained from $\epsilon_{ki}^{(l)}$ by replacing $\Lambda_k(t)$ with $\hat{\Lambda}_k(t)$ under nearby alternative hypothesis. Then, from (13.A5), we obtain a consistent estimator of $\sigma_{l_1 l_2} = \text{cov}(W^{(l_1)}, W^{(l_2)})$ by

$$\hat{\sigma}_{l_1 l_2} = \sum_{k=1}^{2} \sum_{i=1}^{n_k^{(l_1)}} \hat{\epsilon}_{ki}^{(l_1)} \hat{\epsilon}_{ki}^{(l_2)}$$

$$= \sum_{k=1}^{2} p_{3-k}^2 \sum_{i=1}^{n_k^{(l_1)}} \left[\sum_{j=1}^{m_{ki}^{(l_1)}} \left\{ \delta_{ki}^{(l_1)} - \hat{\Lambda}_k \left(X_{kij}^{(l_1)} \right) \right\} \right] \left[\sum_{j=1}^{m_{ki}^{(l_2)}} \left\{ \delta_{ki}^{(l_2)} - \hat{\Lambda}_k \left(X_{kij}^{(l_2)} \right) \right\} \right]$$

$$= \sum_{k=1}^{2} p_{3-k}^2 \sum_{i=1}^{n_k^{(l_1)}} \left\{ D_{ki}^{(l_1)} - \sum_{j=1}^{m_{ki}^{(l_1)}} \hat{\Lambda}_k \left(X_{kij}^{(l_1)} \right) \right\} \left\{ D_{ki}^{(l_2)} - \sum_{j=1}^{m_{ki}^{(l_2)}} \hat{\Lambda}_k \left(X_{kij}^{(l_2)} \right) \right\}.$$

References

Aalen O. Nonparametric inference for a family of counting processes. Annals of Statistics 1978;6(4):701–726.

Clayton D, Cuzick J. Multivariate generalizations of the proportional Hazards model. Journal of the Royal Statistical Society, Series A (General) 1985; 148(2): 82–108.

DeMets DL, Lan KKG. Interim analysis: the alpha spending function approach. Statistics in Medicine 1994; 13: 1341–1352.

Freedman LS. Tables of the number of patients required in clinical trials using the logrank test. Statistics in Medicine 1982;1(2):121–129.

Hasan MT, Choi YH, Briollais L. A sequential approach for clustered survival data in family studies based on a weighted log-rank statistic. Journal of Applied Statistical Science 2011; 18(4): 443–460.

Harper CC, Rocca CH, Thompson KM, et al. Reductions in pregnancy rates in the USA with long-acting reversible contraception: a cluster randomised trial. Lancet 2015;386(9993):562–568.

Howie VM, Schwartz RH. Acute otitis media: one year in general pediatric practice. American Journal of Diseases in Children 1983; 137: 155–158.

Jung SH, Jeong JH. Rank tests for clustered survival data. Lifetime Data Analysis 2003; 9(1): 21–33.

Kim K, Boucher H, Tsiatis AA. Design and analysis of group sequential logrank tests in maximum duration versus information trials. Biometrics 1995; 51(3): 988–1000.

Lan KKG, DeMets DL. Discrete sequential boundaries for clinical trials. Biometrika 1983; 70: 659–663.

Lan KKG, Lachin JM. Implementation of group sequential logrank tests in a maximum duration trial. Biometrics 1990; 46(3): 759–770.

Li J, Jung SH. Sample size calculation for cluster randomization trials with a time-to-event endpoint. Statistics in Medicine 2020; 39(25): 3608–3623.

McNeil AJ. Sampling nested Archimedean copulas. Journal of Statistical Computation and Simulation 2008; 78(6): 567–581.

Nelson W. Hazard plotting for incomplete failure data. Journal of Quality Technology 1969; 1(1): 27–52.

O'Brien PC, Fleming TR. A multiple testing procedure for clinical trials. Biometrics 1979; 35: 549–556.

Peto R, Peto J. Asymptotically efficient rank invariant test procedures (with discussion. Journal of the Royal Statistical Society, Series A 1972; 135: 185–206.

Pocock SJ. Group sequential methods in the design and analysis of clinical trials. Biometrika 1977; 64: 191–199.

Schoenfeld DA. Sample-size formula for the proportional-hazards regression model. Biometrics 1983; 39(2): 499–503.

Simon R. Optimal two-stage designs for phase II clinical trials. Controlled Clinical Trials 1989; 10: 1–10.

Teele DW, Klein JO, Rosner B, et al. Epidemiology of otitis media during the first seven years of life in children in greater Boston. Journal of Infectious Diseases 1989; 160: 89–94.

Tsiatis AA. Repeated significance testing for a general class of statistics used in censored survival analysis. Journal of the American Statistical Association 1982; 77(380): 855–861.

14

Random Number Generation of Clustered Survival Data

Chapters 9–13 discuss statistical testing and sample size methods for paired and clustered survival data. Random number generation of dependent survival data has been a key component of these sections to evaluate the finite sample performance of those statistical methods through simulations. This chapter summarizes various random number generation methods for clustered survival data under cluster randomization and subunit randomization. Paired data are simple example of clustered data under subunit randomization so that we do not consider random number generation of paired survival data case separately.

Moran's Method

Moran (1967) proposed a simple algorithm to generate paired exponential random numbers. This algorithm can be easily modified to generate clustered exponential data. This algorithm is very simple to generate clustered exponential data, but its multivariate distribution functions have infinite number of terms so that it is not appropriate for simulations to evaluate the performance of sample size methods which require specification of bivariate Survival distribution functions. However, it is very convenient to generate clustered survival data to evaluate the performance of test statistics. Lee et al. (2007) proposed a Bayesian method to analyze paired survival data with Moran's model.

Under Cluster Randomization

Suppose that $(U_1, ..., U_m)$ and $(V_1, ..., V_m)$ are mutually independent, but each random vector has a multivariate normal distribution with marginally 0 mean and variance 1, and exchangeable structure with correlation coefficient $\sqrt{\rho}$. Define $T_j = (U_j^2 + V_j^2)/(2\lambda)$. Then, $(T_1, ..., T_m)$ are random variables that have marginally exponential distribution with failure rate λ and exchangeable structure with correlation coefficient ρ.

DOI: 10.1201/9781003221951-14

Under Subunit Randomization

Suppose that $(U_{11}, ..., U_{1,m_1}, U_{21}, ..., U_{2,m_2})$ and $(V_{11}, ..., V_{1,m_1}, V_{21}, ..., V_{2,m_2})$ are mutually independent, but each random vector has a multivariate normal distribution with marginal means of 0, variances of 1, and correlation coefficients, $\text{corr}(U_{kj}, U_{kj'}) = \text{corr}(V_{kj}, V_{kj'}) = \sqrt{\rho_w}$ for $j \neq j'$ and $\text{corr}(U_{1j}, U_{2j'}) = \text{corr}(V_{1j}, V_{2j'}) = \sqrt{\rho_b}$. Then, for the new random vector $(T_{11}, ..., T_{1,m_1}, T_{21}, ..., T_{2,m_2})$ with $T_{kj} = 0.5(U_{kj}^2 + V_{kj}^2)/\lambda_k$, $(T_{kj}, j = 1, ..., m_k, k = 1, 2)$ are marginally exponential random variables with hazard rate λ_k and correlation coefficients $\text{corr}(T_{kj}, T_{kj'}) = \rho_w$ for $j \neq j'$ and $\text{corr}(T_{1j}, T_{2j'}) = \rho_b$. Note that ρ_w and ρ_b are intracluster correlation coefficients (ICCs) among subunits within each group and between different groups, respectively.

Sequential Random Number Generation using Conditional Survival Functions

Suppose that random vector $(T_1, ..., T_m)$ has a joint survival function $S(t_1, ..., t_m)$. Then we generate $(T_1, ..., T_m) = (t_1, ..., t_m)$ sequentially by generating $u_1, ..., u_m$ IID $U(0, 1)$ random variables and solving $S(t_1) = u_1$ with respect to t_1, and $S(t_j | t_1, ..., t_{j-1}) = u_j$ with respect to t_j for $j = 2, ..., m$. Note that

$$\begin{aligned}
&P(T_1 \geq t_1, T_2 \geq t_2, ..., T_m \geq t_m) \\
&\quad = P\{S^{-1}(U_1) \geq t_1, S^{-1}(U_2|t_1) \geq t_2, ..., S^{-1}(U_m|t_1, ..., t_{m-1}) \geq t_m\} \\
&\quad = P\{U_1 \geq S(t_1), U_2 \geq S(t_2|t_1), ..., U_m \geq S(t_m|t_1, ..., t_{m-1})\} \\
&\quad = S(t_1) \times S(t_2|t_1) \times \cdots \times S(t_m|t_1, ..., t_{m-1}) \\
&\qquad\qquad \text{since } U_1, ..., U_m \sim \text{ IID } N(0, 1) \\
&\quad = S(t_1, ..., t_m)
\end{aligned}$$

Hence, $(T_1, ..., T_m)$ has joint survival function $S(t_1, ..., t_m)$.

For example, for Clayton and Cuzick's (1985) model with exponential marginal distributions with hazard rates λ_j for T_j, the joint survival function of is given as

$$S(t_1, ..., t_m) = \left\{ \sum_{j=1}^{m} \exp(\lambda_j t_j / \theta) - (m - 1) \right\}^{-\theta},$$

where $\theta = 1/2(1/\tau - 1) > 0$ and $\tau \in [0, 1]$ is the Kendall's tau with 0 meaning no relationship and 1 meaning a perfect relationship between paired survival times.

For this distribution, the conditional survival function of T_j given $T_1 = t_1, ..., T_{j-1} = t_{j-1}$ is

$$S(t_j|t_1, ..., t_{j-1}) = \frac{\partial^{j-1} S(t_1, ..., t_j)}{\partial t_1 \cdots \partial t_{j-1}} \Big/ \frac{\partial^{j-1} S(t_1, ..., t_{j-1})}{\partial t_1 \cdots \partial t_{j-1}}$$

$$= \left(\frac{\sum_{j'=1}^{j} e^{\lambda_j t_{j'}/\theta} - j + 1}{\sum_{j'=1}^{j-1} e^{\lambda j t_{j'}/\theta} - j + 2} \right)^{-\theta - j + 1}.$$

Then, for IID $U(0,1)$ random variables $u_1, .., u_m$, survival times $(T_1, ..., T_m) = (t_1, ..., t_m)$ are sequentially generated by solving the equations $u_1 = S(t_1) = \exp(-\lambda_1 t_1)$ and, for $j = 2, ..., m$,

$$u_j = S(t_j|t_1, ..., t_{j-1})$$

with respect to $t_1, ..., t_m$. That is, for $1 \leq j \leq m$, we have

$$t_j = \frac{\theta}{\lambda_j} \log\{j - 1 - e_{j-1} + (e_{j-1} - j + 2) u_j^{-1/(\theta + j - 1)}\}. \tag{14.1}$$

where $e_0 = 0$ and $e_j = e_{j-1} + \exp(\lambda_j t_j / \theta)$ for $j = 1, ..., m - 1$.

Under Cluster Randomization

Suppose that random vector $(T_1, ..., T_m)$ has Clayton and Cuzick's model with exponential marginal distributions with hazard rates λ. From (14.1), for IID $U(0,1)$ random variables $u_1, .., u_m$, clustered survival times $(T_1, ..., T_m) = (t_1, ..., t_m)$ are sequentially generated

$$t_j = \frac{\theta}{\lambda} \log\{j - 1 - e_{j-1} + (e_{j-1} - j + 2) u_j^{-1/(\theta + j - 1)}\}$$

for $j = 1, ..., m$, where $e_0 = 0$ and $e_j = e_{j-1} + \exp(\lambda t_j / \theta)$.

Under Subunit Randomization

Suppose that random vector $(T_{11}, ..., T_{1,m_1}, T_{21}, ..., T_{2,m_2})$ has Clayton and Cuzick's model with exponential marginal distributions with hazard rates λ_k for T_{kj}. Then, from (14.1), for IID $U(0,1)$ random variables $(u_{11}, ..., u_{1,m_1}, u_{21}, ..., u_{2,m_2})$, clustered survival times

$$(T_{11}, ..., T_{1,m_1}, T_{21}, ..., T_{2,m_2}) = (t_{11}, ..., t_{1,m_1}, t_{21}, ..., t_{2,m_2})$$

are sequentially generated by

$$t_{1j} = \frac{\theta}{\lambda_1} \log\{j - 1 - e_{1,j-1} + (e_{1,j-1} - j + 2) u_{1j}^{-1/(\theta + j - 1)}\}$$

for $j = 1, ..., m_1$, and

$$t_{2j} = \frac{\theta}{\lambda_2} \log\{m_1 + j - 1 - e_{2,j-1} + (e_{2,j-1} - j + 2)u_{2j}^{-1/(\theta+m_1+j-1)}\}$$

for $j = 1, ..., m_2$, where $e_{10} = 0$, $e_{1j} = e_{1,j-1} + \exp(\lambda_1 t_{1j}/\theta)$ for $j = 1, ..., m_1$, $e_{20} = e_{1,m_1}$, and $e_{2j} = \sum_{j_1=1}^{m_1} \exp(\lambda_1 t_{1j_1}/\theta) + \sum_{j_2=1}^{j} \exp(\lambda_2 t_{2j_2}/\theta)$ for $j = 1, ..., m_2$.

Gamma-Exponential Frailty Model

Subunits with a gamma frailty share a frailty with a common frailty $V \sim \Gamma(\kappa, 1/\kappa)$ with probability density function of

$$f_V(v) = \frac{\kappa^\kappa}{\Gamma(\kappa)} v^{\kappa-1} \exp(-\kappa v).$$

Here, κ determines the ICC of the clustered data. We have $\Gamma(\kappa) = (\kappa - 1)!$ if κ is a positive integer and

$$\Gamma(\kappa) = \int_0^\infty v^{\kappa-1} e^{-v} dv$$

for $\kappa > 0$. Further, $\Gamma(\kappa) = (\kappa - 1)\Gamma(\kappa - 1)$. We investigate the gamma-exponential frailty model with $\kappa > 2$ in this section. Read Appendix B about gamma-exponential frailty model.

Using these results, we can show that

$$E(V^{-1}) = \frac{\kappa}{\kappa - 1} \quad \text{and} \quad E(V^{-2}) = \frac{\kappa^2}{(\kappa - 1)(\kappa - 2)}. \tag{14.2}$$

Given a gamma frailty $V = v$, T_1 and T_2 have independent exponential distribution with, for $j = 1, 2$, hazard rate $v\lambda_j$, survival function

$$S_j(t|v) = P(T_j \geq t|V = v) = \exp(-v\lambda_j t)$$

and, for $l = 1, 2$,

$$E(T_j^l|v) = l(v\lambda_j)^{-l}. \tag{14.3}$$

From (14.2) and (14.3), we have

$$E(T_j) = E_V E(T_j|V) = \frac{1}{\lambda_j} E(V^{-1}) = \frac{\kappa}{\lambda_j(\kappa - 1)} \tag{14.4}$$

and

$$E(T_j^2) = E_V E(T_j^2|V) = \frac{2\kappa^2}{\lambda_j^2(\kappa \quad 1)(\kappa \quad 2)}.$$

Hence,

$$\text{var}(T_j) = \frac{\kappa^3}{\lambda_j^2(\kappa-1)^2(\kappa-2)}.$$

Given $V = v$, T_1 and T_2 are independent so that from (14.2) we have

$$E(T_1T_2|V) = E(T_1|V)E(T_2|V) = \frac{V^{-2}}{\lambda_1\lambda_2}.$$

Hence, from (14.2), we have

$$E(T_1T_2) = E_V\{E(T_1T_2|V) = \frac{\kappa^2}{\lambda_1\lambda_2(\kappa-1)(\kappa-2)}$$

and, by combining this with (14.4),

$$\text{cov}(T_1,T_2) = \frac{\kappa^2}{\lambda_1\lambda_2(\kappa-1)(\kappa-2)} - \frac{\kappa^2}{\lambda_1\lambda_2(\kappa-1)^2}$$

$$= \frac{\kappa^2}{\lambda_1\lambda_2(\kappa-1)^2(\kappa-2)}.$$

Therefore, $\rho = \text{corr}(T_1,T_2) = \text{cov}(T_1,T_2)/\sqrt{\text{var}(T_1)\text{var}(T_2)} = 1/\kappa$.

Now we derive the joint distribution function of $(T_1,...,T_m)$ to be used in sample size calculation. Given $V = v$, T_j are independent exponential random variables with hazard rate $v\lambda_j$ so that

$$S(t_1,...,t_m|v) = P(T_1 \geq t_1,...,T_m \geq t_m|v) = \exp\left(-v\sum_{j=1}^{m}\lambda_j t_j\right)$$

Hence, the joint survivor function $S(t_1,...,t_m) = P(T_1 \geq t_1,...,T_m \geq t_m)$ of $(T_1,...,T_m)$ is obtained by

$$S(t_1,...,t_m) = E_V S(t_1,...,t_m|V) = \frac{\kappa^\kappa}{\Gamma(\kappa)}\int_0^\infty v^{\kappa-1}\exp\{-(\kappa+\sum_{j=1}^{m}\lambda_j t_j)v\}$$

$$= \left(\frac{\kappa}{\kappa+\sum_{j=1}^{m}\lambda_j t_j}\right)^\kappa. \quad (14.5)$$

The first and second moments of (T_1,T_2) can be derived directly using this (unconditional) survival function too.

NOTE: As an effort not to change the hazard rate of the exponential survival distribution, we multiply a common frailty with $E(V) = 1$ to it. However, the marginal distribution of T_j is not an exponential distribution.

Under Cluster Randomization

Given a gamma frailty $V = v$, the clustered survival times $(T_1, ..., T_m)$ have IID exponential distribution with hazard rate $v\lambda$. Then, from above results, we have

$$S(t|v) = P(T_j \geq t|V = v) = \exp(-v\lambda t)$$

$$E(T_j) = \frac{\kappa}{\lambda(\kappa - 1)}$$

$$\text{var}(T_j) = \frac{\kappa^3}{\lambda^2(\kappa - 1)^2(\kappa - 2)}$$

$$\text{cov}(T_j, T_{j'}) = \frac{\kappa^2}{\lambda^2(\kappa - 1)^2(\kappa - 2)}$$

for $j \neq j'$, and the ICC is $\rho = 1/\kappa$.

By (14.5), the joint survivor function of $(T_1, ..., T_m)$ is given as

$$S(t_1, ..., t_m) = \left(\frac{\kappa}{\kappa + \lambda \sum_{j=1}^{m} t_j}\right)^{\kappa}.$$

We generate $(T_1, ..., T_m)$ as follows.

(1) Generate $V = v$ from $\Gamma(\kappa, 1/\kappa)$ distribution, and $U_1, ..., U_2 \sim$ IID $U(0, 1)$.

(2) Generate T_j by solving $S(t|v) = U_j$ with respect to t, i.e.,

$$T_j = -\frac{\log U_j}{v\lambda}.$$

Under Subunit Randomization

Suppose that $(T_{11}, ..., T_{1,m_1}, T_{21}, ..., T_{2,m_2})$ have a gamma-exponential frailty model. Given $V = v$, T_{kj} follows exponential distribution with hazard rate $v\lambda_k$. Then, we have

$$S_k(t|v) = P(T_{kj} \geq t|V = v) = \exp(-v\lambda_k t)$$

$$E(T_{kj}) = \frac{\kappa}{\lambda_k(\kappa - 1)}$$

$$\text{var}(T_{kj}) = \frac{\kappa^3}{\lambda_k^2(\kappa - 1)^2(\kappa - 2)}$$

$$\text{cov}(T_{kj}, T_{kj'}) = \frac{\kappa^2}{\lambda_k^2(\kappa - 1)^2(\kappa - 2)}$$

for $j \neq j'$,

$$\text{cov}(T_{1j}, T_{2j'}) = \frac{\kappa^2}{\lambda_1\lambda_2(\kappa-1)^2(\kappa-2)}.$$

Hence, between arm ICC ρ_b and within arm ICC ρ_w are identical, i.e., $\rho_b = \rho_w = 1/\kappa$.

By (14.5), the joint survivor function of $(T_{11}, ..., T_{1,m_1}, T_{21}, ..., T_{2,m_2})$ is given as

$$S(t_{11}, ..., t_{1,m_1}, t_{21}, ..., t_{2,m_2}) = \left(\frac{\kappa}{\kappa + \sum_{k=1}^{2} \lambda_k \sum_{j=1}^{m_k} t_{kj}}\right)^{\kappa}.$$

We generate $(T_{11}, ..., T_{1,m_1}, T_{21}, ..., T_{2,m_2})$ as follows.

(1) Generate $V = v$ from $\Gamma(\kappa, 1/\kappa)$ distribution, and $(U_{11}, \ldots, U_{1,m_1}, U_{21}, ..., U_{2,m_2}) \sim$ IID $U(0, 1)$.

(2) Generate T_{kj} by solving $S_k(t|v) = U_{kj}$ with respect to t, i.e.,

$$T_{jk} = -\frac{\log U_{kj}}{v\lambda_k}.$$

References

Clayton D, Cuzick J. Multivariate generalizations of the proportional Hazards model. Journal of the Royal Statistical Society, Series A (General) 1985;148(2): 82–108.

Lee JY, Kim J, Jung SH. Bayesian analysis of paired survival data using a bivariate exponential distribution. Lifetime Data Analysis 2007; 13: 119–137.

Moran PAP. Testing for correlation between non-negative variates. Biometrika 1967; 54: 385–394.

15

Cox's Regression for Clustered Survival Data

Cox's (1972) proportional hazards model (PHM) has been used widely in the analysis of independent survival data because of its easy estimation, robustness, and high efficiency. Lee, Wei, and Amato (1992) extended Cox's (1972) PHM to clustered survival data. In this chapter, we briefly review Lee, Wei, and Amato (1992). In a clinical trial collecting clustered survival data, the primary analysis may be to compare treatment arms using the rank tests that are investigated in Chapters 10–12 as a univariate analysis. In a secondary analysis, however, we often compare treatment arms adjusting for other prognostic factors, such as baseline characteristics, using a regression method.

In a clinical trial to evaluate the drug sorbinil, an aldose reductase inhibitor, for diabetic retinopathy, 497 patients with insulin-dependent diabetes mellitus were randomly assigned to take oral sorbinil or placebo (Sorbinil Retinopathy Trials Research Group, 1993). One of the endpoints in the study was the time to occurrence of severe visual loss in each eye (subunits). Since the oral treatment affects the whole body of the patient (cluster) and the two eyes share the physiology of each patient, the observations from the two eyes of each patient are likely to be dependent. This study is a cluster randomization trial.

Another example is from the Diabetic Retinopathy Study by the National Eye Institute to evaluate the photocoagulation treatment for proliferative diabetic retinopathy (Diabetic Retinopathy Study Research Group 1981). Treatment by photocoagulation was randomly assigned to one eye (subunit) of each patient (cluster), with the other eye serving as an untreated control. One of the study objectives was to investigate whether the time to severe visual loss of the treated eye is longer than that of the control. Since the two eyes of each patient share the same physiology, the observations from the two eyes of each patient are likely to be dependent. Some of the covariates to be adjusted for are the presence or absence of macular edema of the eye, age, duration of diabetes, and the type of diabetes at the randomization. This is a typical example of a trial with subunit randomization. This study used a paired design via subunit randomization for an ethical reason. That is, in the absence of knowledge of whether treatment was beneficial or harmful, this

DOI: 10.1201/9781003221951-15

design gave each patient the best chance of retaining vision in at least one eye.

Lee et al.'s (1992) modified Cox's PHM provides a multivariate analysis method appropriate for these trials accounting for possible dependency of survival data from subunits of each cluster.

Cox's PHM for Clustered Survival Data

Suppose that there are n independent clusters and cluster $i (= 1, ..., n)$ consists of m_i subunits. The asymptotic theory in this chapter is based on large n. For subunit j of cluster i, T_{ij} denotes the survival time which is assumed to be independent of censoring time C_{ij}. From a trial, we observe $X_{ij} = \min(T_{ij}, C_{ij})$ together with the event indicator $\delta_{ij} = I(T_{ij} \leq C_{ij})$. Let $z_{ij} = (z_{ij1}, ..., z_{ijp})^T$ denote the covariates including the treatment allocation and known prognostic factors, such as baseline characteristics. The resulting data are summarized by $\{(X_{ij}, \delta_{ij}, z_{ij}), j = 1, ..., m_i, i = 1, ..., n\}$. For subunit j of cluster i, let $Y_{ij}(t) = I(X_{ij} \geq t)$ and $N_{ij}(t) = \delta_{ij} I(X_{ij} \leq t)$ denote the at-risk and event processes, respectively.

Given z_{ij}, the marginal hazard function for T_{ij} is given as

$$\lambda_{ij}(t) = \lambda_0(t) \exp(\beta^T z_{ij}), \tag{15.1}$$

where $\beta = (\beta_1, ..., \beta_p)^T$ is the vector of regression coefficients and $\lambda_0(t)$ is the unknown baseline hazard function.

Define

$$S_0(\beta, t) = \sum_{i=1}^{n} \sum_{j=1}^{m_i} Y_{ij}(t) \exp(\beta^T z_{ij})$$

$$S_1(\beta, t) = \sum_{i=1}^{n} \sum_{j=1}^{m_i} Y_{ij}(t) z_{ij} \exp(\beta^T z_{ij})$$

and

$$S_2(\beta, t) = \sum_{i=1}^{n} \sum_{j=1}^{m_i} Y_{ij}(t) z_{ij}^{\otimes 2} \exp(\beta^T z_{ij}),$$

where $a^{\otimes 2} = aa^T$. Ignoring the intracluster dependency, the Cox's partial score function is

$$U(\beta) = \sum_{i=1}^{n} \sum_{j=1}^{m_i} \int_0^{\infty} \left\{ z_{ij} - \frac{S_1(\beta, t)}{S_0(\beta, t)} \right\} dN_{ij}(t) \tag{15.2}$$

and the partial information is

$$A(\beta) = -\frac{\partial U(\beta)}{\partial \beta} = \sum_{i=1}^{n} \sum_{j=1}^{m_i} \int_0^{\infty} \left\{ \frac{S_2(\beta, t)}{S_0(\beta, t)} - \frac{S_1(\beta, t)^{\otimes 2}}{S_0(\beta, t)^2} \right\} dN_{ij}(t).$$

The regression estimator $\hat{\beta} = (\hat{\beta}_1, ..., \hat{\beta}_p)$ of model (15.1) is the solution to $U(\beta) = 0$ that is obtained by the Newton-Raphson method, $\hat{\beta}^{(l)} = \hat{\beta}^{(l-1)} - A^{-1}(\hat{\beta}^{(l-1)})U(\hat{\beta}^{(l-1)})$, where $\hat{\beta}^{(l)}$ is the estimator at the lth iteration. Lee et al. (1992) show that $\hat{\beta} = (\hat{\beta}_1, ..., \hat{\beta}_p)$ is a consistent estimator of β. If the survival data are independent, $A^{-1}(\hat{\beta})$ is a variance estimator of $\hat{\beta}$. For clustered survival data, however, it is not a valid variance estimator of $\hat{\beta}$.

From (15.2),

$$U(\beta) = \sum_{i=1}^{n} \sum_{j=1}^{m_i} \int_0^\infty \left\{ z_{ij} - \frac{S_1(\beta, t)}{S_0(\beta, t)} \right\} dM_{ij}(t), \tag{15.3}$$

where $dM_{ij}(t) = dN_{ij}(t) - Y_{ij}(t)\exp(\beta^T z_{ij}) d\Lambda_0(t)$ and $\Lambda_0(t) = \int_0^t \lambda_0(s)ds$ is the baseline cumulative hazard function. Due to intracluster dependency, $M_{ij}(t)$ are not martingales, but $n^{-1/2}\sum_{i=1}^n \sum_{j=1}^{m_i} M_{ij}(t)$ converges to a 0-mean Gaussian process in probability. Hence, by the central limit theorem applied to (15.3), $n^{-1/2}U(\beta)$ converges to the normal distribution with mean 0 and variance V that can be consistently estimated by

$$\hat{V} = \frac{1}{n}\sum_{i=1}^{n} \hat{\epsilon}_i^{\otimes 2}$$

$\hat{\epsilon}_i = \sum_{j=1}^{m_i} \int_0^\infty \{z_{ij} - S_1(\hat{\beta}, t)/S_0(\hat{\beta}, t)\} d\hat{M}_{ij}(t)$, $d\hat{M}_{ij}(t) = dN_{ij}(t) - Y_{ij}(t)\exp(\hat{\beta}^T z_{ij}) d\hat{\Lambda}_0(t)$, and $\hat{\Lambda}_0(t) = \sum_{i=1}^n \sum_{j=1}^{m_i} \int_0^t S_0^{-1}(\hat{\beta}, s) dN_{ij}(s)$ is the Breslow's (1972) estimators of $\Lambda_0(t)$.

Since $\sqrt{n}(\hat{\beta} - \beta) = nA^{-1}(\beta)n^{-1/2}U(\beta) + o_p(1)$, $\sqrt{n}(\hat{\beta} - \beta)$ converges to the normal distribution with mean 0 and variance-covariance matrix Σ that can be consistently estimated by $\hat{\Sigma} = n^2 A^{-1}(\hat{\beta})\hat{V} A^{-1}(\hat{\beta})$.

In summary, Lee et al. (1992) consistently estimate the regression coefficients by assuming that the survival times are independent, but their variances are estimated using the generalized estimating equation method that is by Liand and Zeger (1986).

By model (15.1), the survival function $S(t|z) = P(T \geq t|z)$ of a subunit with covariate value z is given as

$$\hat{S}(t|z) = \exp\{-\hat{\Lambda}_0(t)\exp(\hat{\beta}^T z)\}.$$

The asymptotic normality of $\hat{S}(t|z)$ can be derived using the delta-method. Furthermore, the median survival time of a subunit with covariate value z can be estimated by solving the equation $\hat{S}(t|z) = 1/2$ with respect to t.

Example

Lee et al. (1992) apply the above methods to the Diabetic Retinopathy Study that was introduced above. This study enrolled $n = 742$ patients with proliferative diabetic retinopathy were enrolled in the study between 1972 and 1975. For each patient, one eye was randomized into the treatment by photocoagulation and the other to an untreated control. Three covariates are included in their analysis: $z_{ij1} = 1$ if eye j is treated by photocoagulation and 0 otherwise; $z_{ij2} = 1$ if macular edema was pre-existing in eye j at baseline and 0 otherwise; $z_{ij3} = 1$ if eye j had questionable macular edema before the study and 0 otherwise. The estimates of regression coefficients are $(\hat{\beta}_1, \hat{\beta}_2, \hat{\beta}_3) = (-0.628, -0.717, -0.343)$ and their variance estimates are $(\hat{\sigma}_1^2, \hat{\sigma}_2^2, \hat{\sigma}_3^2) = (0.012, 0.041, 0.045)$. Hence, the standardized test statistics are $(Z_1, Z_2, Z_3) = (-5.733, -3.541, -1.617)$ and two-sided p-values are $(p_1, p_2, p_3) = (0.000, 0.000, 0.106)$. Note that photocoagulation is significantly superior to no treatment and patients with pre-existing macular edema at baseline have longer failure time.

References

Breslow NE. Discussion of the paper by D. R. Cox. Journal of Royal Statistical Society B 1972; 34: 216–217.

Cox DR. Regression models and life-tables (with discussion). Journal of Royal Statistical Society B 1972; 34: 187–220.

Diabetic Retinopathy Study Research Group. Diabetic retinopathy study. Investigative Ophthalmology and Visual Science 1981; 21(2): 149–226.

Lee EW, Wei LJ, Amato DA. (1992). Cox-type regression analysis for large numbers of small groups of correlated failure time observations. In Survival Analysis: State of the Art, J. P. Klein and P. K. Goel (eds), 237–247. Dordrecht: Kluwer.

Liang KY and Zeger SL. Longitudinal data analysis using generalized linear models. Biometrika 1986; 73: 13–22.

Sorbinil Retinopathy Trial Research Group. The Sorbinil Retinopathy Trial: Neuropathy results. Neurology 1993; 43: 1141–1149.

16

Design and Analysis of Individually Randomized Group-Treatment Trials

Individually randomized group-treatment (IRGT) trials are composite of traditional independent subject randomization and cluster randomization. In an IRGT trial, the control arm is to treat patients individually, whereas the experimental arm is to treat patients using a group training, education, or treatment to increase the treatment effect by close interactions with patients. As a result, the outcome data of the control arm are independent as in traditional trials, but those in the experimental arm are correlated within each group, called cluster as in cluster randomization trials. Hence, two arms in IRGT trials have different dependency structures. Unlike standard cluster randomization trials, clusters of IRGT trials are usually organized after randomization. But statistically, they have identical statistical issues between the two types of trials, i.e., accounting for the dependency within each cluster.

The number of IRGT trials is growing (Pals et al. 2008), but design and analysis methods for them are still in need. Turner et al. (2017a,b) discuss statistical issues and analysis methods for IRGT trials that have been developed by then. Roberts and Roberts (2005) propose a sample size method for continuous outcomes and Moerbeek and Wong (2008) propose sample size methods for IRGT trials with binary and continuous outcome variables, and Wang, Turner, and Li (2024) propose a sample size method for IRGT trials collecting longitudinal data. These methods assume constant cluster sizes. Candel and Van Breukelen (2009) investigate the relative efficiency of test statistics between constant cluster size cases and varying cluster size cases based on a random effect model that can cover continuous outcomes and binary outcomes for both cluster randomization and subunit randomization trials, but do not propose a sample size formula for these types of trials.

Oftentimes in IRGT trials, the number of clusters is given in advance and cluster sizes grow during accrual period. Even when we assume identical cluster sizes at the time of study design, the attained cluster sizes may vary-due to the random allocation to different clusters post-randomization. As shown by Candel and Van Breukelen (2009), the power of the statistical tests depends on the mean and variance of cluster size distribution for trials with clusters so that it is important to accurately reflect the expected cluster size distribution in sample size calculations.

DOI: 10.1201/9781003221951-16

Suppose that arm 1 is a control arm and arm 2 is an experimental arm. n_k patients are randomized into arm $k = (1, 2)$ and $n = n_1 + n_2$ denotes the total number of patients. Arm 2 has ν_2 clusters so that each patient in arm 2 will be assigned to one of the clusters after randomization. Let m_i denote the number of patients (subunits) assigned to cluster $i (= 1, ..., \nu_2)$, by which we have $n_2 = \sum_{i=1}^{\nu_2} m_i$. For the large sample approximation, we assume that ν_2 is large, i.e., $\nu_2/n \to \psi(> 0)$ as $n \to \infty$.

In this chapter, we discuss two-sample testing methods and their sample size calculation methods for IRGT trials with binary, continuous, or time-to-event endpoints.

IRGT Trials with Binary Data

Moerbeek and Weng Kee Wong (2008) propose analysis and sample size methods for IRGT trials with binary outcome variables. They present a generalized estimating equation (GEE, Liang and Zeger 1986) type test statistic and its sample size formula assuming that cluster sizes in arm 2 are constant. In this section, we consider the same type of test statistic and present its sample size formula when cluster sizes are either constant or random.

Modified Chi-Squared Test

Suppose that we have observations $(x_{11}, ..., x_{1,n_1})$ from subjects in arm 1, and $\{(x_{2i1}, ..., x_{2i,m_i}), i = 1, ..., \nu_2\}$ from subjects in arm 2 with $p_1 = E(x_{1i})$ and $p_2 = E(x_{2i'j})$. Consistent estimators of the expected values are given as

$$\hat{p}_1 = \frac{1}{n_1} \sum_{i=1}^{n_1} x_{1i}$$

and

$$\hat{p}_2 = \frac{1}{n_2} \sum_{i=1}^{\nu_2} \sum_{j=1}^{m_i} x_{2ij}.$$

Under H_0, we have

$$\sqrt{n}(\hat{p}_1 - \hat{p}_2) = n^{-1/2} \left(\sum_{i=1}^{n_1} \epsilon_{1i} - \sum_{i=1}^{\nu_2} \epsilon_{2i} \right). \tag{16.1}$$

where

$$\epsilon_{1i} = \frac{n}{n_1}(x_{1i} - p_1)$$

and

$$\epsilon_{2ij} = \frac{n}{n_2} \sum_{j=1}^{m_i} (x_{2ij} - p_2).$$

Since $\epsilon_{11}, ..., \epsilon_{1,n_1}, \epsilon_{21}, ..., \epsilon_{2,\nu_2}$ are independent 0-mean random variables, by the central limit theorem, $\sqrt{n}(\hat{p}_1 - \hat{p}_2)$ converges to $N(0, \sigma^2)$ under H_0. From (16.1), a consistent estimator of σ^2 is obtained by

$$\hat{\sigma}^2 = \frac{1}{n}\left(\sum_{i=1}^{n_1} \hat{\epsilon}_{1i}^2 + \sum_{i=1}^{\nu_2} \hat{\epsilon}_{1i}^2\right),$$

where

$$\hat{\epsilon}_{1i} = \frac{n}{n_1}(x_{1i} - \hat{p})$$

$$\hat{\epsilon}_{2ij} = \frac{n}{n_2}\sum_{j=1}^{m_i}(x_{2ij} - \hat{p})$$

and $\hat{p} = (n_1\hat{p}_1 + n_2\hat{p}_2)/n$. That is,

$$\hat{\sigma}^2 = \frac{n}{n_1^2}\sum_{i=1}^{n_1}(x_{1i} - \hat{p})^2 + \frac{n}{n_2^2}\sum_{i=1}^{\nu_2}\{\sum_{j=1}^{m_i}(x_{2ij} - \hat{p})\}^2. \tag{16.2}$$

A modified χ^2-test statistic is given as Z^2 with

$$Z = \frac{\sqrt{n}(\hat{p}_1 - \hat{p}_2)}{\hat{\sigma}}.$$

We reject H_0 if $|Z| > z_{1-\alpha}$, where $z_{1-\alpha/2}$ is the $100(1 - \alpha/2)$ percentile of $N(0, 1)$ distribution.

Sample Size Calculation for the Modified Chi-Squared Test

Let $a_k = n_k/n$ denote the allocation proportion for arm k. We derive a sample size formula for the modified t-test. Let $s_k^2 = p_k(1-p_k)$, and $\text{corr}(x_{2ij}, x_{2ij'}) = \rho$ for $j \neq j'$. From (16.2), $\hat{\sigma}^2$ converges to

$$\sigma^2 = s_1^2/p_1 + s_2^2/p_2\{1 + (\bar{\bar{m}}/\bar{m} - 1)\rho\}.$$

Furthermore, under H_1, the expected value of $\hat{p}_k$ is p_k. Hence, for given n, the power of the modified t-test is given as

$$\begin{aligned} 1 - \beta =& P(|Z| \geq z_{1-\alpha/2}|H_1) \\ \approx& P\left(\frac{\sqrt{n}\{(\hat{p}_1 - \hat{p}_2) - (p_1 - p_2)\}}{\sigma} \geq z_{1-\alpha/2} - \frac{\sqrt{n}(p_1 - p_2)}{\sigma}|H_1\right). \end{aligned} \tag{16.3}$$

Since $\sqrt{n}((\hat{p}_1 - \hat{p}_2 - p_1 + p_2)/\sigma$ is $N(0, 1)$ under H_1, from (16.3), we have

$$1 - \beta = \bar{\Phi}\left(z_{1-\alpha/2} - \frac{\sqrt{n}(p_1 - p_2)}{\sigma}\right). \tag{16.4}$$

By solving (16.4) with respect to n, we obtain the sample size

$$n = \frac{\sigma^2(z_{1-\alpha/2} + z_{1-\beta})^2}{(p_1 - p_2)^2}.$$

IRGT Trials with Continuous Data

Moerbeek and Weng Kee Wong (2008) propose analysis and sample size methods for IRGT trials with continuous outcome variables. They present a GEE type test statistic and its sample size formula assuming that cluster sizes in arm 2 are constant. In this section, we consider the same type of test statistic and present its sample size formula when cluster sizes are either constant or random.

Modified t-Test

Suppose that we have observations $(x_{11}, ..., x_{1,n_1})$ from subjects in arm 1, and $\{(x_{2i1}, ..., x_{2i,m_i}), i = 1, ..., \nu_2\}$ from subjects in arm 2 with $\mu_1 = E(x_{1i})$ and $\mu_2 = E(x_{2i'j})$. Consistent estimators of the expected values are given as

$$\hat{\mu}_1 = \frac{1}{n_1}\sum_{i=1}^{n_1} x_{1i}$$

and

$$\hat{\mu}_2 = \frac{1}{n_2}\sum_{i=1}^{\nu_2}\sum_{j=1}^{m_i} x_{2ij}.$$

Under H_0, we have

$$\sqrt{n}(\hat{\mu}_1 - \hat{\mu}_2) = n^{-1/2}\left(\sum_{i=1}^{n_1}\epsilon_{1i} - \sum_{i=1}^{\nu_2}\epsilon_{1i}\right), \tag{16.5}$$

where

$$\epsilon_{1i} = \frac{n}{n_1}(x_{1i} - \mu_1)$$

and

$$\epsilon_{2ij} = \frac{n}{n_2}\sum_{j=1}^{m_i}(x_{2ij} - \mu_2).$$

Since $\epsilon_{11}, ..., \epsilon_{1,n_1}, \epsilon_{21}, ..., \epsilon_{2,\nu_2}$ are independent 0-mean random variables, by the central limit theorem, $\sqrt{n}(\hat{\mu}_1 - \hat{\mu}_2)$ converges to $N(0, \sigma^2)$ under H_0. From (16.5), a consistent estimator of σ^2 is obtained by

$$\hat{\sigma}^2 = \frac{1}{n}\left(\sum_{i=1}^{n_1}\hat{\epsilon}_{1i}^2 + \sum_{i=1}^{\nu_2}\hat{\epsilon}_{2i}^2\right),$$

where

$$\hat{\epsilon}_{1i} = \frac{n}{n_1}(x_{1i} - \hat{\mu})$$

$$\hat{\epsilon}_{2i} = \frac{n}{n_2}\sum_{j=1}^{m_i}(x_{2ij} - \hat{\mu})$$

and $\hat{\mu} = (n_1\hat{\mu}_1 + n_2\hat{\mu}_2)/n$. That is,

$$\hat{\sigma}^2 = \frac{n}{n_1^2}\sum_{i=1}^{n_1}(x_{1i} - \hat{\mu})^2 + \frac{n}{n_2^2}\sum_{i=1}^{\nu_2}\{\sum_{j=1}^{m_i}(x_{2ij} - \hat{\mu})\}^2. \tag{16.6}$$

A modified t-test statistic is given as

$$Z = \frac{\sqrt{n}(\hat{\mu}_1 - \hat{\mu}_2)}{\hat{\sigma}}.$$

We reject H_0 if $|Z| > z_{1-\alpha}$.

Sample Size Calculation for the Modified t-Test

We derive a sample size formula for the modified t-test. Let $p_k = n_k/n$ denote the allocation proportion for arm k, $\text{var}(x_{1i}) = \text{var}(x_{2i'j}) = s^2$, and $\text{corr}(x_{2ij}, x_{2ij'}) = \rho$ for $j \neq j'$. From (16.6), $\hat{\sigma}^2$ converges to

$$\sigma^2 = s^2\{1 + p_1(\bar{\bar{m}}/\bar{m} - 1)\rho\}/(p_1p_2).$$

Furthermore, under H_1, the expected value of $\hat{\mu}_k$ is μ_k. Hence, for given n, the power of the modified t-test is given as

$$\begin{aligned} 1 - \beta =& P(|Z| \geq z_{1-\alpha/2}|H_1) \\ \approx& P\left(\frac{\sqrt{n}\{(\hat{\mu}_1 - \hat{\mu}_2) - (\mu_1 - \mu_2)\}}{\sigma} \geq z_{1-\alpha/2} - \frac{\sqrt{n}(\mu_1 - \mu_2)}{\sigma}|H_1\right) \end{aligned} \tag{16.3}$$

Since $\sqrt{n}(\hat{\mu}_1 - \hat{\mu}_2 - \mu_1 + \mu_2)/\sigma$ is $N(0,1)$ under H_1, from (16.3), we have

$$1 - \beta = \bar{\Phi}\left(z_{1-\alpha/2} - \frac{\sqrt{n}(\mu_1 - \mu_2)}{\sigma}\right). \tag{16.7}$$

By solving (16.7) with respect to n, we obtain the sample size

$$n = \frac{\sigma^2(z_{1-\alpha/2} + z_{1-\beta})^2}{(\mu_1 - \mu_2)^2}.$$

IRGT Trials with Survival Data

In this section, we propose a modified log-rank test and its sample size calculation method for IRGT trials with time-to-event endpoints by modifying the log-rank test of Jung and Jeong (2003) and its sample size method of Li and Jung (2020) that are reviewed in Chapter 11. The proposed log-rank test is so robust that it does not require any assumptions except that survival time and censoring time are independent for each individual. The censoring times of subjects in each cluster of experimental arm may be correlated or even common. Cluster sizes may be either constant or random. The sample size of the log-rank test modified for IRGT trials depends on the marginal survival and censoring distributions of two arms, bivariate survival and censoring distributions and cluster size distribution of experimental arm. The bivariate censoring distribution can be fully specified by the univariate censoring distribution for popular trial designs. The sample size method allows the cases where the number of clusters is given and cluster sizes grow during accrual period, or cluster sizes are given (whether constant or random) and the number of clusters grows over accrual period. We also propose optimal allocation proportions minimizing the total sample size in the presence of intracluster dependency or the total cost when two arms have different cost for treatment per subject. Simulations are conducted to evaluate the performance of the proposed testing and sample size methods. The sample size method is demonstrated with an example mimicking a real IRGT trial.

Rank Test for IRGT

Suppose that arm 1 is a control arm and arm 2 is an experimental arm, n_k patients are randomized into arm $k = (1, 2)$, and $n = n_1 + n_2$ denotes the total number of patients. Let $p_k = n_k/n$ denote the allocation proportion for arm k. Arm 2 has ν_2 clusters so that each patient in arm 2 will be assigned to one of the clusters after randomization. Let m_i denote the number of patients assigned to cluster $i(= 1, ..., \nu_2)$, by which we have $n_2 = \sum_{i=1}^{\nu_2} m_i$. For the large sample approximation, we assume that ν_2 is large, i.e., $\nu_2 = O_p(n)$.

$T_{k1}, ..., T_{k,n_k}$ are survival times of patient i in arm k with survival function (SF) $S_k(t) = P(T_{kj} \geq t)$ and cumulative hazard function $\Lambda_k(t) = -\log S_k(t)$. We want to test $H_0 : \Lambda_1(t) = \Lambda_2(t)$ against $H_1 : \Lambda_1(t) \neq \Lambda_2(t)$.

Survival times are subject to censoring so that we observe (X_{ki}, δ_{ki}) from patient i in arm k, where X_{ki} is the minimum of survival time T_{ki} and censoring time C_{ki} and δ_{ki} is the event indicator taking 1 if the patient has an event and 0 otherwise. We assume that censoring times are independent of survival times.

For patient i in arm k, let $N_{ki}(t) = \delta_{ki} I(X_{ki} \leq t)$ and $Y_{ki}(t) = I(X_{ki} \geq t)$ denote the event and at-risk processes, respectively, $N_k(t) = \sum_{i=1}^{n_k} N_{ki}(t)$,

$N(t) = N_1(t) + N_2(t)$, $Y_k(t) = \sum_{i=1}^{n_k} Y_{ki}(t)$, and $Y(t) = Y_1(t) + Y_2(t)$. The weighted rank statistic for testing $H_0 : \Lambda_1(t) = \Lambda_2(t)$ against $H_1 : \Lambda_1(t) \neq \Lambda_2(t)$ is given as

$$W = \sqrt{n} \int_0^\infty H(t)\{d\hat{\Lambda}_1(t) - d\hat{\Lambda}_2(t)\}, \tag{16.8}$$

where $\hat{\Lambda}_k(t) = \int_0^t Y_k^{-1}(s)dN_k(s)$ is the Nelson-Aalen estimator (Nelson 1969, Aalen 1978) of $\Lambda_k(t)$ and $H(t)$ is a predictable process of bounded variation that is uniformly convergent to a square integrable function $h(t)$. For example, $H(t) = n^{-1}Y_1(t)Y_2(t)/Y(t)$ for the log-rank statistic (Peto and Peto 1972), $H(t) = n^{-2}Y_1(t)Y_2(t)$ for the Gehan-Wilcoxon test (Gehan 1965), and $H(t) = n^{-1}\hat{S}^-(t)Y_1(t)Y_2(t)/Y(t)$ for the Prentice-Wilcoxon test (Prentice 1978), where $Y(t) = Y_1(t) + Y_2(t)$ and $\hat{S}^-(t)$ is the left-continuous version of the Kaplan-Meier (1958) estimate from the pooled sample $\{(X_{kj}, \delta_{kj}), j = 1, ..., n_k, k = 1, 2\}$. When individuals within clusters in arm 2 are independent, the asymptotic distribution of the test statistics is well developed, refer to Gill (1980) and Fleming and Harrington (2011).

Since the patients of arm 2 are clustered after randomization, their survival times will be dependent within each cluster, whereas those in arm 1 stay independent. In order to account for this, we change the notations for arm 2 patients slightly. Let (X_{2ij}, δ_{2ij}) denote the survival data for patient $j(= 1, ..., m_i)$ in cluster $i(= 1, ..., \nu_2)$ of arm 2, and $N_{2ij}(t)$ and $Y_{2ij}(t)$ are redefined from $N_{2i'}(t)$ and $Y_{2i'}$ accordingly. By the new arrangement, we have $N_2(t) = \sum_{i=1}^{\nu_2}\sum_{j=1}^{m_i} N_{2ij}(t)$ and $Y_2(t) = \sum_{i=1}^{\nu_2}\sum_{j=1}^{m_i} Y_{2ij}(t)$.

Under H_0, W is expressed as

$$W = \sqrt{n}\{\sum_{i=1}^{n_1}\int_0^\infty H(t)Y_1^{-1}(t)dM_{1i}(t) - \sum_{i=1}^{\nu_2}\int_0^\infty H(t)Y_2^{-1}(t)dM_{2i}(t)\},$$

where $M_{1i}(t) = \int_0^t \{dN_{1j}(t) - Y_{1j}(t)d\Lambda_1(t)\}$, $M_{2i}(t) = \sum_{j=1}^{m_i} M_{2ij}(t)$, and $M_{2ij}(t) = \int_0^t \{dN_{2ij}(t) - Y_{2ij}(t)d\Lambda_2(t)\}$.

Let $G(t) = P(C_{ki} \geq t)$ denote the SF of the censoring variable. Then, $n_k^{-1}Y_k(t)$ and $H(t)$ uniformly converge to $y_k(t) = S_k(t)G(t)$ and $h(t)$, respectively. Read Ying and Wei (1994) about the uniform convergence of $n_2^{-1}Y_2(t)$ with clustered data. Hence, under H_0, we have

$$\begin{aligned} W &= \frac{1}{\sqrt{n}}\left\{\sum_{i=1}^{n_1}\int_0^\infty \frac{h(t)}{p_1 y_1(t)} dM_{1i}(t) - \sum_{i=1}^{\nu_2}\int_0^\infty \frac{h(t)}{p_2 y_2(t)} dM_{2i}(t)\right\} + o_p(1) \\ &= \frac{1}{\sqrt{n}}\left(\sum_{i=1}^{n_1}\epsilon_{1i} - \sum_{i=1}^{\nu_2}\epsilon_{1i}\right), \end{aligned}$$

where

$$\epsilon_{ki} = \int_0^\infty \frac{h(t)}{p_k y_k(t)} dM_{ki}.$$

As in Appendix A, under H_0, W is asymptotically normal with mean 0 and variance σ^2 that can be consistently estimated by

$$\hat{\sigma}^2 = n^{-1}\left(\sum_{i=1}^{n_1}\hat{\epsilon}_{1i}^2 + \sum_{i=1}^{\nu_2}\hat{\epsilon}_{2i}\right)^2,$$

where $\hat{\epsilon}_{ki}$ are obtained from $\hat{\epsilon}_{ki}$ by replacing $h(t)$, $p_k y_k(t)$, and $\Lambda_k(t)$ with $H(t)$, $n^{-1}Y_k(t)$, and $\hat{\Lambda}(t) = \int_0^t Y^{-1}(t)dN(t)$, the Nelson-Aalen (Nelson 1969; Aalen 1978) estimator from the pooled data, respectively. We reject H_0 if $|W|/\hat{\sigma} > z_{1-\alpha/2}$, where $z_{1-\alpha/2}$ is the $100(1-\alpha/2)$ percentile of $N(0,1)$ distribution.

Sample Size Calculation for the Log-Rank Test

We derive a sample size formula for the log-rank test with $H(t) = Y_1(t)Y_2(t)/\{nY(t)\}$, i.e.,

$$W = \frac{1}{\sqrt{n}}\int_0^\infty \left\{\frac{Y_2(t)}{Y(t)}dN_1(t) - \frac{Y_1(t)}{Y(t)}dN_2(t)\right\}.$$

Sample size formula for other weighted rank tests can be similarly derived.

The power of the log-rank test for IRGT trials depends the distribution of cluster sizes m_i in arm 2 so that we have to specify the cluster size distribution for a sample size calculation. Cluster sizes m_i in arm 2 may be either random or constant. Let $\bar{m} = E(m_i)$ and $\bar{\bar{m}} = E(m_i^2)$ denote the first and second moments, respectively, of cluster size distribution. If cluster sizes are constant with $m_i = m$, then we have $\bar{m} = m$ and $\bar{\bar{m}} = m^2$. Note that $n_2/\nu_2 - \nu_2^{-1}\sum_{i=1}^{\nu_2} m_i$ converges to $\bar{m}$.

For a sample size formula of W, we need to derive the distribution of W under $H_1 : \Lambda_1(t) \neq \Lambda_2(t)$. As shown in Appendix A, the asymptotic distribution of W under H_1 depends on the bivariate distributions of survival times and censoring times between two patients in each cluster of arm 2 as well as their marginal distributions for two arms.

Suppose that, for arm $k(=1,2)$, patients have marginal hazard function $\lambda_k(t) = \partial\Lambda_k(t)/\partial t$, and two patients in each cluster of arm 2 have a bivariate SF

$$S_2(t_1,t_2) = P(T_{2ij} \geq t_1, T_{2ij'} \geq t_2)$$

and joint probability density function $f_2(t_1,t_2) = \partial^2 S_2(t_1,t_2)/\partial t_1\partial t_2$. Further, for arm 2, we define the joint hazard function

$$\lambda_2(t_1,t_2) = f_2(t_1,t_2)/S_2(t_1,t_2)$$

and two conditional hazard functions

$$\lambda_{2(1|2)}(t_1,t_2) = \lim_{\epsilon\to 0}\frac{P(t_1 \leq T_{2ij} < t_1+\epsilon, T_{2ij'} \geq t_2)}{P(T_{2ij} \geq t_1, T_{2ij'} \geq t_2)} = -\frac{\partial S_2(t_1,t_2)/\partial t_1}{S_2(t_1,t_2)}$$

and

$$\lambda_{2(2|1)}(t_1,t_2)=\lim_{\epsilon\to 0}\frac{P(T_{2ij}\geq t_1, t_2\leq T_{2ij'}<t_2+\epsilon)}{P(T_{2ij}\geq t_1, T_{2ij'}\geq t_2)}=-\frac{\partial S_2(t_1,t_2)/\partial t_2}{S_2(t_1,t_2)}$$

for $j\neq j'$. For two subunits $j\neq j'$ in a cluster of arm 2, let $G(t_1,t_2)=P(C_{2ij}\geq t_1, C_{2ij'}\geq t_2)$ denote the bivariate SF of the clustered censoring times.

As $n\to\infty$, $\nu_2^{-1}\sum_{i=1}^{\nu_2}m_i$ and $\nu_2^{-1}\sum_{i=1}^{\nu_2}m_i^2$ converges to $\bar{m}$ and $\bar{\bar{m}}$, respectively. From Appendix A, under H_1, W is asymptotically normal with mean $\omega\sqrt{n}$ and variance

$$\sigma^2=\sigma_1^2+\sigma_2^2+(\bar{\bar{m}}/\bar{m}-1)c_2=\sigma_1^2+\sigma_2^2\{1+(\bar{\bar{m}}/\bar{m}-1)\rho\},$$

where

$$\omega=p_1p_2\int_0^\infty\frac{S_1(t)S_2(t)G(t)}{p_1S_1(t)+p_2S_2(t)}\{d\Lambda_1(t)-d\Lambda_2(t)\}$$

$$\sigma_k^2=p_kp_{k-3}^2\int_0^\infty\frac{S_k(t)S_{3-k}(t)^2G(t)}{\{p_1S_1(t)+p_2S_2(t)\}^2}d\Lambda_k(t)$$

$$c_2=p_1^2p_2\int_0^\infty\int_0^\infty\frac{S_1(t_1)S_1(t_2)S_2(t_1,t_2)G(t_1,t_2)}{\{p_1S_1(t_1)+p_2S_2(t_1)\}\{p_1S_1(t_2)+p_2S_2(t_2)\}}dA_2(t_1,t_2)$$

$$\begin{aligned}dA_2(t_1,t_2)=&\{\lambda_2(t_1,t_2)-\lambda_{2(1|2)}(t_1,t_2)\lambda_2(t_2)\\&-\lambda_{2(2|1)}(t_1,t_2)\lambda_2(t_1)+\lambda_2(t_1)\lambda_2(t_2)\}dt_1dt_2\end{aligned}$$

and

$$\rho=\frac{c_2}{\sigma_2^2}=\frac{\int_0^\infty\int_0^\infty\frac{S_1(t_1)S_1(t_2)S_2(t_1,t_2)G(t_1,t_2)}{\{p_1S_1(t_1)+p_2S_2(t_1)\}\{p_1S_1(t_2)+p_2S_2(t_2)\}}dA_2(t_1,t_2)}{\int_0^\infty\frac{S_1^2(t)S_2(t)G(t)}{\{p_1S_1(t)+p_2S_2(t)\}^2}d\Lambda_2(t)}$$

denotes the intracluster correlation coefficient (ICC) of arm 2.

Hence, the power of the log-rank test is given as

$$1-\beta=P\left(\frac{|W|}{\hat{\sigma}}\geq z_{1-\alpha/2}|H_1\right)\approx P\left(\frac{W-\omega\sqrt{n}}{\sigma}\geq z_{1-\alpha/2}-\frac{\omega\sqrt{n}}{\sigma}|H_1\right). \tag{16.9}$$

Since $(W-\omega\sqrt{n})/\sigma$ is $N(0,1)$ under H_1, from (16.9), we have

$$1-\beta=\bar{\Phi}\left(z_{1-\alpha/2}-\frac{\omega\sqrt{n}}{\sigma}\right), \tag{16.10}$$

where $\bar{\Phi}(\cdot)$ is the SF of $N(0,1)$ distribution. By solving (16.10) with respect to n, we obtain the sample size

$$n=\frac{\sigma^2(z_{1-\alpha/2}+z_{1-\beta})^2}{\omega^2}. \tag{16.11}$$

From Appendix B, under the nearby alternative hypothesis with where $S_1(t) \approx S_2(t)$, we have $\omega = p_1 p_2 d(\Delta - 1) \approx p_1 p_2 d \log \Delta$ and $\sigma^2 = p_1 p_2 d \times \text{DE}$ so that we have

$$\frac{\sigma^2}{\omega^2} = \frac{\text{DE}}{p_1 p_2 d (\log \Delta)^2}$$

and (16.11) is simplified to

$$n = \frac{(z_{1-\alpha/2} + z_{1-\beta})^2}{p_1 p_2 d (\log \Delta)^2} \text{DE}, \tag{16.12}$$

where $\Delta = \Lambda_1(t)/\Lambda_2(t)$ is the hazard ratio, $d = p_1 d_1 + p_2 d_2$, $d_k = -\int_0^\infty G(t) dS_k(t)$ is the probability that a patient in arm k experiences an event during the study, and

$$\text{DE} = 1 + p_1 \rho(\bar{\bar{m}}/\bar{m} - 1) \tag{16.13}$$

is the design effect factor indicating the increase of sample size due to the ICC in arm 2 that is expressed as

$$\rho = d^{-1} \int_0^\infty \int_0^\infty S_2(t_1, t_2) G(t_1, t_2) dA_2(t_1, t_2).$$

If the survival times of arm 2 are independent, then we have $\rho = 0$ and $\text{DE} = 1$ so that $D = n \times d$ in (16.12) is reduced to the formula for required number of events by Schoenfeld (1983) for the log-rank test with independent survival data. Furthermore, the design effect for CRTs $\text{DE}_c = 1 + \rho(\bar{\bar{m}}/\bar{m} - 1)$ by Li and Jung (2020) is larger than that of IRGT trials (16.13) so that IRGT trials are more powerful than CRTs.

When n patients are recruited, the last cluster of arm 2 may not have been filled up yet. In this case, we propose to randomize patients between two arms until the last cluster of arm 2 is filled in. In (16.12), the expected number of clusters in arm 2 is $p_2[n/\bar{m}]$, where $[x]$ is the round-up of x. By rounding up the expected number of clusters in arm 2, the total number of patients randomized is likely to be slightly larger than n calculated by (16.12).

Distributional Assumptions for Sample Size Calculation

Note that the sample size of the log-rank test modified for IRGT trials depends on the bivariate distributions of censoring and survival times, and cluster size distribution of arm 2. For IRGT trials, however, the bivariate censoring distribution function can be fully specified by its univariate distribution function as described below. In this section, we consider some survival and censoring distributions for sample size calculations.

Censoring Distribution

In IRGT trials, patients are randomized between two arms, and only those randomized into arm 2 will be clustered for treatment. In this sense, whichever arm they are assigned to, all patients are recruited independently so that we have $G(t_1, t_2) = G(t_1)G(t_2)$ if there are no loss to follow-up (i.e., administrative censoring only) or dependent loss to follow-up within each cluster. If there exists loss to follow-up, however, the censoring times of patients in arm 2 may be possibly correlated within each cluster. If it is the case, we can model the bivariate censoring distribution for arm 2 accounting for the expected cluster-specific loss to follow-up at the study design stage. In this chapter, we consider administrative censoring only so that $G(t_1, t_2) = G(t_1)G(t_2)$ for arm 2 patients.

If patients are recruited with a constant rate over an accrual period a and followed for additional period b after completion of accrual, then the censoring distribution is $U(b, a + b)$ so that we have

$$G(t) = I(t < a + b) - \frac{t - b}{a} I(b \le t < a + b).$$

Survival Distribution

For arm 1, we assume exponential distribution with hazard rate λ_1. We may use any multivariate survival distribution for arm 2 for sample size calculation. But, for sample size calculations in this chapter, we consider the Clayton and Cuzick's (1985) frailty model with an exponential marginal distribution whose bivariate SF is given as

$$S_2(t_1, t_2) = \{\exp(\lambda_2 t_1/\theta) + \exp(\lambda_2 t_2/\theta) - 1\}^{-\theta},$$

where $\theta = 1/(2\tau) - 1/2$ and $\tau \in [0, 1]$ is the Kendall's tau, 0 meaning no relationship and 1 meaning a perfect relationship between paired survival times. For this joint survival distribution, we have the joint hazard function

$$\lambda_2(t_1, t_2) = \frac{\lambda_2^2(1 + 1/\theta)e^{(t_1+t_2)\lambda_2/\theta}}{(e^{\lambda_2 t_1/\theta} + e^{\lambda_2 t_2/\theta} - 1)^2}$$

and two conditional hazard functions

$$\lambda_{2(1|2)}(t_1, t_2) = \frac{\lambda_2 e^{\lambda_2 t_1/\theta}}{e^{\lambda_2 t_1/\theta} + e^{\lambda_2 t_2/\theta} - 1}$$

$$\lambda_{2(2|1)}(t_1, t_2) = \frac{\lambda_2 e^{\lambda_2 t_2/\theta}}{e^{\lambda_2 t_1/\theta} + e^{\lambda_2 t_2/\theta} - 1}$$

and

$$dA_2(t_1, t_2) = \lambda_2^2 \left\{ \frac{(1 + 1/\theta)e^{(t_1+t_2)\lambda_2/\theta}}{(e^{\lambda_2 t_1/\theta} + e^{\lambda_2 t_2/\theta} - 1)^2} - \frac{e^{\lambda_2 t_1/\theta} + e^{\lambda_2 t_2/\theta}}{e^{\lambda_2 t_1/\theta} + e^{\lambda_2 t_2/\theta} - 1} + 1 \right\} dt_1 dt_2. \tag{16.14}$$

Hence, for the Clayton and Cuzick's model with an exponential marginal distribution and independent $U(b, a+b)$ censoring assumption, we have

$$\omega = p_1 p_2(\lambda_1 - \lambda_2) \int_0^{a+b} \frac{e^{-(\lambda_1+\lambda_2)t}(1 - a^{-1}[t-b]_+)}{p_1 e^{-\lambda_1 t} + p_2 e^{-\lambda_2 t}} dt$$

$$\sigma_k^2 = p_k p_{k-3}^2 \lambda_k \int_0^{a+b} \frac{e^{-(\lambda_k+2\lambda_{3-k})t}(1 - a^{-1}[t-b]_+)}{(p_1 e^{-\lambda_1 t} + p_2 e^{-\lambda_2 t})^2} dt$$

and

$$c_2 = p_1^2 p_2 \int_0^{a+b} \int_0^{a+b} \frac{e^{-\lambda_1(t_1+t_2)}\{e^{\lambda_2 t_1/\theta} + e^{\lambda_2 t_2/\theta} - 1\}^{-\theta}}{(p_1 e^{-\lambda_1 t_1} + p_2 e^{-\lambda_2 t_1})(p_1 e^{-\lambda_1 t_2} + p_2 e^{-\lambda_2 t_2})}$$

$$\times (1 - a^{-1}[t_1 - b]_+)(1 - a^{-1}[t_2 - b]_+) dA_2(t_1, t_2)$$

for formula (16.11), and

$$d_k = 1 - (1 - e^{-a\lambda_k}) \frac{e^{-b\lambda_k}}{a\lambda_k}$$

and $\rho = c_2/d$ with

$$c_2 = p_1^2 p_2 \int_0^{a+b} \int_0^{a+b} \frac{(1 - a^{-1}[t_1 - b]_+)(1 - a^{-1}[t_2 - b]_+)}{\{\exp(\lambda_2 t_1/\theta) + \exp(\lambda_2 t_2/\theta) - 1\}^{\theta}} dA_2(t_1, t_2)$$

for formula (16.12). Here, $[x]_+ = x \times I(x > 0)$ and $dA_2(t_1, t_2)$ in (16.14) is used for the both sample size formulas.

When Number of Clusters is Given

So far, we have assumed that clusters and their subunits are recruited over accrual period a. Oftentimes in an IRGT trial, however, all of clusters are recruited before opening the trial so that number of clusters ν_2 is predetermined together with their relative sizes. Furthermore, it is easier to estimate the accrual rate r for a new trial based on the number of patients who have visited the clinics participating in the trial recently, rather than to specify an accrual period a. Let γ_i denote the relative size of cluster $i(= 1, ..., \nu_2)$ with $\sum_{i=1}^{\nu_2} \gamma_i = 1$. In this case, $p_k r$ patients will be randomized into arm k during a unit time of accrual period. And, $p_2 r$ patients of arm 2 will be randomly allocated to ν_2 clusters with the proportions of γ_i per unit time period so that accrual rate of cluster i in arm 2 is $r_i = p_2 r \gamma_i$. So, for an accrual period a, the number of patients in arm 1 will be $n_1 = p_1 a r$ and the number of patients in cluster i of arm 2 will be a function of a given as $m_i(a) = [a \times r_i] = [p_2 a r \gamma_i]$ so that

$$\bar{m}(a) = \nu_2^{-1} \sum_{i=1}^{\nu_2} m_i(a) = \frac{p_2 a r}{\nu_2}$$

and

$$\bar{\bar{m}}(a) = \nu_2^{-1}\sum_{i=1}^{\nu_2} m_i^2(a) = \frac{p_2^2 a^2 r^2 \sum_{i=1}^{\nu_2}\gamma_i^2}{\nu_2}.$$

Also, in the left hand size of (16.12), $n \approx ar$, and $d = d(a)$ and $\rho = \rho(a)$ are functions of unknown parameter a. By plugging these functions of a in (16.12), we have

$$a \times r = \frac{(z_{1-\alpha/2} + z_{1-\beta})^2}{p_1 p_2 d(a)(\log\Delta)^2}\text{DE}(a), \tag{16.15}$$

where $\text{DE}(a) = 1 + p_1\rho(a)\{\bar{\bar{m}}(a)/\bar{m}(a) - 1\}$. Note that, in $\text{DE}(a)$, $\bar{\bar{m}}(a)/\bar{m}(a) = p_2 ar\sum_{i=1}^{\nu_2}\gamma_i^2$. The required accrual period $a = a^*$ is obtained by solving equation (16.15), and the total number of patients is $n = a^* \times r$. By rounding up $m_i(a)$ values to $\lceil p_2 ar\gamma_i \rceil$, the final sample size may be slightly increased.

Optimal Designs

One may want to find $p = p_1$ minimizing the total sample size n. In (16.12), sample size n depends on $p = p_1$ through

$$Q_1(p) = \frac{1 + p\rho(\bar{\bar{m}}/\bar{m} - 1)}{p(1-p)}.$$

In fact, $d = pd_1 + (1-p)d_2$ in (16.12) also depends on p, but $d_1 \approx d_2$ under the nearby alternative hypothesis so that d is approximately free of p. By some simple calculations, we find that $Q_1(p)$ is minimized at

$$p = \frac{-1 + \sqrt{1 + \rho(\bar{\bar{m}}/\bar{m} - 1)}}{\rho(\bar{\bar{m}}/\bar{m} - 1)}. \tag{16.16}$$

As $p = p_1$ changes, however, d and ρ changes a little so that the p value minimizing n is slightly different from that given in (16.16). It is easy to numerically find p minimizing n directly without any approximation.

On the other hand, the cost per patient may be different between two arms. In this case, we may want to find the allocation proportion $p = p_1$ minimizing the total cost for the study. Let η_k denote the cost per patient for arm k and $\eta = \eta_2/\eta_1$ the relative cost between two arms. For a given $p = p_1$, the total cost is

$$C(p) = \eta_1 n_1 + \eta_2 n_2 = \eta_1 n\{p + \eta(1-p)\}.$$

By plugging n from (16.12) in this equation and removing the factors free of p, we can find the optimal p minimizing

$$Q_2(p) = \frac{\{p + (1-p)\eta\}\{1 + p\rho(\bar{\bar{m}}/\bar{m} - 1)\}}{p(1-p)\{pd_1 + (1-p)d_2)\}}.$$

From $Q_2(p)$, we find that optimal allocation proportion $p = p_1$ depends on c, cluster size distribution, and bivariate survival distribution through ICC ρ

of arm 2. We can use a numerical method to identify the p value minimizing $Q_2(p)$.

Numerical Studies

Simulations

Our sample size formula is derived using an asymptotic theory. We conduct extensive simulations to evaluate the finite sample properties of our proposed test statistic and sample size formulas.

Survival times for arm 1 $t_{11}, ..., t_{1,n_1}$ are generated from independent exponential distribution with hazard rate λ_1, i.e., for independent and identically distributed (IID) $U(0,1)$ random variables $u_{11}, ..., n_{1,n_1}$, $t_{1i} = -\lambda_1^{-1} \log u_{1i}$.

We assume that clustered survival times for arm 2 have the Clayton and Cuzick's model with an exponential marginal distribution whose joint SF for a cluster with size m is given as

$$S_2(t_1, ..., t_m) = \left\{ \sum_{j=1}^{m} \exp(\lambda_2 t_j/\theta) - (m-1) \right\}^{-\theta}.$$

For this distribution, the conditional SF of t_j given $(t_1, ..., t_{j-1})$ is

$$S_2(t_j|t_1, ..., t_{j-1}) = \frac{\partial^{j-1} S_2(t_1, ..., t_j)}{\partial t_1 \cdots \partial t_{j-1}} \Big/ \frac{\partial^{j-1} S_2(t_1, ..., t_{j-1})}{\partial t_1 \cdots \partial t_{j-1}}$$

$$= \left(\frac{\sum_{j'=1}^{j} e^{\lambda_2 t_{j'}/\theta} - j + 1}{\sum_{j'=1}^{j-1} e^{\lambda_2 t_{j'}/\theta} - j + 2} \right)^{-\theta-j+1}.$$

For IID $U(0,1)$ random variables $u_1, .., u_m$, survival times $(t_1, ..., t_m)$ for a cluster in arm 2 are sequentially generated by solving the equations $u_1 = S_2(t_1) = \exp(-\lambda_2 t_1)$ and $u_j = S_2(t_j|t_1, ..., t_{j-1})$ for $j \geq 2$ with respect to $t_1, ..., t_m$. That is, starting from $e_0 = 0$ and $t_1 = -\lambda_2^{-1} \log u_1$, calculate e_j and then t_{j+1} using algorithm $e_j = e_{j-1} + \exp(\lambda_2 t_j/\theta)$ and

$$t_{j+1} = \frac{\theta}{\lambda_2} \log\{j - e_j + (e_j - j + 1) u_{j+1}^{-1/(\theta+j)}\}$$

for $1 \leq j \leq m-1$.

In this simulation study, we assume that cluster sizes in arm 2 are fixed at $m_i = 10$ or $m_i = 15$, or random with a discrete uniform distribution between 8 and 12, denoted as $U(8,12)$ or a discrete uniform distribution between 13 and 17, denoted as $U(13,17)$. Note that $m_i = 10$ and $U(8,12)$ have the same mean $\bar{m} = 10$, but different variances 0 and 2, respectively, and $m_i = 15$ and $U(8,12)$ have the same mean $\bar{m} = 15$, but different variances 0 and 2, respectively. We set $\alpha = 0.05$; $1 - \beta = 0.8, 0.85$, or 0.9; $p_1 = p_2 = 1/2$ for

TABLE 16.1

Table 1. Sample size n (and simulation results of empirical type error rate $\hat{\alpha}$ and power $1-\hat{\beta}$) in parenthesis) under various design settings. Cluster sizes are constant, $m_i = 10$ or 15, or random with discrete uniform distribution, $U(8,12)$ or $U(13,17)$, and the hazard rates are $\lambda_1 = \lambda_2 = 0.5$ under H_0 and $\lambda_2 = 0.3$ or 0.35 under H_1

$1-\beta$	m_i	λ_2	$\tau = 0.1$	$\tau = 0.2$	$\tau = 0.3$
0.8	10	0.3	251(0.060, 0.821)	335(0.069, 0.780)	418(0.067, 0.790)
		0.35	518(0.054, 0.797)	704(0.059, 0.806)	886(0.064, 0.801)
	$U(8,12)$	0.3	252(0.067, 0.842)	337(0.067, 0.800)	421(0.070, 0.801)
		0.35	520(0.057, 0.803)	708(0.059, 0.808)	892(0.055, 0.805)
	15	0.3	298(0.069, 0.793)	428(0.077, 0.808)	558(0.073, 0.784)
		0.35	622(0.055, 0.802)	912(0.061, 0.800)	1195(0.061, 0.794)
	$U(13,17)$	0.3	298(0.069, 0.833)	430(0.070, 0.810)	560(0.070, 0.799)
		0.35	624(0.069, 0.799)	915(0.068, 0.792)	1199(0.057, 0.787)
0.85	10	0.3	287(0.067, 0.853)	383(0.068, 0.854)	478(0.070, 0.834)
		0.35	592(0.057, 0.853)	805(0.059, 0.850)	1013(0.056, 0.839)
	$U(8,12)$	0.3	288(0.067, 0.858)	385(0.067, 0.827)	481(0.066, 0.838)
		0.35	594(0.056, 0.843)	810(0.058, 0.842)	1020(0.059, 0.832)
	15	0.3	340(0.065, 0.853)	490(0.068, 0.859)	638(0.065, 0.847)
		0.35	712(0.057, 0.841)	1044(0.057, 0.843)	1367(0.058, 0.846)
	$U(13,17)$	0.3	341(0.071, 0.860)	491(0.075, 0.834)	640(0.067, 0.846)
		0.35	713(0.062, 0.849)	1047(0.053, 0.837)	1372(0.060, 0.841)
0.9	10	0.3	336(0.065, 0.897)	448(0.062, 0.892)	560(0.064, 0.897)
		0.35	693(0.058, 0.908)	942(0.056, 0.894)	1186(0.059, 0.900)
	$U(8,12)$	0.3	337(0.062, 0.911)	451(0.067, 0.901)	563(0.066, 0.896)
		0.35	696(0.055, 0.900)	948(0.059, 0.905)	1194(0.054, 0.892)
	15	0.3	398(0.070, 0.900)	573(0.072, 0.907)	746(0.066, 0.886)
		0.35	833(0.056, 0.896)	1221(0.061, 0.895)	1600(0.049, 0.901)
	$U(13,17)$	0.3	399(0.070, 0.911)	575(0.063, 0.896)	749(0.066, 0.893)
		0.35	835 (0.057, 0.908)	1225(0.061, 0.901)	1605(0.055, 0.889)

balanced allocations; $\lambda_1 = 0.5$, and $\lambda_2 = 0.5$ under H_0 and $\lambda_2 = 0.3$ or 0.35 under H_1. Kendall's $\tau = 0.1, 0.2$, or 0.3; $(a, b) = (3, 2)$.

At first, we calculate the required sample size n using (16.12) under each design setting of $(\alpha, 1-\beta, \lambda_1, \lambda_2, \tau, p_1, a, b)$ and cluster size distribution. Once a sample size is calculated, we generate a sample of IRGT data under H_1 and apply the log-rank test (16.8) with $H(t) = Y_1(t)Y_2(t)/\{nY(t)\}$. A total of 5,000 samples are generated under the same design setting and the empirical power $1-\hat{\beta}$ is estimated by the proportion of simulation samples rejecting H_0 out of the 5,000 samples. If the empirical power is close to the nominal level, $1-\beta$, then we will conclude that the calculated power is accurately powered. In order to evaluate the finite sample performance of the log-rank statistic, we also generate 5,000 samples of size n under H_0 and estimate the empirical type I error rate $\hat{\alpha}$.

TABLE 16.2

Sample size n (and p_1) for (a) $p_1 = 1/2$, (b) for p minimizing n, and (c) to (f) for p minimizing the total cost with relative cost $c = c_2/c_1 = 5/4, 3/2, 7/4$, and 2, respectively, for $1 - \beta = 0.8$

m_i	λ_2	τ	(a)	(b) min n	(c) $c = 5/4$	(d) $c = 3/2$	(e) $c = 7/5$	(f) $c = 2$
10	0.3	0.1	251	249(0.43)	250(0.48)	252(0.51)	254(0.53)	256(0.54)
		0.2	285	325(0.39)	326(0.44)	328(0.46)	331(0.48)	335(0.50)
		0.3	351	397(0.36)	398(0.41)	401(0.43)	404(0.45)	409(0.47)
	0.35	0.1	518	508(0.43)	510(0.46)	513(0.48)	518(0.50)	524(0.52)
		0.2	629	670(0.37)	672(0.41)	678(0.44)	685(0.46)	689(0.47)
		0.3	786	819(0.34)	822(0.38)	827(0.40)	834(0.42)	843(0.44)
$U(8, 12)$	0.3	0.1	253	251(0.42)	251(0.48)	253(0.50)	256(0.53)	258(0.54)
		0.2	288	328(0.39)	330(0.44)	332(0.46)	335(0.48)	339(0.50)
		0.3	356	402(0.35)	402(0.40)	406(0.43)	410(0.45)	414(0.47)
	0.35	0.1	522	512(0.42)	514(0.46)	517(0.48)	522(0.50)	528(0.52)
		0.2	637	677(0.37)	679(0.41)	683(0.43)	689(0.45)	697(0.47)
		0.3	797	829(0.34)	832(0.38)	837(0.40)	845(0.42)	855(0.44)
15	0.3	0.1	298	292(0.40)	292(0.45)	295(0.48)	298(0.50)	301(0.52)
		0.2	360	406(0.35)	407(0.40)	410(0.43)	414(0.45)	419(0.47)
		0.3	463	513(0.33)	515(0.37)	520(0.40)	525(0.42)	531(0.44)
	0.35	0.1	622	600(0.40)	602(0.43)	606(0.45)	611(0.47)	618(0.49)
		0.2	809	841(0.33)	842(0.37)	850(0.40)	858(0.42)	868(0.44)
		0.3	1053	1063(0.30)	1066(0.34)	1072(0.36)	1081(0.38)	1093(0.40)
$U(13, 17)$	0.3	0.1	299	293(0.40)	294(0.45)	296(0.48)	299(0.50)	303(0.52)
		0.2	362	408(0.35)	409(0.40)	413(0.43)	416(0.45)	421(0.47)
		0.3	466	516(0.33)	518(0.37)	521(0.39)	528(0.42)	534(0.44)
	0.35	0.1	625	603(0.39)	605(0.43)	608(0.45)	614(0.47)	621(0.49)
		0.2	814	845(0.34)	847(0.37)	854(0.40)	862(0.42)	873(0.44)
		0.3	1060	1069(0.30)	1072(0.34)	1079(0.36)	1088(0.38)	1100(0.40)

Table 16.1 summarizes the simulation results. As expected, sample size increases in $1 - \beta$, τ, mean cluster size $\bar{m}$ (e.g., $m_i = 10$ vs. $m_i = 15$), and variance of cluster size distribution (e.g., $m_i = 10$ vs. $m_i \sim U(8, 12)$), and decreases in hazard ratio $\Delta = \lambda_1/\lambda_2$. The sample sizes maintain the nominal power well overall. If the calculated sample size is small and is slightly larger than a multiple of the cluster size, e.g., $n = 251$ for $(1 - \beta, m_i, \lambda_2, \tau) = (0.8, 10, 0.3, 0.1)$, the empirical power can be higher than the nominal level. This is because the trial will continue randomizing patients until the last cluster of arm 2 is completely filled and its impact will be large when the total sample size is small. Under H_0, the log-rank test tends to be slightly anti-conservative when sample size is small. In summary, the calculated sample sizes are appropriately powered and the log-rank test controls type I error rate accurately overall.

Optimal Allocation Proportions

We identify optimal allocation proportion p_1 and the corresponding sample size n under the design settings considered for simulations of Table 16.1. To identify the proportion minimizing total cost, we consider relative cost of $\eta = \eta_2/\eta_1$ of $5/4$, $3/2$, $7/4$, and 2. Table 16.2 lists optimal sample size n (together with the optimizing p_1 value in the parentheses) under the settings. For comparison, Table 16.2 also lists n for $p_1 = p_2 = 1/2$ that are listed in Table 16.1. Since the optimal allocation proportion does not depend on the nominal power, only $1 - \beta = 0.8$ is considered here. From Table 16.2, we find that p_1 value minimizing the total sample size n decreases in τ. In other words, if the ICC of arm 2 is high, then the optimal allocation randomizes much less patients to arm 1. On the other hand, as the cost of arm 2 relative to that of arm 1 increases, the allocation proportion p_1 minimizing the total cost tends to increase from the p_1 value minimizing n. That is, the p_1 value just minimizing n assigns too many patients to arm 2 so that the p_1 value minimizing the total cost moves toward the balanced allocation with $p_1 = 1/2$ if the relative cost for arm 2 is high.

Example

Harper et. al. (2015) conducted a CRT to study interventions for reducing unintended pregnancy for young women. They performed the study in 40 clinics across United States, of which 20 clinics were randomly assigned to receive a specialized training on intrauterine devices or progestin implants (arm 2) and the other 20 clinics to receive a standard care (arm 1). If the standard care does not need a group training, we can consider an IRGT design for this trial. Suppose that only the experimental arm has $\nu_2 = 20$ clusters while the control arm of standard care has independent individuals, with a balanced allocation, i.e., $p_1 = p_2 = 1/2$. The 20 training groups have similar recruiting capacity so that we assume $\gamma_i = 1/\nu_2 = 1/20$ for $i = 1, ..., \nu_2$. The 1-year pregnancy-free probability for the control arm is known to be 80%, and we want to calculate the required accrual period and the sample size to detect a hazard ratio of $\Delta = \lambda_1/\lambda_2 = 2$ with a power of $1 - \beta = 90\%$. The expected annual accrual rate for the whole study is $r = 200$ and all participating women will be followed until an unexpected pregnancy or for additional $b = 1$ year after completion of accrual. Assuming exponential survival distributions, we have $\lambda_1 = -\log(0.8) = 0.223$ and, under H_1, $\lambda_2 = \lambda_1/\Delta = 0.112$. Assuming $\tau = 0.05$, corresponding to $\theta = 9.5$ and $\text{corr}(T_{2ij}, T_{2ij'}) = 0.1$, we need an expected accrual period of $a = 1.76$ years and a total sample size of $n = 353$ from (16.15) for the log-rank test with two-sided $\alpha = 0.05$. From 5,000 simulations we observe an empirical type I error rate of 0.051 and power of 0.892. By rounding up m_i values using $m_i(a) = [p_2 a r \gamma_i]$, the final sample size is slightly increased to $n = 361$ by a balanced randomization. The allocation proportion minimizing the total sample size is $p_1 = 0.58$ with $n = 345$. If the cost for arm 2 is 50% higher than that of arm 1, i.e., $\eta = 1.5$, then the allocation proportion minimizing the total cost is $p_1 = 0.64$ with $n = 353$. Note that this numerical study is slightly different from those for Tables 16.1 and 16.2. Accrual rate r is given and the number of clusters for arm 2 is fixed here, while accrual period a and cluster sizes are given and the required number of clusters for arm 2 is calculated in the simulations for Tables 16.1 and 16.2.

Discussion

As shown through numerical studies, the sample size depends on many design parameters including the survival and censoring distributions, and ICC and cluster size distribution of arm 2. The sample size calculation of an IRGT trial should be based on the best estimate of these design parameters reflecting the basic design of the new trial.

In designing a new IRGT trial, we propose to use a sample size robust to possible mis-specification of these parameters. As a common example, when all participating clusters are expected to have similar recruiting capacity, we may assume constant cluster sizes at the sample size calculation. When the trial is conducted, however, the attained cluster sizes may vary slightly due to randomization. In this case, the calculated sample size will be slightly underpowered by the increased variance of cluster size distribution. Accounting for possible loss to follow-up and any possible discrepancy between the design parameters specified for sample size calculation and the true or attained ones, we propose to increase the calculated sample size by 5% to 10%.

Appendix A: Limiting distribution of the log-rank statistic under H_1

We derive the distribution of W under $H_1 : \Lambda_1(t) \neq \Lambda_2(t)$. By definition of the log-rank test is

$$W = \frac{1}{\sqrt{n}} \int_0^\infty \left\{ \frac{Y_2(t)}{Y(t)} dN_1(t) - \frac{Y_1(t)}{Y(t)} dN_2(t) \right\}$$

so that we have

$$W = \frac{1}{\sqrt{n}} \int_0^\infty \frac{Y_2(t)}{Y(t)} \{dN_1(t) - Y_1(t) d\Lambda_1(t)\} - \frac{1}{\sqrt{n}} \int_0^\infty \frac{Y_1(t)}{Y(t)} \{dN_2(t) - Y_2(t) d\Lambda_2(t)\}$$

$$+ \frac{1}{\sqrt{n}} \int_0^\infty \frac{Y_1(t) Y_2(t)}{Y(t)} \{d\Lambda_1(t) - d\Lambda_2(t)\}. \quad (16.A1)$$

Since $n_k^{-1}Y_k(t)$ uniformly converge to $y_k(t) = S_k(t)G(t)$, from (16.A1), we have

$$W = \frac{p_2}{\sqrt{n}}\sum_{i=1}^{n_1}\int_0^\infty \frac{y_2(t)}{y(t)}dM_{1i}(t) - \frac{p_1}{\sqrt{n}}\sum_{i=1}^{\nu_2}\int_0^\infty \frac{y_1(t)}{y(t)}dM_{2i}(t) + \omega\sqrt{n} + o_p(1), \tag{16.A2}$$

where $y(t) = p_1y_1(t) + p_2y_2(t)$ and

$$\omega = p_1p_2\int_0^\infty \frac{y_1(t)y_2(t)}{y(t)}\{d\Lambda_1(t) - d\Lambda_2(t)\}$$

$$= p_1p_2\int_0^\infty \frac{S_1(t)S_2(t)G(t)}{p_1S_1(t) + p_2S_2(t)}\{d\Lambda_1(t) - d\Lambda_2(t)\}. \tag{16.A3}$$

Since the patients in the two arms are independent, the first two terms of (16.A2) are independent. Further, $M_{11}, ..., M_{1,n_1}$ are independent 0-mean martingales so that the variance of the first term of (16.A2) is given as

$$\sigma_1^2 = p_1p_2^2\int_0^\infty \frac{y_1(t)y_2(t)^2}{y(t)^2}d\Lambda_1(t)$$

$$= p_1p_2^2\int_0^\infty \frac{S_1(t)S_2(t)^2G(t)}{\{p_1S_1(t) + p_2S_2(t)\}^2}d\Lambda_1(t). \tag{16.A4}$$

By Ying and Wei (1994), $n^{-1/2}\sum_{i=1}^{\nu_2} M_{2i}(t)$ converges weakly to a Gaussian process $U_2(t)$. As in Lee, Wei, and Ying (1993), we can show that the second term of (16.A2) converge a.s. to $\int_0^\infty y_1(t)/y(t)\}dU_2(t)$. Hence, by the standard central limit theorem for sum of independent random variables, the second term of (16.A2) converges to a normal distribution with mean 0 and variance

$$\text{var}\left\{\int_0^\infty \frac{y_1(t)}{y(t)}dM_{2i}(t)\right\} = \int_0^\infty \frac{y_1^2(t)}{y^2(t)}Y_{2i}d\Lambda_2(t)$$

$$+2\int_0^\infty\int_0^\infty \frac{y_1(t_1)y_1(t_2)}{y(t_1)y(t_2)}\sum_{1\le j<j'\le m_i} Y_{i(j,j')}(t_1,t_2)dA_2(t_1,t_2),$$

where $Y_{2i}(t) = \sum_{j=1}^{m_i} Y_{2ij}(t)$, $Y_{i(j,j')}(t_1,t_2) = I(X_{2ij} \ge t_1, X_{2ij'} \ge t_2)$ for $j \ne j'$ and

$$\begin{aligned} dA_2(t_1,t_2) =&\{\lambda_2(t_1,t_2) - \lambda_{2(1|2)}(t_1,t_2)\lambda_2(t_2) \\ &- \lambda_{2(2|1)}(t_1,t_2)\lambda_2(t_1) + \lambda_2(t_1)\lambda_2(t_2)\}dt_1dt_2 \end{aligned}$$

by similar arguments of Li and Jung (2020).

So, the variance of the second term of (16.A5) is

$$v_2 = \frac{p_1^2}{n}\int_0^\infty \frac{y_1^2(t)}{y^2(t)}Y_2(t)d\Lambda_2(t)$$

$$+\frac{p_1^2}{n}\int_0^\infty\int_0^\infty \frac{y_1(t_1)y_1(t_2)}{y(t_1)y(t_2)}\sum_{i=1}^{\nu_2}\sum_{1\le j<j'\le m_i} Y_{i(j,j')}(t_1,t_2)dA_2(t_1,t_2).$$

We can show that

$$\frac{\sum_{i=1}^{\nu_2}\sum_{1\le j<j'\le m_i} Y_{i(j,j')}(t_1,t_2)}{\sum_{i=1}^{\nu_2} m_i(m_i-1)}$$

uniformly converge to $y_2(t_1,t_2) = S_2(t_1,t_2)G(t_1,t_2)$ as in Lin and Ying (1993), and we have $\nu_2^{-1}\sum_{i=1}^{\nu_2} m_i(m_i-1) \to \bar{\bar{m}} - \bar{m}$ and $\nu_2/n = (\nu_2/n_2)(n_2/n) \to p_2/\bar{m}$.

Hence,

$$v_2 = \sigma_2^2 + (\bar{\bar{m}}/\bar{m} - 1)c_2, \qquad (16.A5)$$

where

$$\sigma_2^2 = p_1^2 p_2 \int_0^\infty \frac{y_1^2(t)y_2(t)}{y^2(t)} d\Lambda_2(t) = p_1^2 p_2 \int_0^\infty \frac{S_1^2(t)S_2(t)G(t)}{\{p_1S_1(t)+p_2S_2(t)\}^2} d\Lambda_2(t) \qquad (16.A6)$$

and

$$c_2 = p_1^2 p_2 \int_0^\infty\int_0^\infty \frac{y_1(t_1)y_1(t_2)}{y(t_1)y(t_2)} y_2(t_1,t_2)dA_2(t_1,t_2)$$

$$= p_1^2 p_2 \int_0^\infty\int_0^\infty \frac{S_1(t_1)S_1(t_2)S_2(t_1,t_2)G(t_1,t_2)}{\{p_1S_1(t_1)+p_2S_2(t_1)\}\{p_1S_1(t_2)+p_2S_2(t_2)\}} dA_2(t_1,t_2). \qquad (16.A7)$$

Note that the ICC in arm 2 is expressed as

$$\rho = \frac{c_2}{\sigma_2^2} = \frac{\int_0^\infty\int_0^\infty \frac{S_1(t_1)S_1(t_2)S_2(t_1,t_2)G(t_1,t_2)}{\{p_1S_1(t_1)+p_2S_2(t_1)\}\{p_1S_1(t_2)+p_2S_2(t_2)\}} dA_2(t_1,t_2)}{\int_0^\infty \frac{S_1^2(t)S_2(t)G(t)}{\{p_1S_1(t)+p_2S_2(t)\}^2} d\Lambda_2(t)}. \qquad (16.A8)$$

From (16.A4) and (16.A5), under H_1, $\text{var}(W) = \sigma^2$ is given as

$$\sigma^2 = \sigma_1^2 + \sigma_2^2 + (\bar{\bar{m}}/\bar{m} - 1)c_2 = \sigma_1^2 + \sigma_2^2\{1 + (\bar{\bar{m}}/\bar{m} - 1)\rho\}.$$

Appendix B: Limiting distribution of the log-rank statistic under the nearby alternative hypothesis

We simplify the asymptotic mean ω and variance σ^2 of W under the nearby alternative hypothesis, where $S_1(t) \approx S_2(t)(= S(t))$. Under the nearby alternative hypothesis, ω in (16.A3) is simplified to

$$\omega = p_1p_2(\Delta - 1)\int_0^\infty S(t)G(t)d\Lambda(t) = p_1p_2(\Delta - 1),$$

where $\Delta = \lambda_1/\lambda_2$, $\Lambda(t) = -\log S(t)$, and $d = \int_0^\infty G(t)dS(t)$ is the probability that a patients experiences an event during study. We propose to calculate d by $p_1 d_1 + p_2 d_2$ with $d_k = \int_0^\infty G(t)dS_k(t)$. Hence, we have

$$\omega = p_1 p_2 (\Delta - 1)d.$$

By the Taylor expansion, we have $\Delta - 1 \approx \log \Delta$ so that we have

$$\omega = p_1 p_2 d \log \Delta.$$

From (16.A4) and (16.A6), we have

$$\sigma_k^2 = p_k p_{3-k}^2 \int_0^\infty S(t)G(t)d\Lambda(t) = -p_k p_{3-k}^2 \int_0^\infty G(t)dS(t) = p_k p_{3-k}^2 d$$

under the nearby alternative hypothesis.

From (16.A7),

$$c_2 = p_1^2 p_2 \int_0^\infty \int_0^\infty S_2(t_1, t_2)G(t_1, t_2)dA_2(t_1, t_2).$$

Hence, we have

$$\sigma^2 = p_1 p_2^2 d + p_1^2 p_2 d\{1 + (\bar{\bar{m}}/\bar{m} - 1)\rho\} = p_1 p_2 d\{1 + p_1 \rho(\bar{\bar{m}}/\bar{m} - 1)\},$$

where the ICC in (16.A8) is reduced

$$\rho = \frac{c_2}{\sigma_2^2} = d^{-1} \int_0^\infty \int_0^\infty S_2(t_1, t_2)G(t_1, t_2)dA_2(t_1, t_2).$$

References

Aalen O. Nonparametric inference for a family of counting processes. Annals of Statistics 1978;6(4):701–726.

Candel MJ, Van Breukelen GJ. Varying cluster sizes in trials with clusters in one treatment arm: sample size adjustments when testing treatment effects with linear mixed models. Statistics in Medicine 2009; 28(18): 2307–2324.

Clayton D, Cuzick J. Multivariate generalizations of the proportional Hazards model. Journal of the Royal Statistical Society, Series A (General) 1985;148(2): 82–108.

Fleming TR, Harrington DP. Counting Processes and Survival Analysis. Hoboken, NJ: John Wiley & Sons; 2011.

Gehan EA. A generalized Wilcoxon test for comparing arbitrarily singly-censored samples. Biometrika 1965; 52(1–2): 203–224.

Gill RD. Censoring and Stochastic Integrals. Mathematical Centre Tracts 124, Mathematisch Centrum: Amsterdam, 1980.

Harper CC, Rocca CH, Thompson KM, et al. Reductions in pregnancy rates in the USA with long-acting reversible contraception: a cluster randomised trial. Lancet. 2015;386(9993):562–568.

Jung SH, Jeong JH. Rank tests for clustered survival data. Lifetime Data Analysis 2003; 9(1): 21–33.
Kaplan EL, Meier P. Nonparametric estimator from incomplete observations. Journal of the American Statistical Association 1958; 53: 457–481.
Lakatos E. Sample sizes based on the log-rank statistic in complex clinical trials. Biometrics 1988; 44(1): 229–241.
Lee EW, Wei LJ, Ying Z. Linear regression analysis for highly stratified failure time data. Journal of American Statistical Association 1993; 88(422): 557–565.
Li J, Jung SH. Sample size calculation for cluster randomization trials with a time-to-event endpoint. Statistics in Medicine 2020; 39(25): 3608–3623.
Lin DY, Ying Z. A Simple Nonparametric Estimator of the Bivariate Survival function under univariate censoring. Biometrika 1993; 80: 573–581.
Moerbeek M, Wong WK. Sample size formulae for trials comparing group and individual treatments in a multilevel model. Statistics in Medicine 2008; 27: 2850–2864.
Nelson W. Hazard plotting for incomplete failure data. Journal of Quality Technology 1969; 1(1): 27–52.
Pals SL, Murray DM, Alfano CM, Shadish WR, Hannan PJ, Baker WL. Individually randomized group treatment trials: a critical appraisal of frequently used design and analytic approaches. American Journal of Public Health 2008; 98(8): 1418–1424.
Peto R, Peto J. Asymptotically efficient rank invariant test procedures (with discussion. Journal of the Royal Statistical Society, Series A 1972; 135: 185–206.
Prentice RL. Linear rank tests with right censored data. Biometrika 1978; 65: 167–179.
Roberts C, Roberts SA. Design and analysis of clinical trials with clustering effects due to treatment. Clinical Trials 2005; 2(2): 152–162.
Schoenfeld DA. Sample-size formula for the proportional-hazards regression model. Biometrics 1983; 39(2): 499–503.
Turner EL, Li F, Gallis JA, Prague M, Murray DM. Review of recent methodological developments in group-randomized trials: Part 1—design. American Journal of Public Health 2017; 107(6): 907–915.
Turner EL, Prague M, Gallis JA, Li F, Murray DM. Review of recent methodological developments in group-randomized trials: part 2—analysis. American Journal of Public Health 2017; 107(7): 1078–1086.
Wang X, Turner EL, Li F. Designing individually randomized group treatment trials with repeated outcome measurements using generalized estimating equations. Statistics in Medicine 2024; 43: 358–378.
Ying Z, Wei LJ. The Kaplan-Meier estimate for dependent failure time observations. Journal of Multivariate Analysis 1994; 50: 17–29.

17

Analysis of Medical Tests I: Comparison of Concordance Rates with Clustered Data

In this chapter, we investigate statistical testing methods to compare agreement between two medical tests. In gold standard comparison problems, one is interested in whether the agreement between a new method with a gold standard is better than the agreement between an old method (also called control) with the gold standard. The measurements for the two methods and the gold standard are made from each site of subjects. In this case, the measurements from multiple sites within each subject tend to be correlated, and an analysis result without adjusting for the potential dependency will be biased. We are interested in testing the equality of the correlated concordance rates between two medical tests with a common gold standard. We consider binary and categorical variable types for measurements. In the example study of categorical variable type measurements, there is no gold standard.

Concordance Rates of Clustered Binary Data

For binary data, the degree of agreement is often quantified by Cohen's Kappa coefficient (1960). However, the Kappa coefficient has been criticized because of its unexpected behavior due to its dependence on disease prevalence and marginal distributions (Maclure and Willett, 1987; Feinstein and Cicchetti, 1990; Cichetti and Feinstein 1990; Cook, 1998). It is possible that Kappa may be low even though there are high levels of observed agreement due to low prevalence of the disease. Therefore, the intuitive omnibus indices, such as concordance, observed agreement or overall agreement, still remain attractive due to their easy understanding and interpretation by clinicians.

Cicchetti and Feinstein (1990) advocated using two separate indices, positive agreement and negative agreement, to summarize agreement in the positive and negative decisions. Meier (2006) and Biswas (2006) from the FDA advocated the use of positive percent agreement (PPA) and negative percent agreement (NPA) for comparing a new method to a reference standard (imperfect gold standard) or a non-reference standard. The PPA is

DOI: 10.1201/9781003221951-17

defined as the percent of observed agreement on positive value between the new method and the standard given the standard is positive and the NPA is the percent of observed agreement on negative value given the standard is negative. Therefore the concordance rate is the weighted average of the PPA and NPA with weights of the marginal probabilities of the standard method. The PPA and NPA are analogous to sensitivity and specificity concepts in assessing diagnostic accuracy where the standard is the perfect gold standard.

If the choice of omnibus index for summarizing agreement is Kappa, sample size computation, interval estimates, comparison of Kappas have been well developed in the literatures for both independent and dependent samples (e.g., Donner and Eliasziw, 1992; Cantor, 1996; Donner, 1999; Lin, Williamson and Lipsitz, 2003; Nam, 2006). If the choice of omnibus index for summarizing agreement is concordance, sample size computation or comparisons of independent concordance rates can be easily carried out for independent samples due to easy computation of standard errors of the estimated concordance rates. However, there is not much research on sample size computation where the interest is comparing the correlated concordance rates in dependent samples such as data come from binary measurements by several methods on multiple sites of the same subject, e.g., eyes, ears or teeth. In this section, we discuss a statistical testing method on concordance rates with clustered binary data and its sample size calculation method that was proposed by Jung et al. (2008).

Statistical Testing to Compare Concordance Rates

Suppose that measurements by new method ($k = 1$), old method ($k = 2$), and gold standard are made from each site of study subjects. For site $j(= 1, ..., m_i)$ of subject $i(= 1, ..., n)$, let binary variables y_{kij} and g_{ij} denote the measurements by methods $k(= 1, 2)$ and gold standard, respectively, each of which taking 1 if the measurement is positive and 0 otherwise. Also, let $x_{kij} = I(y_{kij} = g_{ij})$ denote the binary random variables taking 1 if the measurement by method k concords with that by the gold standard and 0 otherwise. Let $p_k = E(x_{kij}) = P(y_{kij} = g_{ij})$ denote the concordance rate of method k with the gold standard. Note that $PPA_k = P(y_{kij} = g_{ij}|g_{ij} = 1)$ and $NPA_k = P(y_{kij} = g_{ij}|g_{ij} = 0)$ with $p_k = PPA_k \times P(g_{ij} = 1) + NPA_k \times P(g_{ij} = 0)$. Thus the methods developed here can be easily modified for PPA_k or NPA_k.

The large sample theory in this chapter is based on large n with $\max_{i=1}^{n} m_i \leq c(< \infty)$. A consistent and unbiased estimator for the concordance rate for method k is given by

$$\hat{p}_k = \frac{\sum_{i=1}^{n} \sum_{j=1}^{m_i} x_{kij}}{M},$$

where $M = \sum_{i=1}^{n} m_i$ denotes the total number of sites (subunits) with measurements.

Let $\delta = p_1 - p_2$. Then, we have

$$\sqrt{n}(\hat{p}_1 - \hat{p}_2 - \delta) = \frac{1}{\sqrt{n}}\sum_{i=1}^{n}\epsilon_i,$$

where $\epsilon_i = \sum_{j=1}^{m_i}(x_{1ij} - x_{2ij} - \delta)$. Since $\epsilon_1, ..., \epsilon_n$ are independent 0-mean random variables, by the central limit theorem, $\sqrt{n}(\hat{p}_1 - \hat{p}_2 - \delta)$ is approximately normal with mean 0 and variance σ^2 that can be consistently estimated by

$$\hat{\sigma}^2 = \frac{1}{m}\sum_{i=1}^{n}\left\{\sum_{j=1}^{m_i}\hat{\epsilon}_i\right\}^2,$$

where $\epsilon_i = \sum_{j=1}^{m_i}(x_{1ij} - x_{2ij} - \hat{\delta})$ and $\hat{\delta} = \hat{p}_1 - \hat{p}_2$.

Hence, we reject $H_0 : p_1 - p_2 = \delta_0$ in favor of $H_a : p_1 - p_2 \neq \delta_0$ when

$$\frac{\sqrt{n}|\hat{p}_1 - \hat{p}_2 - \delta_0|}{\hat{\sigma}} > z_{1-\alpha/2}, \tag{17.1}$$

where $z_{1-\alpha/2}$ is the $100(1 - \alpha/2)$ percentile of the $N(0, 1)$ distribution. Dukalski et al. (2003) use a similar statistic for non-inferiority testing on clustered binary data.

Power and Sample Size Calculation

We want to calculate the sample size under a specific alternative hypothesis $H_1 : p_1 - p_2 = \delta_1$. Let $\bar{m} = E(m_i)$ and $\bar{\bar{m}} = E(m_i^2)$ denote the first and second moments for the distribution of the number of sites per subject.

For a sample size formula, we have to derive the distribution of test statistic under H_1. At first, we derive the limit of the variance estimator $\hat{\sigma}^2$. Let $\epsilon_{kij} = x_{kij} - p_k$ for $k = 1, 2$. Note that ϵ_{1ij} and $\epsilon_{2ij'}$ are correlated. By the definition of $\hat{\sigma}^2$, we have

$$\hat{\sigma}^2 = \frac{1}{n}\sum_{i=1}^{n}\left\{\sum_{j=1}^{m_i}(\epsilon_{1ij} - \epsilon_{2ij})\right\}^2 + o_p(1) = \frac{1}{n}\sum_{i=1}^{n}E\left\{\sum_{j=1}^{m_i}(\epsilon_{1ij} - \epsilon_{2ij})\right\}^2 + o_p(1). \tag{17.2}$$

Let $\sigma_k^2 = E(\epsilon_{kij}^2) = p_k(1 - p_k)$, and $\rho_{kk'}$ and $\rho'_{kk'}$ denote the correlation coefficients of concordance variables x_{kij} between methods k and k' in the same site and in the different sites, respectively, of each subject, i.e., $\rho_{12} = \text{corr}(x_{1ij}, x_{2ij})$ and $\rho'_{kk'} = \text{corr}(x_{kij}, x_{k'ij'})$ for $j \neq j'$. Note that $\rho_{11} = \rho_{22} = 1$. Noting that $n^{-1}\sum_{i=1}^{n} m_i \to \bar{m}$ and $n^{-1}\sum_{i=1}^{n} m_i^2 \to \bar{\bar{m}}$, from (17.2), we have

$$\sigma^2 = \bar{m}(\sigma_1^2 + \sigma_2^2 - 2\sigma_1\sigma_2\rho_{12}) + (\bar{\bar{m}} - \bar{m})(\sigma_1^2\rho'_1 + \sigma_2^2\rho'_{22} - 2\sigma_1\sigma_2\rho'_{12}).$$

Since $p(x_{1ij} = 1, x_{2ij} = 1) \leq \min(p_k, p_{k'})$, we have

$$\rho_{12} \leq \frac{\min(p_1, p_2) - p_1p_2}{\sqrt{p_1p_2q_1q_2}}.$$

Similarly, we have

$$\rho'_{kk'} \le \frac{\min(p_k, p_{k'}) - p_k p_{k'}}{\sqrt{p_k p_{k'} q_k q_{k'}}}.$$

Without loss of generality, suppose that $\delta = \delta_1 - \delta_0 < 0$. Usually, $\delta_0 = 0$. Under $H_1 : p_1 - p_2 = \delta_1$, the power of our test is

$$1 - \beta = P\left(\frac{|\sqrt{n}(\hat{p}_1 - \hat{p}_2 - \delta_0)|}{\hat{\sigma}} > z_{1-\alpha/2}|\delta_1\right)$$

$$\approx P\left(\frac{\sqrt{n}(\hat{p}_1 - \hat{p}_2 - \delta_1)}{\sigma} + \frac{\delta\sqrt{n}}{\sigma} < -z_{1-\alpha/2}|\delta_1\right)$$

$$= \bar{\Phi}\left(z_{1-\alpha/2} + \frac{\delta\sqrt{n}}{\sigma}\right),$$

where $\bar{\Phi}(\cdot)$ is the survivor function of $N(0,1)$. Hence, the sample size, or the required number of subjects, is obtained as

$$n = \frac{\bar{\sigma}^2(z_{1-\alpha/2} + z_{1-\beta})^2}{\bar{m}\delta^2}. \tag{17.3}$$

where

$$\bar{\sigma}^2 = \bar{m}^{-1}\sigma^2 = (\sigma_1^2 + \sigma_2^2 - 2\sigma_1\sigma_2\rho_{12}) + (\bar{\bar{m}}/\bar{m} - 1)(\sigma_1^2\rho'_1 + \sigma_2^2\rho'_{22} - 2\sigma_1\sigma_2\rho'_{12}). \tag{17.4}$$

Note that $M = \bar{m}n$ is the required number of subunits.

Assuming that $p_1 \approx p_2$ (so that $\sigma_1^2 \approx \sigma_2^2$), from (17.3) and (17.4), the correlation coefficients $\sigma'_{kk'}$ for $k, k' = 1, 2$ have a similar impact on n. If $\bar{\bar{m}}/\bar{m}$ is larger than 2, these correlation coefficients have a larger impact on n than ρ_{12} does. In other words, even though the mean cluster size $\bar{m}$ is identical, if the variance of cluster size distribution is large, then the sample size is more sensitive to the dependency among the sites within each cluster than the dependency of the measurements by two methods within each site.

If cluster sizes are constant $m_i = m$, then we have $\bar{m} = m$, $\bar{\bar{m}} = m^2$ so that (17.3) is simplified to

$$n = \frac{\bar{\sigma}^2(z_{1-\alpha/2} + z_{1-\beta})^2}{m\delta^2}$$

with

$$\bar{\sigma}^2 = \sigma_1^2 + \sigma_2^2 - 2\sigma_1\sigma_2\rho_{12} + (m-1)(\sigma_1^2\rho'_{11} + \sigma_2^2\rho'_{22} - 2\sigma_1\sigma_2\rho'_{12}).$$

A sample size is calculated as follows.

1. Specify $(\alpha, 1-\beta, p_1, p_2)$ together with the correlation coefficients ρ_{12}, $\rho_{kk'}$, and $\rho'_{kk'}$, and the first and second moments of cluster size distribution, $\bar{m}$ and $\bar{\bar{m}}$.

2. Calculate $\bar{\sigma}^2$ by (17.4)
3. Obtain the required sample size n by (17.3)

Simulation Studies

At first, we consider the setting of an eye study with $m_i = 2$ with $\bar{m} = 2$ and $\bar{\bar{m}} = 4$. We set $\alpha = 0.05$; $1 - \beta = 0.8$ or 0.9; $(p_1, p_2) = (.7, .8)$, (.7,.9), or (.8,.9); $\rho_{12} = 0.2$ or 0.4; $\rho'_{11} = \rho'_{22} = 0.2$ or 0.4; $\rho'_{12} = 0.2$ or 0.4. For each set design parameter values, we calculate n. And then we generate 5,000 simulation data $(x_{kij}, k = 1, 2; 1 \leq i \leq n; j = 1, 2)$ of size n under the setting of sample size calculation, and apply the statistical test (17.1) to each sample. Empirical power, $1 - \hat{\beta}$, is calculated by the proportion of simulation samples rejecting $H_0 : p_1 = p_2$ among 5,000 simulation samples. If the calculated sample size is accurate, then we expect $1 - \hat{\beta}$ to be close to the nominal $1 - \beta$. In order to evaluate the small sample performance of the testing (17.1), we also generate 5,000 simulation samples of size n under H_0 with all design parameter values fixed except that $p_2 = p_1$, and estimate the empirical type I error probability, $\hat{\alpha}$. The correlated binary data are generated by dichotomizing multivariate normal random variables as described in Chapter 6.

Table 17.1 reports the sample size n and $(\hat{\alpha}, 1 - \hat{\beta})$ under each setting. Each combination of $(p_1, p_2, \rho_{12}, \rho'_{kk}, \rho'_{12})$ that does not define a positive definite correlation matrix for a multivariate normal distribution is excluded. As implied by (17.3) and (17.4), sample size increases as $1 - \beta$ and ρ'_{kk} increase, and as $|p_1 - 1/2|$, $\delta = |p_1 - p_2|$, ρ_{12}, and ρ'_{12} decrease. Note that some settings have the same sample sizes although they have different correlation coefficients. For example, when $(p_1, p_2) = (0.8, 0.9)$, $(\rho_{12}, \rho'_{kk}, \rho'_{12}) = (0.2, 0.2, 0.2)$, (0.2,0.4,0.4) and (0.4,0.4,0.2) have the same n since $\bar{\sigma}^2$, from (17.4), is identical for these settings. The empirical type I error probability $\hat{\alpha}$ is very close to the nominal $\alpha = 5\%$ level over all so that the test statistic based on large sample approximation seems to perform accurately with practical sample sizes. The empirical power $1 - \hat{\beta}$ is close to the corresponding nominal level $1 - \beta$ for each setting too.

In the second set of numerical studies, we consider a setting of tooth study, where each patient contribute between $m_i = 1$ and 4 teeth to the study with probabilities of $(f(1), f(2), f(3), f(4)) = (0.1, 0.5, 0.3, 0.1)$. Under the distribution, we have $\bar{m} = 2.4$ and $\bar{\bar{m}} = 6.4$. Other design parameters are set at the same values as those for the first simulations. Table 17.2 summarizes the sample size n and $(\hat{\alpha}, 1 - \hat{\beta})$ under each setting. We observe very similar results from those of the first set of numerical studies.

TABLE 17.1

Sample size and simulations results, $n(\hat{\alpha}, 1-\hat{\beta})$, under various settings of $(p_1, p_2, \rho, 1-\beta)$ for eye studies with $m = 2$. $\hat{\alpha}$ is estimated under $H_0 : p_1 = p_2$

ρ_{12}	ρ'_{kk}	ρ'_{12}	$1-\beta = 0.8$	$1-\beta = 0.9$
$(p_1, p_2) = (0.7, 0.9)$				
0.2	0.2	0.2	25(0.041, 0.781)	33(0.047, 0.898)
		0.4	20(0.041, 0.787)	26(0.045, 0.919)
	0.4	0.2	31(0.046, 0.795)	41(0.038, 0.895)
		0.4	26(0.042, 0.819)	34(0.049, 0.925)
0.4	0.2	0.2	20(0.035, 0.786)	26(0.049, 0.920)
	0.4	0.2	26(0.041, 0.811)	34(0.041, 0.919)
		0.4	20(0.034, 0.785)	27(0.041, 0.947)
$(p_1, p_2) = (0.7, 0.8)$				
0.2	0.2	0.2	117(0.046, 0.781)	157(0.052, 0.898)
		0.4	88(0.050, 0.797)	118(0.046, 0.902)
	0.4	0.2	146(0.048, 0.786)	196(0.048, 0.896)
		0.4	117(0.048, 0.802)	157(0.052, 0.893)
0.4	0.2	0.2	88(0.053, 0.791)	118(0.049, 0.900)
		0.4	60(0.037, 0.802)	80(0.047, 0.913)
	0.4	0.2	117(0.049, 0.797)	157(0.052, 0.894)
		0.4	89(0.050, 0.796)	119(0.050, 0.905)
$(p_1, p_2) = (0.8, 0.9)$				
0.2	0.2	0.2	81(0.049, 0.810)	109(0.051, 0.904)
		0.4	62(0.044, 0.819)	82(0.051, 0.904)
	0.4	0.2	100(0.049, 0.804)	134(0.049, 0.904)
		0.4	81(0.047, 0.808)	109(0.049, 0.914)
0.4	0.2	0.2	62(0.038, 0.806)	82(0.051, 0.906)
		0.4	43(0.040, 0.807)	57(0.049, 0.914)
	0.4	0.2	81(0.046, 0.816)	109(0.051, 0.915)
		0.4	63(0.044, 0.823)	84(0.049, 0.928)

Example

Retinopathy of Prematurity (ROP) is a disease of the retina that affects infants born prematurely. It consists of abnormal retinal vessels that grow at the border between vascular and avascular retina. Abnormal dilation and tortuosity of the retinal blood vessels in the posterior, central retina is called plus disease. Plus disease is one of the most important prognostic indicators in ROP , and it is the primary criterion for laser treatment (Schaffer et al. 1993; ETRPCG 2003). A retinal image study is designed to investigate if a new computer-assisted method is better than the standard visual method by eye examiners to diagnose plus disease from infants with ROP. The image of each eye is read by computer, an examiner, and three experts. The consensus by three experts will be used as a gold standard. The concordance rate for the standard visual method is expected to be about 85%. An improvement to 92.5% in concordance rate for the computer-aided method will be of interest. Under $H_a : (p_1, p_2) = (0.925, 0.85)$, we have $\sigma_1^2 = 0.925 \times (1 - 0.925) = 0.069375$ and $\sigma_2^2 = 0.85 \times (1 - 0.85) = 0.1275$. In this case, $\delta = 0.925 - 0.85 = 0.075$.

Without a pilot data, it is difficult to project the correlation coefficient, $\rho_{kk'}$ and $\rho'_{kk'}$. The correlation coefficients would be non-negative in nature, and theoretically, ρ_{12} and ρ'_{12} should be smaller than

$$\min\left(\sqrt{\frac{p_1q_2}{p_2q_1}}, \sqrt{\frac{p_2q_1}{p_1q_2}}\right).$$

(see, e.g., Jung and Ahn 2005). The upper limit is about .68 under the design setting. As an approximation, we assume that all the correlation coefficients are the same and are located about the center of this range, i.e., 0.34. Hence, $\sigma^2 = 0.136$. Finally for two-sided $\alpha = 0.05$ and $n = 95$, we have

$$z_{1-\alpha/2} - \frac{|\delta|\sqrt{2n}}{\sigma} = 1.96 - \frac{0.075\sqrt{2 \times 95}}{0.34} = -0.8423,$$

which corresponds to 80% of power.

As observed from the simulations, the sample size is sensitive to the true correlation values. We propose a two-stage study design for a sample size recalculate in the middle of a study based on the estimated correlation coefficients using the data from the first stage. A study with a sample size recalculation can be carried out as follows.

1. Suppose that $m_i = 2$. Specify the input variables $(\alpha, 1 - \beta, p_1, p_2, \rho_{12}, \rho'_{11}, \rho'_{12}, \rho'_{22})$, and calculate the initial sample size n_1.
2. Accrue $n_1/2$ patients, and, using the data $(x_{kij}, k = 1, 2; i = 1, ..., n_1/2; j = 1, 2)$, estimate

$$\hat{\rho}_{12} = \frac{\hat{p}_{12} - \hat{p}_1\hat{p}_2}{\hat{\sigma}_1\hat{\sigma}_2}$$

$$\hat{\rho}'_{kk'} = \frac{\hat{p}'_{kk'} - \hat{p}_k\hat{p}_{k'}}{\hat{\sigma}_k\hat{\sigma}_{k'}}$$

for $k \neq k'$, where

$$\hat{p}_{12} = \frac{\sum_{i=1}^{n_1/2}\sum_{j=1}^{2} x_{1ij}x_{2ij}}{n_1}$$

$$\hat{p}'_{kk} = \frac{2\sum_{i=1}^{n_1/2} x_{ki1}x_{ki2}}{n_1}$$

$$\hat{p}'_{12} = \frac{\sum_{i=1}^{n_1/2}(x_{1i1}x_{2i2} + x_{1i2}x_{2i1})}{n_1}$$

for $k = 1, 2$.

3. Calculate sample size n_2 using $(\hat{\rho}_{12}, \hat{\rho}'_{11}, \hat{\rho}'_{12}, \hat{\rho}'_{22})$ in place of $(\rho_{12}, \rho'_{11}, \rho'_{12}, \rho'_{22})$.
4. For $\gamma > 1$, accrue additional $\min(\gamma n_1, n_2) - n_1/2$ subjects to have a total sample size of $n = \min(\gamma n_1, n_2)$, and conduct a statistical testing using the whole data $(x_{kij}, k = 1, 2; i = 1, ..., n; j = 1, 2)$.

In this procedure, sample size recalculation is conducted when 50% of the initial sample size is accomplished. If the first stage sample size is too small, then the estimates of the correlation coefficients may not be reliable enough; if it is too large, then the first stage sample size may be larger than the recalculated sample size n_2. We want the amount of increase by the final sample size to be no more than γ times the initial sample size. If the amount of the increase is too large for the resources allowed for the study, the investigators may decide to abandon the study. For variations of the procedure, readers may refer to Chapter 14 of Jennison and Turnbull (2000) and the references therein.

In the above example, suppose that the true correlation coefficients are $\rho_{12} = 0.4$, $\rho'_{11} = \rho'_{22} = 0.3$, and $\rho'_{12} = 0.2$. Then, for $(\alpha, 1-\beta, p_1, p_2) = (0.05, 0.8, 0.85, 0.925)$, the required sample size is obtained as $n = 113$. In order to address the performance of the proposed sample size recalculation procedure, we conduct a brief simulation study. At first, we calculate the initial sample size $n_1 = 95$ based on the misspecified correlation coefficients $\rho_{12} = \rho'_{11} = \rho'_{12} = \rho'_{22} = 0.34$. In each simulation, we generate a half of data $\{x_{kij}, k = 1, 2; i = 1, ..., n_1/2 (= 47); j = 1, 2\}$ and estimate the correlation coefficients; recalculate sample size $n = n_2$ using the estimated correlation coefficients; generate additional data $\{x_{kij}, k = 1, 2; i = 48, ..., n; j = 1, 2\}$; apply testing (17.1) to the combined data of size n. From 5,000 simulations, the average of the final sample size n is obtained as $\bar{n} = 116.3$, which is close to 113 that would be obtained if we used the true correlation coefficients from the beginning. The empirical power is obtained as 0.787, which is close to the nominal power $1 - \beta = 0.8$. In these simulations, we do not limit the amount of increase by the recalculated sample size. When we limit the increase at a maximum of 30% of the initial sample size (i.e. $\gamma = 1.3$), we obtain $\bar{n} = 105.8$ and an empirical power of 0.764.

Concordance Rates of Clustered Categorical Data

There are different types of device trials depending on the use of device and the study objectives. In this section, we discuss the statistical methods proposed by Liu et al. (2021) to design and analyze a trial on a device based on artificial intelligence (AI) technology for the diagnosis of breast cancer (Zhang and Sejdic 2019). This trial collects measurements with (both ordinal and nominal) categorical variable type.

TABLE 17.2

Sample size and simulations results, $n(\hat{\alpha}, 1-\hat{\beta})$, under various settings of $(p_1, p_2, \rho, 1-\beta)$ for tooth studies with $(f(1), f(2), f(3), f(4)) = (.1, .5, .3, .1)$. $\hat{\alpha}$ is estimated under $H_0 : p_1 = p_2$

ρ_{12}	ρ'_{kk}	ρ'_{12}	$1-\beta = 0.8$	$1-\beta = 0.9$
$(p_1, p_2) = (0.7, 0.9)$				
0.2	0.2	0.2	21(0.047, 0.783)	28(0.045, 0.904)
0.2	0.4	0.2	29(0.045, 0.799)	39(0.047, 0.909)
		0.4	22(0.044, 0.820)	29(0.049, 0.931)
0.4	0.2	0.2	17(0.041, 0.804)	22(0.038, 0.912)
	0.4	0.2	25(0.049, 0.828)	33(0.051, 0.932)
		0.4	17(0.040, 0.783)	23(0.042, 0.938)
$(p_1, p_2) = (0.7, 0.8)$				
0.2	0.2	0.2	98(0.054, 0.788)	131(0.049, 0.907)
	0.4	0.2	138(0.053, 0.786)	185(0.051, 0.897)
		0.4	98(0.054, 0.796)	131(0.045, 0.907)
0.4	0.2	0.2	74(0.046, 0.799)	99(0.051, 0.895)
	0.4	0.2	114(0.052, 0.802)	153(0.045, 0.902)
		0.4	74(0.049, 0.813)	99(0.049, 0.910)
$(p_1, p_2) = (0.8, 0.9)$				
0.2	0.2	0.2	68(0.050, 0.799)	90(0.050, 0.909)
	0.4	0.2	95(0.052, 0.805)	127(0.049, 0.906)
		0.4	69(0.047, 0.826)	92(0.049, 0.922)
0.4	0.2	0.2	52(0.050, 0.824)	69(0.049, 0.912)
	0.4	0.2	79(0.040, 0.816)	106(0.049, 0.917)
		0.4	53(0.044, 0.830)	71(0.048, 0.933)

Imaging technologies play a major role in the diagnosis of breast cancer. The reading and interpretation of imaging requires intensive medical training and significant clinical experience. With the advance of big data analysis methods, machine learning and AI-based imaging systems are currently under active development (D'Orsi et al. 2013). If an AI-based imaging device can read the image as accurately as experienced radiologists, it may be able to help radiologists increase the accuracy of their reading, manage their workloads, or possibly replace radiologists in remote clinics that would not have an experienced radiologist available for consultation.

In the assessment of breast lesions, the BI-RADS reporting system and classification are widely used (D'Orsi et al. 2013). This system includes categories between 1 and 5 (benign to malignant) with a key diagnostic transition subdivided into categories 4a (low suspicion of malignancy), 4b (moderate suspicion), and 4c (high suspicion, greater than 50% likelihood but less than 95% likelihood of malignancy). Furthermore, the BI-RADS lexicon covers radiological descriptive features that are important in diagnostic assessments, and these vary by modality. Examples of ultrasound lexicon used in AI-based classifications is given in Table 17.3. The earlier approaches to breast ultrasound technology concentrated on the extraction of features of lesions such

TABLE 17.3

Examples of ultrasound lexicon

Ground Truth	Lesion Type
Shape	Oval
	Round
	Irregular
Margin	Circumscribed
	Indistinct
	Angular
	Microlobulated
	Spiculated
Orientation	Parallel
	Not parallel
Echo pattern	Anechoic
	Hypoechoic
	Complex cystic and solid
	Isoechoic
	Hyperechoic
	Heterogeneous
Posterior features	No features
	Enhancement
	Shadowing
	Combined pattern

as size, shape, texture, and boundaries within a clustering or classification or rule-based decision making algorithms (Liu et al. 2010; Cheng et al. 2010; Shan et al. 2012; Wu et al. 2012). More recent developments in AI, machine learning, and deep learning systems have utilized layers of convolution neural network models, a variety of approaches and extensive training sets to produce differentiated output classifications (O'Connell et al. 2022; Wu et al. 2019).

Since BI-RADS reporting system does not have a gold standard, the performance of the device is evaluated by how well its reading concords with those of radiologists. We consider two types of study objectives to evaluate the performance of an AI-based device for the diagnosis of breast cancer. For each study objective, we propose a testing method and its sample size formula. Suppose that we have images from n subjects.

Objective 1: Is the Concordance Rate between the AI-based Device and Radiologists as High as That among Radiologists?

The image of each subject is read by m radiologists and the AI-based device. BI-RADS lexicon does not have a gold standard. In order to validate a device with an AI-based algorithm, we should show that the reading of the device concurs with those with radiologists. For example, for BI-RADS lexicon classification (see in Table 17.3, Shape, two radiologists will be declared to be concurrent for an image if they both read oval, round or irregular. The question is how high the concordance rate should be between the device and the radiologists. The concordance rate among radiologists is used as a reference.

For each category of BI-RADS lexicon classifications, let p_r and p_s denote the concordance rate among radiologists and that between radiologists and the device, respectively. Since the latter cannot be higher than the former, we specify a similarity margin $\delta_1(>0)$. That is, we will not be interested in the AI-based device if $p_s \le p_r - \delta_1$ and will be highly interested in it if $p_s = p_r$. So, we want to test a null hypothesis $H_1 : p_s = p_r - \delta_1$ against the alternative hypothesis $\bar{H}_1 : p_s > p_r - \delta_1$.

Statistical Testing Method

Suppose that there are n patients, and the image of each patient is read by the AI-based device and m radiologists. For subject $i(=1,...,n)$ and radiologist $j(=1,...,m)$, let $r_{ijj'} = 1$ if radiologists j and j' concur and $= 0$ otherwise, and let $s_{ij} = 1$ if radiologist j and the device concur and $= 0$ otherwise. Note that we have $p_r = E(r_{ijj'})$ and $p_s = E(s_{ij})$. Since $r_{ijj'} = r_{ij'j}$ and $r_{ijj} = 1$ for $j, j' = 1,...,m$, the number of informative concordance scores among m radiologists is $m(m-1)/2$ for each image (subject), the concordance rate among radiologists for subject i is estimated by

$$r_i = \frac{\sum_{j=1}^{m-1}\sum_{j'=j+1}^{m} r_{ijj'}}{m(m-1)/2}.$$

On the other hand, for subject i, the concordance rate between the device and m radiologists is estimated by

$$s_i = \frac{\sum_{j=1}^{m} s_{ij}}{m}.$$

Using the images from n subjects, concordance rate among radiologists is estimated by

$$\hat{p}_r = \frac{2}{nm(m-1)}\sum_{i=1}^{n}\sum_{j=1}^{m-1}\sum_{j'=j+1}^{m} r_{ijj'} = \frac{1}{n}\sum_{i=1}^{n} r_i$$

and that between the device and radiologists is estimated by

$$\hat{p}_s = \frac{1}{nm}\sum_{i=1}^{n}\sum_{j=1}^{m} s_{ij} = \frac{1}{n}\sum_{i=1}^{n} s_i.$$

Note that these estimators are unbiased and consistent for large n.

Since $r_1,...,r_n$ are independent random variables with mean p_r, by the central limit theorem for large n,

$$\sqrt{n}(\hat{p}_r - p_r) = \frac{1}{\sqrt{n}}\sum_{i=1}^{n}(r_i - p_r)$$

is asymptotically normal with mean 0 and variance σ_r^2 that can be consistently estimated by

$$\hat{\sigma}_r^2 = \frac{1}{n}\sum_{i=1}^{n}(r_i - \hat{p}_r)^2.$$

Similarly, $s_1, ..., s_n$ are independent random variables with mean p_s so that for large n,

$$\sqrt{n}(\hat{p}_s - p_s) = \frac{1}{\sqrt{n}}\sum_{i=1}^{n}(s_i - p_s)$$

is asymptotically normal with mean 0 and variance σ_s^2 that can be consistently estimated by

$$\hat{\sigma}_s^2 = \frac{1}{n}\sum_{i=1}^{n}(s_i - \hat{p}_s)^2.$$

Since each subject's image is read by the device and radiologists, r_i and s_i are correlated. However, $(s_i - r_i + \delta_1, i = 1, ..., n)$ are independent, with mean 0 under the null hypothesis H_1. Hence, by the central limit theorem under H_1,

$$\sqrt{n}(\hat{p}_s - \hat{p}_r + \delta_1) = \frac{1}{\sqrt{n}}\sum_{i=1}^{n}(s_i - r_i + \delta_1)$$

is asymptotically normal with mean 0 and variance σ_1^2 that can be consistently estimated by

$$\hat{\sigma}_1^2 = \frac{1}{n}\sum_{i=1}^{n}(s_i - r_i + \delta_1)^2.$$

Hence, we reject the null hypothesis $H_1 : p_s \leq p_r - \delta_1$ in favor of the alternative hypothesis $\bar{H}_1 : p_s > p_r - \delta_1$ if $Z_1 > z_{1-\alpha}$, where

$$Z_1 = \frac{\sqrt{n}(\hat{p}_s - \hat{p}_r + \delta_1)}{\hat{\sigma}_1}$$

and $z_{1-\alpha}$ is the $100(1 - \alpha)$ percentile of the standard normal distribution. Note that we use a one-sided test because the hypotheses are one-sided and to avoid an excessive sample size with a small δ_1.

Note that $\hat{p}_r$ and $\hat{p}_s$ are the generalized estimating equation (GEE, Liang and Zeger 1986) estimators of p_r and p_s, respectively, using a working independent correlation structure. Furthermore, the robust estimator of σ_1^2 by the GEE method is given as

$$\tilde{\sigma}_1^2 = \frac{1}{n}\sum_{i=1}^{n}(s_i - r_i + \hat{p}_s - \hat{p}_r)^2.$$

Since $\hat{p}_s - \hat{p}_r$ is a consistent estimator of $p_s - p_r$, $\tilde{\sigma}_1^2$ is asymptotically identical to $\hat{\sigma}_1^2$ under H_1. Hence, Z_1 can be counted as a test statistic based on the GEE method with a working independent correlation.

Power and Sample Size Calculation

We calculate the sample size for the test statistic Z_1 under a specific alternative hypothesis $\bar{H}_1 : p_r = p_s$. An accurate sample size calculation for the statistical test requires specification of correlation coefficients between $r_{ij_1j_2}$ and $r_{ij'_1j'_2}$, between $r_{ij_1j_2}$ and s_{ij}, and between s_{ij} and $s_{ij'}$. The dependency between $r_{ij_1j_2}$ and $r_{ij_1j'_2}$ is expected to be higher than that between $r_{ij_1j_2}$ and $r_{ij'_1j'_2}$ for $j_1 \neq j'_1 \neq j_2 \neq j'_2$ because the former pair includes the same reader j_1 while the latter pair contains four different readers. Similarly, we expect that the dependency between $r_{ij_1j_2}$ and s_{ij_1} is expected to be higher than that between $r_{ij_1j_2}$ and $s_{ij'_1}$ for $j_1, j_2 \neq j'_1$.

For a simplified sample size formula, we just specify $\rho_1 = \text{corr}(r_i, s_i)$. We define the correlation coefficients among the concordance scores $\rho_{r1} = \text{corr}(r_{i12}, r_{i13})$, $\rho_{r2} = \text{corr}(r_{i12}, r_{i34})$, $\rho_{s1} = \text{corr}(r_{i12}, s_{i1}) = \text{corr}(r_{i12}, s_{i2})$, and $\rho_{s2} = \text{corr}(r_{i12}, s_{i3})$, and $\rho_{ss} = \text{corr}(s_{i1}, s_{i2})$. Appendix A shows that we have $\rho_1 = \text{corr}(r_i, s_i)$ is expressed as

$$\rho_1 = \frac{\frac{2}{m}\rho_{s1} + \frac{m-2}{m}\rho_{s2}}{\sqrt{\left(\frac{2}{m(m-1)} + \frac{4(m-2)}{m(m-1)}\rho_{r1} + \frac{(m-2)(m-3)}{m(m-1)}\rho_{r2}\right)\left(\frac{1}{m} + \frac{m-1}{m}\rho_{ss}\right)}}.$$

Under $\bar{H}_1 : p_r = p_s$, $\{(s_i - r_i), i = 1, ..., n\}$ are independent random variables with mean 0 so that $\sqrt{n}(\hat{p}_s - \hat{p}_r)$ is asymptotically normal with mean 0 and variance σ_1^2 that can be consistently estimated by $s_1^2 = \sqrt{n}^{-1}\sum_{i=1}^n (s_i - r_i)^2$. Since $\hat{\sigma}_1^2$ is asymptotically identical to $s_1^2 + \delta_1^2$ under $\bar{H}_1$, it converges to $\sigma_1^2 + \delta_1^2$. Hence, the power for a given sample size n is

$$\begin{aligned}
1 - \beta &= P\left(\frac{\sqrt{n}(\hat{p}_s - \hat{p}_r + \delta_1)}{\hat{\sigma}_1} > z_{1-\alpha} | p_r = p_s\right) \\
&= P\left(\frac{\sqrt{n}(\hat{p}_s - \hat{p}_r) + \delta_1\sqrt{n})}{\sqrt{\sigma_1^2 + \delta_1^2}} > z_{1-\alpha} | p_r = p_s\right) \\
&= P\left(\frac{\sqrt{n}(\hat{p}_s - \hat{p}_r)}{\sigma_1} > \frac{z_{1-\alpha}\sqrt{\sigma_1^2 + \delta_1^2} - \delta_1\sqrt{n}}{\sigma_1} | p_r = p_s\right) \\
&= \bar{\Phi}\left(\frac{z_{1-\alpha}\sqrt{\sigma_1^2 + \delta_1^2} - \delta_1\sqrt{n}}{\sigma_1}\right), \qquad (17.5)
\end{aligned}$$

where $\bar{\Phi}(.)$ is the survivor function of the standard normal distribution and σ_1^2 is the limit of $n^{-1}\sum_{i=1}^n (s_i - r_i)^2$.

By solving the power Equation (17.5) with respect to n, we obtain the required sample size for power $1 - \beta$

$$n = \frac{(z_{1-\alpha}\sqrt{\sigma_1^2 + \delta_1^2} + z_{1-\beta}\sigma_1)^2}{\delta_1^2}, \qquad (17.6)$$

where, as shown in the Appendix B,

$$\sigma_1^2 = \text{var}(s_i) + \text{var}(r_i) - 2\rho_1\sqrt{\text{var}(s_i)\text{var}(r_i)} \tag{17.7}$$

$$\text{var}(s_i) = p_r(1 - p_r)\{1/m + \rho_{ss}(m - 1)/m\}$$

and

$$\text{var}(r_i) = p_r(1 - p_r)\left(\frac{2}{m(m-1)} + \frac{4(m-2)}{m(m-1)}\rho_{r1} + \frac{(m-2)(m-3)}{m(m-1)}\rho_{r2}\right).$$

The process of calculating a required sample size is summarized as follows:

1. Specify $(\alpha, 1 - \beta)$, expected concordance rate among radiologists p_r, similarity margin δ_1 and hypothetical correlation coefficients $\rho_{r1}, \rho_{r2}, \rho_{ss}, \rho_{s1}$ and ρ_{s2}.
2. Calculate σ_1^2 using (17.7).
3. Obtain sample size using (17.6).

It may be difficult to specify the correlation coefficients $\rho_{r1}, \rho_{r2}, \rho_{ss}, \rho_{s1}$ and ρ_{s2}. If pilot data are available, we may estimate them from the pilot data. Otherwise, we may conduct a two-stage trial to estimate these correlation coefficients from the first stage data and recalculate the sample size for the whole trial based on the estimated correlation coefficients.

Objective 2: Is the AI-based Device More Concordant with Experienced Radiologists Than with Junior Radiologists?

As another study objective of the imaging study, we want to test if the reading of the AI-based device agrees more with those of experienced radiologists compared with those of junior radiologists for each BI-RADS lexicon classification category.

Let p_x and p_y denote the concordance rate between the AI-based device and highly experienced radiologists and that between the AI-based device and less experienced radiologists, respectively. We want to test the null hypothesis $H_2 : p_x = p_y$ against the alternative hypothesis $\bar{H}_2 : p_x > p_y$.

Statistical Testing Method

Let m (= 5, say) denote the number of radiologists in each group (highly experienced group and less experienced group). For subject i $(= 1, ..., n)$ and senior radiologist j $(= 1, ..., m)$, let $x_{ij} = 1$ if the reading by senior radiologist j and that by the AI-based device agree and =0 otherwise, and $y_{ij} = 1$ if the reading by less experienced radiologist j $(= 1, ..., m)$ and that by the

AI-based device agree and =0 otherwise. Then, we have $p_x = E(x_{ij})$ and $p_y = E(y_{ij})$. Using the data from subject i, p_x is estimated by

$$\bar{x}_i = \frac{\sum_{j=1}^{m} x_{ij}}{m}$$

and p_y is estimated by

$$\bar{y}_i = \frac{\sum_{j=1}^{m} y_{ij}}{m}.$$

Using the whole data, we estimate p_x and p_y by

$$\hat{p}_x = \frac{1}{nm}\sum_{i=1}^{n}\sum_{j=1}^{m} x_{ij} = \frac{1}{n}\sum_{i=1}^{n}\bar{x}_i$$

and

$$\hat{p}_y = \frac{1}{nm}\sum_{i=1}^{n}\sum_{j=1}^{m} y_{ij} = \frac{1}{n}\sum_{i=1}^{n}\bar{y}_i$$

respectively. Note that those estimates are unbiased.

For large n under H_2, $\sqrt{n}(\hat{p}_x - \hat{p}_y)$ is approximately normal with mean 0 and variance σ_2^2 that can be estimated by

$$\hat{\sigma}_2^2 = \frac{1}{n}\sum_{i=1}^{n}(\bar{x}_i - \bar{y}_i)^2$$

since $(\bar{x}_i - \bar{y}_i, i = 1, ..., n)$ are independent random variables with mean 0 under H_2.

Hence, we reject $H_2 : p_x = p_y$ if $|Z_2| > z_{1-\alpha/2}$, where

$$Z_2 = \frac{\sqrt{n}(\hat{p}_x - \hat{p}_y)}{\hat{\sigma}_2}.$$

Note that we use a standard two-sided test since usually there is no small effect size issue in this case.

Power and Sample Size Calculation

We calculate the sample size under a specific alternative hypothesis $\bar{H}_2 : p_x = p_y + \delta_2$. Since each subject's image is read by all experienced and inexperienced radiologists as well as the device, $\{(x_{ij}, y_{ij}), j = 1, ..., m\}$ are correlated.

For $j \neq j'$, let $\rho_{xx} = corr(x_{ij}, x_{ij'})$ denote the intracluster correlation coefficient (ICC) of concordance scores between the device and highly experienced radiologists and $\rho_{yy} = corr(y_{ij}, y_{ij'})$ denote the ICC of concordance scores between the device and less experienced radiologists. Further, let

$\rho_{xy} = \text{corr}(x_{ij}, y_{ij'})$ for $j, j' = 1, ..., m$ denote the correlation coefficient between the concordance score between the device and a highly experienced radiologist and that between the device and a less experienced radiologist. Let $\rho_2 = corr(x_i, y_i)$. As shown in Appendix C. ρ_2 is a function of ρ_{xx}, ρ_{yy}, and ρ_{xy}.

Under $\bar{H}_2 : p_x - p_y = \delta_2$, $(x_i - y_i - \delta_2, i = 1, ..., n)$ are independent random variables with mean 0 so that $\sqrt{n}(\hat{p}_x - \hat{p}_y - \delta_2)$ is asymptotically normal with mean 0 and variance σ_2^2 that can be consistently estimated by $s_2^2 = \sqrt{n}^{-1} \sum_{i=1}^n (x_i - y_i - \delta_2)^2$. Note that $\hat{\sigma}_2^2$ is asymptotically identical to $s_2^2 + \delta_2^2$ under $\bar{H}_2$ so that it converges to $\sigma_2^2 + \delta_2^2$. Hence, the power for a given sample size n is

$$1 - \beta = P\left(\frac{\sqrt{n}(\hat{p}_x - \hat{p}_y)}{\hat{\sigma}_2} > z_{1-\alpha/2} | p_x = p_y + \delta_2\right)$$

$$= P\left(\frac{\sqrt{n}(\hat{p}_x - \hat{p}_y - \delta_2) + \delta_2\sqrt{n}}{\sqrt{s_2 + \delta_2^2}} > z_{1-\alpha/2} | p_x = p_y + \delta_2\right)$$

$$= P\left(\frac{\sqrt{n}(\hat{p}_x - \hat{p}_y - \delta_2)}{\sigma_2} > \frac{z_{1-\alpha/2}\sqrt{\sigma_2^2 + \delta_2^2} - \delta_2\sqrt{n}}{\sigma_2} | p_x = p_y + \delta_2\right)$$

$$= \bar{\Phi}\left(\frac{z_{1-\alpha/2}\sqrt{\sigma_2^2 + \delta_2^2} - \delta_2\sqrt{n}}{\sigma_2}\right) \tag{17.8}$$

since $\sqrt{n}(\hat{p}_x - \hat{p}_y - \delta_2)/\sigma_2$ is $N(0, 1)$ under $\bar{H}_2$, where σ_2^2 is the limit of $n^{-1} \sum_{i=1}^n (x_i - y_i - \delta_2)^2$ under $\bar{H}_2$.

By solving (17.8) with respect to n, we obtain the required sample size for power $1 - \beta$

$$n = \frac{(z_{1-\alpha/2}\sqrt{\sigma_2^2 + \delta_2^2} + z_{1-\beta}\sigma_2)^2}{\delta_2^2}. \tag{17.9}$$

Appendix D shows that

$$\sigma_2^2 = \text{var}(\bar{x}_i) + \text{var}(\bar{y}_i) - 2\rho_2\sqrt{\text{var}(\bar{x}_i)\text{var}(\bar{y}_i)}, \tag{17.10}$$

where

$$\text{var}(\bar{x}_i) = p_x(1 - p_x)\{1/m + (m-1)/m\rho_{xx}\}$$

and

$$\text{var}(\bar{y}_i) = (p_x - \delta_2)\{1 - p_x + \delta_2)(1/m + (m-1)/m\rho_{yy}\}$$

under $\bar{H}_2$.

The process of calculating the required sample size is summarized as follows:

1. Specify $(\alpha, 1 - \beta)$, expected concordance rate between the AI-based device and a highly experienced radiologist p_x, clinically meaningful

difference in concordance rates δ_2 and correlation coefficients ρ_{xx}, ρ_{yy} and ρ_{xy}.

2. Calculate σ_2^2 using (17.10).
3. Obtain the required sample size using (17.9).

It will be difficult to specify the correlation coefficients ρ_{xx}, ρ_{yy} and ρ_{xy}. If pilot data are available, we may estimate them from the pilot data. Otherwise, we may use a two-stage design to estimate these correlation coefficients from the first stage data and calculate the sample size for the whole trial based on the estimated correlation coefficients.

Numerical Studies and Results

Note that our test statistics and sample size formulas are derived based on large sample approximations. We want to conduct simulation studies to evaluate their finite sample performance.

We consider the type of study objective 1 to test if the concordance rate between an AI-based device and radiologists is as high as that among radiologists. Suppose that each subject's image is read by the AI-based device and $m = 10$ radiologists. We set $\alpha = 0.05$, $1 - \beta = 0.8$ or 0.9, $p_r = 0.3$, 0.5 or 0.7, $\delta_1 = 0.05$ or 0.1 and $\rho_1 = 0.1, 0.3, 0.5$, or 0.7. Assuming $\rho_{s1} = \rho_{s2} + 0.1, \rho_{r1} = \rho_{r2} + 0.1, \rho_{r1} = \rho_{ss} = \rho_{s1} + 0.1$, we calculate the correlation coefficients for a given $\rho = corr(r_i, s_i)$. That is, we obtain $(\rho_{s1}, \rho_{s2}, \rho_{ss}, \rho_{r1}, \rho_{r2}) = (0.101, 0.001, 0.201, 0.201, 0.101)$, (0.16, 0.06, 0.26, 0.26, 0.16), (0.26, 0.16, 0.36, 0.36, 0.26) and (0.48, 0.38, 0.58, 0.58, 0.48) for $\rho_1 = 0.1$, 0.3, 0.5, and 0.7, respectively.

For each design setting, we calculate the required sample size n using formula (17.6) and generate 10,000 simulation data sets of size n under the design setting under H_1 or $\bar{H}_1$. Then, we apply the statistical testing using Z_1 to each simulation data set, and compute the empirical type I error ($\hat{\alpha}$) and power ($1 - \hat{\beta}$) by the proportion of samples that reject H_1 among the 10,000 samples simulated under $H_1 : p_s = p_r - \delta_1$ and $\bar{H}_1 : p_s = p_r$, respectively. The correlated concordance (binary) data are generated by first generating multivariate normal data and then dichotomizing them with corresponding proportion level as discussed in Chapter 6.

Table 17.4 reports the sample size n, empirical type I error rate $\hat{\alpha}$, and power $1 - \hat{\beta}$ under each design setting. We observe that the required sample size increases in $1 - \beta$ and decreases in δ_1 and ρ_1. With other design parameters fixed, we have the same sample sizes for $p_r = 0.3$ and $p_r = 0.7$. We have this result because, from (17.6), the sample size depends on p_r only through $p_r(1 - p_r)$. Since the empirical type I errors are very close to the nominal $\alpha - 0.05$ overall, our test statistic Z_1 controls the type I error rate accurately.

TABLE 17.4

Sample size (empirical type I error rate, empirical power), $n(\hat{\alpha}, 1-\hat{\beta})$, under various design settings of $(p_r, \delta_1, \rho_1, 1-\beta)$ for the type of study objective 1

p_r	δ_1	ρ_1	$1-\beta=0.8$	$1-\beta=0.9$
0.3	0.05	0.1	210(0.044, 0.808)	290(0.051, 0.910)
		0.3	206(0.048, 0.812)	285(0.047, 0.903)
		0.5	200(0.049, 0.805)	275(0.049, 0.910)
		0.7	186(0.054, 0.811)	256(0.056, 0.903)
	0.1	0.1	56(0.041, 0.829)	76(0.045, 0.915)
		0.3	55(0.047, 0.823)	75(0.042, 0.914)
		0.5	53(0.048, 0.822)	73(0.052, 0.921)
		0.7	50(0.061, 0.822)	68(0.060, 0.913)
0.5	0.05	0.1	249(0.047, 0.804)	344(0.048, 0.904)
		0.3	245(0.051, 0.808)	338(0.053, 0.901)
		0.5	237(0.045, 0.812)	327(0.050, 0.907)
		0.7	220(0.053, 0.798)	304(0.050, 0.904)
	0.1	0.1	66(0.052, 0.815)	90(0.048, 0.911)
		0.3	65(0.049, 0.824)	88(0.046, 0.914)
		0.5	63(0.051, 0.831)	86(0.048, 0.912)
		0.7	58(0.054, 0.813)	80(0.054, 0.909)
0.7	0.05	0.1	210(0.052, 0.804)	290(0.054, 0.902)
		0.3	206(0.050, 0.800)	285(0.048, 0.906)
		0.5	200(0.052, 0.802)	275(0.051, 0.906)
		0.7	186(0.055, 0.806)	256(0.049, 0.899)
	0.1	0.1	56(0.055, 0.821)	76(0.054, 0.909)
		0.3	55(0.055, 0.816)	75(0.049, 0.904)
		0.5	53(0.052, 0.814)	73(0.054, 0.911)
		0.7	50(0.060, 0.821)	68(0.058, 0.912)

On the other hand, the empirical powers are close to the corresponding nominal level $1-\beta=0.8$ or 0.9 overall so that we conclude that our sample size formula is accurate too.

Now, we conduct simulations for the type of study objective 1 to test if the AI-based device is more concordant with experienced radiologists than with junior radiologists. We assume that each subject's image is read by $m=5$ experienced radiologists and $m=5$ junior radiologists. We set $\alpha=0.05$, $1-\beta=0.8$ or 0.9, $p_x=0.3$, 0.5, or 0.7, $\delta_2=0.05$ or 0.1, and $\rho_2=0.1$, 0.3, 0.5, or 0.7. Assuming $\rho_{xx}=\rho_{yy}=\rho_{xy}+0.1$, we solve the corresponding correlation coefficients for given $\rho_2=corr(x_i,y_i)$. So, we have $(\rho_{xx},\rho_{yy},\rho_{xy})=(0.13,0.13,0.03)$, $(0.21,0.21,0.11)$, $(0.33,0.33,0.23)$, and $(0.55,0.55,0.45)$ for $\rho_2=0.1$, 0.3, 0.5, and 0.7, respectively. For each design setting, we calculate sample size n using (17.9), and generate 10,000 samples of size n under the design setting and H_2 or $\bar{H}_2$. We apply the test statistic Z_2 to each sample, and calculate the empirical type I error rate and power $(\hat{\alpha}, 1-\hat{\beta})$ under $H_2: p_x=p_y$ and $\bar{H}_2: p_x=p_y+\delta_0$, respectively.

TABLE 17.5

Sample size (empirical type I error rate, empirical power), $n(\hat{\alpha}, 1-\hat{\beta})$, under various design settings of $(p_x, \delta_2, \rho_2, 1-\beta)$ for the type of study objective 2

p_x	δ_2	ρ_2	$1-\beta=0.8$	$1-\beta=0.9$
0.3	0.05	0.1	348(0.052, 0.810)	465(0.052, 0.898)
		0.3	328(0.050, 0.812)	438(0.048, 0.894)
		0.5	298(0.049, 0.807)	397(0.047, 0.900)
		0.7	245(0.053, 0.807)	327(0.048, 0.907)
	0.1	0.1	86(0.054, 0.816)	113(0.050, 0.905)
		0.3	81(0.053, 0.820)	107(0.047, 0.912)
		0.5	74(0.047, 0.825)	98(0.047, 0.914)
		0.7	63(0.053, 0.844)	83(0.048, 0.934)
0.5	0.05	0.1	434(0.050, 0.798)	580(0.048, 0.902)
		0.3	409(0.050, 0.810)	546(0.049, 0.904)
		0.5	370(0.049, 0.806)	495(0.052, 0.905)
		0.7	304(0.054, 0.802)	406(0.050, 0.905)
	0.1	0.1	111(0.053, 0.816)	148(0.053, 0.909)
		0.3	105(0.047, 0.814)	140(0.051, 0.909)
		0.5	96(0.050, 0.811)	127(0.052, 0.911)
		0.7	79(0.052, 0.829)	105(0.050, 0.913)
0.7	0.05	0.1	382(0.051, 0.803)	511(0.052, 0.900)
		0.3	360(0.052, 0.797)	481(0.048, 0.901)
		0.5	327(0.046, 0.804)	436(0.055, 0.902)
		0.7	269(0.047, 0.811)	359(0.053, 0.909)
	0.1	0.1	103(0.050, 0.815)	136(0.049, 0.914)
		0.3	97(0.054, 0.817)	129(0.049, 0.912)
		0.5	89(0.050, 0.821)	117(0.050, 0.917)
		0.7	74(0.048, 0.840)	98(0.045, 0.925)

Table 17.5 summarizes the required sample size n, and empirical type I error rate and power, $(\hat{\alpha}, 1-\hat{\beta})$, under each design setting. We observe that the required sample size increases in $1-\beta$ and decreases in δ_2 and ρ_2. Since the empirical type I errors are very close to the nominal $\alpha = 0.05$ overall, our test statistic Z_2 controls the type I error accurately. On the other hand, the empirical powers are close to the corresponding nominal level $1-\beta = 0.8$ or 0.9 overall so that we conclude that our sample size formula is accurate too.

Appendix A. Derivation of ρ_1

Since $r_i = \{m(m-1)/2\}^{-1}\sum_{j=1}^{m-1}\sum_{j'=j+1}^{m} r_{ijj'}$ and $s_i = m^{-1}\sum_{j=1}^{m} s_{ij}$, we have

$$\rho_1 = \text{corr}(r_i, s_i) = \frac{\text{cov}(r_i, s_i)}{\sqrt{\text{var}(r_i)\text{var}(s_i)}}.$$

Here

$$\text{cov}(r_i, s_i) = \text{cov}\left(\frac{\sum_{j=1}^{m-1}\sum_{j'=j+1}^{m} r_{ijj'}}{m(m-1)/2}, \frac{\sum_{j=1}^{m} s_{ij}}{m}\right)$$

$$= \frac{2}{m^2(m-1)} cov\left(\sum_{j=1}^{m-1}\sum_{j'=j+1}^{m} r_{ijj'}, \sum_{j=1}^{m} s_{ij}\right)$$

$$= \frac{2}{m^2(m-1)}\left\{m(m-1)\text{cov}(r_{ij_1j_2}, s_{ij_1}) + \frac{m(m-1)(m-2)}{2}\text{cov}(r_{ij_1j_2}, s_{ij_1'})\right\}$$

$$= \frac{2}{m}\text{cov}(r_{i12}, s_{i1}) + \frac{m-2}{m}\text{cov}(r_{i12}, s_{i3})$$

$$\text{var}(r_i) = \frac{4}{m^2(m-1)^2}\text{var}(\sum_{j=1}^{m-1}\sum_{j'=j+1}^{m} r_{ijj'})$$

$$= \frac{4}{m^2(m-1)^2}\left\{\frac{m(m-1)}{2}\text{var}(r_{ij_1j_2}) + m(m-1)(m-2)\text{cov}(r_{ij_1j_2}, r_{ij_1j_2'})\right.$$

$$\left. + \frac{m(m-1)(m-2)(m-3)}{4}\text{cov}(r_{ij_1j_2}, r_{ij_1'j_2'})\right\}$$

$$= \frac{2}{m(m-1)} var(r_{i12}) + \frac{4(m-2)}{m(m-1)} cov(r_{i12}, r_{i13}) + \frac{(m-2)(m-3)}{m(m-1)} cov(r_{i12}, r_{i34})$$

and

$$\text{var}(s_i) = \frac{1}{m^2}\{m\text{var}(s_{i1}) + m(m-1)\text{cov}(s_{i1}, s_{i2})\}$$

$$= \frac{1}{m}\text{var}(s_{i1}) + \frac{m-1}{m}\text{cov}(s_{i1}, s_{i2}).$$

Hence,

$$\rho_1 = \frac{\frac{2}{m}\text{cov}(r_{i12}, s_{i1}) + \frac{m-2}{m}\text{cov}(r_{i12}, s_{i3})}{\sqrt{\{\frac{2}{m(m-1)}\text{var}(r_{i12}) + \frac{4(m-2)}{m(m-1)}\text{cov}(r_{i12}, r_{i13}) + \frac{(m-2)(m-3)}{m(m-1)}\text{cov}(r_{i12}, r_{i34})\}}}$$

$$\times \frac{1}{\sqrt{\{\frac{1}{m}\text{var}(s_{i1}) + \frac{m-1}{m} cov(s_{i1}, s_{i2})\}}}$$

$$= \frac{\frac{2}{m}\rho_{s1} + \frac{m-2}{m}\rho_{s2}}{\sqrt{\{\frac{2}{m(m-1)} + \frac{4(m-2)}{m(m-1)}\rho_{r1} + \frac{(m-2)(m-3)}{m(m-1)}\rho_{r2}\}(\frac{1}{m} + \frac{m-1}{m}\rho_{ss})}}.$$

Appendix B. The Limit of $\hat{\sigma}_1^2$ under $\bar{H}_1$

The limit of $\hat{\sigma}_1^2 = n^{-1}\sum_{i=1}^{n}(s_i - r_i)^2$ is its expected value $\sigma_1^2 = E(s_i - r_i)^2$. Since $E(s_i - r_i) = p_s - p_r = 0$ under $\bar{H}_1 : p_r = p_s$, $E(s_i - r_i)^2 = \text{var}(s_i - r_i) = \text{var}(s_i) + \text{var}(r_i) - 2\rho_1\sqrt{\text{var}(s_i)\text{var}(r_i)}$ where $\rho_1 = \text{corr}(r_i, s_i)$,

$$\text{var}(s_i) = \frac{1}{m^2}var\left(\sum_{j=1}^{m} s_{ij}\right) = \frac{1}{m^2}\left\{m\text{var}(s_{ij}) + m(m-1)\text{cov}\left(s_{ij}, s_{ij'}\right)\right\}$$

$$= \frac{1}{m}\text{var}(s_{ij}) + \frac{m-1}{m}\rho_{ss}\text{var}(s_{ij}) = p_s(1-p_s)\left(\frac{1}{m} + \frac{m-1}{m}\rho_{ss}\right)$$

and

$$\text{var}(r_i) = var\left(\frac{1}{m(m-1)/2}\sum_{j_1=1}^{m-1}\sum_{j_2=j+1}^{m} r_{ij_1j_2}\right)$$

$$= \left\{\frac{1}{m(m-1)/2}\right\}^2\left\{\frac{m(m-1)}{2}\text{var}(r_{i12}) + m(m-1)(m-2)\text{cov}(r_{i12}, r_{i13})\right.$$

$$\left. + \frac{m(m-1)(m-2)(m-3)}{4}\text{cov}(r_{i12}, r_{i34})\right\}$$

$$= \left(\frac{2}{m(m-1)}\text{var}(r_{i12}) + \frac{4(m-2)}{m(m-1)}\rho_{r1}\text{var}(r_{i12}) + \frac{(m-2)(m-3)}{m(m-1)}\rho_{r2}\text{var}(r_{i12})\right)$$

$$= p_r(1-p_r)\left\{\frac{2}{m(m-1)} + \frac{4(m-2)}{m(m-1)}\rho_{r1} + \frac{(m-2)(m-3)}{m(m-1)}\rho_{r2}\right\}$$

since $s_{ij} \sim \text{Bernoulli}(p_s)$ and $r_{ij_1j_2} \sim \text{Bernoulli}(p_r)$.

Appendix C. Derivation of ρ_2

Since $x_i = m^{-1}\sum_{j=1}^{m} x_{ij}$ and $y_i = m^{-1}\sum_{j=1}^{m} y_{ij}$,

$$\rho_2 = \text{corr}(x_i, y_i) = \frac{\text{cov}(x_i, y_i)}{\sqrt{\text{var}(x_i)\text{var}(y_i)}}.$$

Here,

$$\text{cov}(x_i, y_i) = \text{cov}\left(\frac{\sum_{j=1}^{m} x_{ij}}{m}, \frac{\sum_{j=1}^{m} y_{ij}}{m}\right) = \text{cov}(x_{ij}, y_{ij})$$

$$\text{var}(x_i) = \frac{1}{m}\text{var}(x_{i1}) + \frac{m-1}{m}\text{cov}(x_{i1}, x_{i2})$$

and, similarly,

$$\text{var}(y_i) = \frac{1}{m}\text{var}(y_{i1}) + \frac{m-1}{m}\text{cov}(y_{i1}, y_{i2}).$$

Hence,

$$\rho_2 = \frac{\text{cov}(x_{i1}, y_{i1})}{\sqrt{\{\frac{1}{m}\text{var}(x_{i1}) + \frac{m-1}{m}\text{cov}(x_{i1}, x_{i2})\}\{\frac{1}{m}\text{var}(y_{i1}) + \frac{m-1}{m}\text{cov}(y_{i1}, y_{i2})\}}}$$

$$= \frac{\rho_{xy}}{\sqrt{(\frac{1}{m} + \frac{m-1}{m}\rho_{xx})(\frac{1}{m} + \frac{m-1}{m}\rho_{yy})}}.$$

Appendix D. The Limit of $\hat{\sigma}_2^2$ under $\bar{H}_2$

The limit of $\hat{\sigma}_2^2 = n^{-1}\sum_{i=1}^{n}(x_i - y_i - \delta_2)^2$ is $\sigma_2^2 = E(x_i - y_i - \delta_2)^2$. Since $E(x_i - y_i - \delta_2) = p_x - p_y - \delta_2 = 0$ under $\bar{H}_2 : p_x = p_y + \delta_0$, $E(x_i - y_i - \delta_2)^2 = \text{var}(x_i - y_i - \delta_2) = \text{var}(x_i - y_i) = \text{var}(x_i) + \text{var}(y_i) - 2\rho_2\sqrt{\text{var}(x_i)\text{var}(y_i)}$. Here, $\rho_2 = \text{corr}(x_i, y_i)$,

$$\text{var}(x_i) = \frac{1}{m^2}\{m\text{var}(x_{i1}) + m(m-1)\text{cov}(x_{i1}, x_{i2})\}$$

$$= \frac{\text{var}(x_{i1})}{m} + \frac{m-1}{m}\rho_{xx}\text{var}(x_{i1})) = p_x(1-p_x)\left(\frac{1}{m} + \frac{m-1}{m}\rho_{xx}\right)$$

and, similarly,

$$\text{var}(y_i) = p_y(1-p_y)\left(\frac{1}{m} + \frac{m-1}{m}\rho_{yy}\right)$$

$$= (p_x - \delta_0)(1 - p_x + \delta_0)\left(\frac{1}{m} + \frac{m-1}{m}\rho_{yy}\right)$$

since $x_{ij} \sim Bernoulli(p_x), y_{ij} \sim Bernoulli(p_y)$.

References

Biswas B. (2006). Assessing agreement for diagnostic devices. presentation at FDA/Industry Statistics Workshop, September 28–29, 2006.

Cantor AB. Sample-size calculations for Cohen's Kappa. Psychological Methods 1996; 1: 150–153.

Cheng HD, Shan J, Ju W, Guo Y, Zhang L. Automated breast cancer detection and classification using ultrasound images: a survey. Pattern Recognition 2010; 43: 299–317.

Cichetti DV, Feinstein AR. High agreement but low kappa: resolving the paradoxes. Journal of Epidemiology 1990; 43: 551–5558.

Cohen J. A coefficient of agreement for nominal scales. Educational and Psychological Measurement 1960; 20: 37–46.

Cook RJ. (1998). Kappa and its dependence on marginal rates. In: The Encyclopedia of biostatistics, P. Armitage, T. Colton, eds., pp. 2166–2168, New York: Wiley.

Donner A. (1999). Sample size requirements for interval estimation of the intraclass kappa statistic. Communications in Statistics - Simulation 1999; 28: 415–429.

Donner A, Eliasziw M. A goodness-of-fit approach to inference procedures for the Kappa statistic: confidence interval construction, significance-testing and sample size estimation. Statistics in Medicine 1992; 11: 1511–1519.

D'Orsi CJ et al. ACR BI-RADS® Atlas, Breast Imaging Reporting and Data System. American College of Radiology: Reston, VA, USA, 2013.

Dukalski VL, Palesch YY, Lipsitz SR, Rust PF. Analysis of clustered matched-pair data for a non-inferiority study design. Statistics in Medicine 2003; 22: 279–290.

Early Treatment for Retinopathy of Prematurity Cooperative Group. Revised indications for the treatment of retinopathy of prematurity: Results of the early treatment of retinopathy of prematurity randomized trial. Archives of Ophthalmology 2003; 121: 1684–1694.

Feinstein AR, Cicchetti DV. High agreement but low kappa: The problems of two paradoxes. Journal of Epidemiology 1990; 43: 543–549.

Jennison C, Turnbull BW. (2000). Group sequential methods with applications to clinical trials. Boca Raton, Florida: CRC Press Inc.

Jung SH, Ahn C. (2005). Sample size for a two-group comparison of repeated binary measurements using GEE. Statistics in Medicine 2005; 24: 2583–2596.

Jung SH, Barnhart HX, Sohn I, Stinnett SS, Wallace DK. Sample size for comparing correlated concordance rates. Journal of Biopharmaceutical Statistics 2008; 18: 359–369.

Liang KY, Zeger S. Longitudinal data analysis using generalized linear models. Biometrika 1986; 73: 13–22.

Lin HM, Williamson JM, Lipsitz SR. Calculating power for the comparison of dependent kappa coefficients. Applied Statistics 2003; 52: 391–404.

Liu B., Cheng H.D., Huang J., Tian J., Tang X., Liu J. Fully automatic and segmentation-robust classification of breast tumors based on local texture analysis of ultrasound images. Pattern Recognition 2010; 43: 280–298.

Liu L, Parker KJ, Jung SH. Design and Analysis Methods for Trials with AI-based Diagnostic Devices. Journal of Personalized Medicine 2021; 11(11): 1150.

Maclure M, Willett WC. Misinterpretation and misuse of the kappa statistic. American Journal of Epidemiology 1987; 126: 161–169.

Meier K. (2006). Revising FDA's "Statistical guidance on reporting results from studies evaluating diagnostic tests", presentation at FDA/Industry Statistics Workshop, September 28–29, 2006.

Nam J. Assessment on homogeneity tests for kappa statistics under equal prevalence across studies in reliability. Statistics in Medicine 2006; 25: 1521–1531.

O'Connell AM, Bartolotta TV, Orlando A, Jung SH, Baek J, Parker KJ. Diagnostic performance of an artificial intelligence system in breast ultrasound. Journal of Ultrasound in Medicine 2022; 41(1): 97–105.

Schaffer DB, Palmer EA, Plotsky DF, et al., for the Cryotherapy for Retinopathy of Prematurity Cooperative Group. Prognostic factors in the natural course of retinopathy of prematurity. Ophthalmology 1993; 100: 230–237.

Shan J, Cheng HD, Wang Y. Completely automated segmentation approach for breast ultrasound images using multiple-domain features. Ultrasound in Medicine & Biology 2012; 38: 262–275.

Wu WJ, Lin SW, Moon WK. Combining support vector machine with genetic algorithm to classify ultrasound breast tumor images. Computerized Medical Imaging Graphics 2012; 36: 627–633.

Wu GG, Zhou LQ, Xu JW, Wang JY, Wei Q, Deng YB, Cui XW, Dietrich CF. Artificial intelligence in breast ultrasound. World Journal of Radiology 2019; 11: 19–26.

Zhang Z, Sejdic E. Radiological images and machine learning: trends, perspectives, and prospects. Computers in Biology and Medicine 2019; 108: 354–370.

18

Comparison of Binary Medical Tests and ROC Curves with Clustered Data

Many new medical tests have been developed with recent advances in biotechnology such as, physical and visual exams, diagnostic imaging, genetic testing, chemical and cellular analysis. Medical tests can be used for various purposes including diagnosis, prognosis, risk prediction, and disease screening. In the early development stage of a medical test, the original data type is continuous. Once a new biomarker is discovered, it is dichotomized or categorized for easy clinical use by classifying patients associated with a clinical outcome. In the first section of this chapter, we investigate statistical methods to compare the performance of two binary medical tests. In the second section, we investigate paired ROC curve methods to compare the performance of two continuous biomarkers. In the third section, we extend the paired ROC method to an ROC method with pair data from multiple sites of each subject, called clustered paired data. These two-sample testing methods can be easily extended to K-sample testing.

Comparison of Binary Tests with Clustered Data

Among frequently used parameters measuring the performance of binary tests are accuracy, sensitivity, specificity, positive predictive value, and negative predictive value. Sensitivity is the probability of a positive test among subjects with disease (cases), and specificity is the probability of a negative test among healthy subjects (controls). On the other hand, positive predictive value (PPV) is the probability of having the disease, given that the test is positive, and negative predictive value (NPV) is the probability of not having the disease, given that the test is negative. McNemar's (1947) test can be used to test equality of the sensitivity or specificity for two tests evaluated on the same subjects, see Chapter 2. However, relatively little attention has been paid to the comparison between paired PPVs or NPVs. Wang et al. (2006) presented a test statistic and its power calculation to compare the PPVs (and of two NPVs in a similar way) of two binary tests. They used the

DOI: 10.1201/9781003221951-18

delta method to derive the asymptotic normality of the log ratio or the difference of two PPVs. Leisenring et al. (2000) implemented the generalized estimating equations to solve this problem. They proposed a score statistic and a Wald statistic derived from a marginal regression model. Kosinski (2013) proposed a weighted generalized score statistic for simpler computation. His statistic reduces to the score statistic in the independent sample situation. Moskowitz et al. (2006) derived sample size formula for the log ratio of two PPVs and they used the multinomial Poisson transformation which transforms the likelihood of the data into a Poisson likelihood with additional parameters to avoid a complicated variance form obtained by the delta method. These methods do not allow clustered data.

Although well established, sensitivity and specificity have some deficiencies in clinical use. This arises mainly from the fact that sensitivity and specificity are population measures, i.e., they summarize the characteristics of the test over a population. When we consider the results of a diagnostic test from a patient's perspective, however, PPV and NPV are much more important than the population level parameters, sensitivity and specificity.

This study was motivated by a real project (Um 2015) to compare the performance of two diagnostic tests to determine the metastatic status of lymph nodes for lung cancer patients. Mediastinoscopy has been a diagnostic standard, but its sensitivity and negative predictive value are not very high. Furthermore, the technique is invasive and the morbidity and mortality rates are known to be about 2% and 0.08%, respectively (Porte et al. 1998, Silvestri et al. 2015). Endobronchial ultrasound-guided transbronchial needle aspiration (EBUS) is a less invasive intervention with broader visual scope so that the investigators would like to compare the new method, EBUS, to the existing diagnostic tool, mediastinoscopy. Both diagnostic tests are conducted for some chosen lymph nodes of each patient so that the resulting data have clustered paired structure, where pairs are two diagnostic tests from each lymph node site (subunit) and clusters are patients contributing multiple sites. The study was designed to show the non-inferiority of the new test compared to the standard test, but it was shown to be even superior in some operating characteristics.

Rao and Scott (1992) proposed a method accounting for the clustering effect multiplying an inflation factor to the variance estimator for independent data. Jung et al. (2001) proposed a sample size calculation method for an optimal estimator of binomial proportion from clustered binary data with random cluster sizes. Hu et al. (2001) derived a sample size formula for sensitivity and specificity of diagnostic tests using the sign test for dependent multiple observations per subject under common correlation model. These methods mainly deal with single sample proportion estimator and the focus has been given on sensitivity or specificity. In addition, Katsis (2004) applied a Bayesian approach to the sample size for two dependent binomial populations using a Dirichlet prior on the proportions.

In this section, we investigate the simple statistical testing method, proposed by Kwak et al. (2013), to compare two binary medical tests on sensitivity, specificity, accuracy, PPV, and NPV using clustered binary data.

Statistical Testing Methods

Suppose that there are two diagnostic tests to be compared. From site $j(= 1, ..., m_i)$ of subject i, we observe binary random variables d_{ij} denoting the disease status, taking 0 for non-disease and 1 for disease, and x_{kij} denoting the outcome of diagnostic test $k(= 1, 2)$, taking 0 for negative and 1 for positive. Thus, the resulting data are summarized as $\{(d_{ij}, x_{1ij}, x_{2ij}), 1 \leq j \leq m_i, 1 \leq i \leq n\}$. Let p_k denote the sensitivity, specificity, accuracy, PPV, or NPV for medical test $k(= 1, 2)$. We assume that $\max_i m_i \leq c(< \infty)$ and a positive diagnostic outcome provides evidence of disease. The asymptotic theory is applied for large n.

For each operational characteristic of diagnostic tests, we propose a consistent estimator $\hat{p}_k$ for p_k and derive the asymptotic normality of $\sqrt{n}(\hat{p}_1 - \hat{p}_2)$ using clustered binary data. Hence, we reject $H_0 : p_1 = p_2$ in favor of $H_1 : p_1 \neq p_2$ if the absolute value of $Z = \sqrt{n}(\hat{p}_1 - \hat{p}_2)/\hat{\sigma}$ is larger than $z_{1-\alpha/2}$, where $\hat{\sigma}^2$ is a variance estimator of $\sqrt{n}(\hat{p}_1 - \hat{p}_2)$ and $z_{1-\alpha/2}$ is the $100(1-\alpha/2)$ percentile of the standard normal distribution.

Sensitivity and Specificity

An unbiased estimator of the sensitivity for diagnostic test $k(= 1, 2)$, p_k, is given by

$$\hat{p}_k = \frac{\sum_{i=1}^{n}\sum_{j=1}^{m_i} x_{kij}d_{ij}}{\sum_{i=1}^{n}\sum_{j=1}^{m_i} d_{ij}}.$$

Let $D = \sum_{i=1}^{n}\sum_{j=1}^{m_i} d_{ij}$ denote the total number of diseased sites across all n subjects. We have

$$\sqrt{n}(\hat{p}_k - p_k) = \frac{\sqrt{n}}{D}\sum_{i=1}^{n}\sum_{j=1}^{m_i}(x_{kij} - p_k)d_{ij}.$$

Since subjects are independent, given the disease status of the patients, $\epsilon_{ki} = \sum_{j=1}^{m_i}(x_{kij} - p_k)d_{ij}$ are independent 0-mean random variables. By the central limit theorem for large n, $\sqrt{n}(\hat{p}_k - p_k)$ is asymptotically normal with mean 0 and variance σ_k^2 that can be consistently estimated by

$$\hat{\sigma}_k^2 = \frac{n}{D^2}\sum_{i=1}^{n}\left\{\sum_{j=1}^{m_i}(x_{kij} - \hat{p}_k)d_{ij}\right\}^2.$$

Hence, we can estimate a confidence interval of p_k by $\hat{p}_k \pm z_{1-\alpha/2}\hat{\sigma}_k/\sqrt{n}$.

Furthermore, for the difference in sensitivity between two diagnostic tests, we have

$$\sqrt{n}(\hat{p}_1 - \hat{p}_2) = \frac{\sqrt{n}}{D} \sum_{i=1}^{n} \sum_{j=1}^{m_i} (x_{1ij} - x_{2ij}) d_{ij}.$$

Under $H_0 : p_1 = p_2$, $\epsilon_i = \sum_{j=1}^{m_i} (x_{1ij} - x_{2ij}) d_{ij}$ are independent 0-mean random variables. Hence, under H_0, $\sqrt{n}(\hat{p}_1 - \hat{p}_2)$ is approximately normal with mean 0 and variance σ^2 that can be consistently estimated by

$$\hat{\sigma}^2 = \frac{n}{D^2} \sum_{i=1}^{n} \left\{ \sum_{j=1}^{m_i} (x_{1ij} - x_{2ij}) d_{ij} \right\}^2 .$$

The inference on specificities can be derived from that on sensitivities by replacing d_{ij} and x_{kij} with $1 - d_{ij}$ and $1 - x_{kij}$, respectively.

Accuracy

In the previous chapter, we have investigated comparison of concordance rates. Accuracy is identical to concordance when the gold standard is disease status. For site j of patient i, the testing result by diagnostic method k is accurate if $y_{kij} \equiv I(x_{kij} = d_{ij}) = x_{kij} d_{ij} + (1 - x_{kij})(1 - d_{ij})$ equals 1, and inaccurate if y_{kij} equals 0. An unbiased and consistent estimator of the accuracy for method k, $p_k = P(x_{kij} = d_{ij})$, is given as

$$\hat{p}_k = \frac{1}{M} \sum_{i=1}^{n} \sum_{j=1}^{m_i} y_{kij},$$

where $M = \sum_{i=1}^{n} m_i$ denotes the total number of sites across all n subjects. From

$$\sqrt{n}(\hat{p}_k - p_k) = \frac{\sqrt{n}}{M} \sum_{i=1}^{n} \sum_{j=1}^{m_i} (y_{kij} - p_k),$$

$\epsilon_{ki} = \sum_{j=1}^{m_i} (y_{kij} - p_k)$ are independent 0-mean random variables for $i = 1, ..., n$. Hence, $\sqrt{n}(\hat{p}_k - p_k)$ is approximately normal with mean 0 and variance σ_k^2 that can be consistently estimated by

$$\hat{\sigma}_k^2 = \frac{n}{M^2} \sum_{i=1}^{n} \left\{ \sum_{j=1}^{m_i} (y_{kij} - \hat{p}_k) \right\}^2$$

For the difference in accuracy between two diagnostic tests, we have

$$\sqrt{n}(\hat{p}_1 - \hat{p}_2) = \frac{\sqrt{n}}{M} \sum_{i=1}^{n} \epsilon_i,$$

where $\epsilon_i = \sum_{j=1}^{m_i}(y_{1ij} - y_{2ij}), i = 1, \ldots, n$ are independent 0-mean random variables under $H_0 : p_1 = p_2$. Hence, under H_0, $\sqrt{n}(\hat{p}_1 - \hat{p}_2)$ is approximately normal with mean 0 and variance σ^2 that can be consistently estimated by

$$\hat{\sigma}^2 = \frac{n}{M^2}\sum_{i=1}^{n}\left\{\sum_{j=1}^{m_i}(y_{1ij} - y_{2ij})\right\}^2.$$

PPV and NPV

Noting that the PPV of diagnostic test k is defined by

$$p_k = P(d_{ij} = 1|x_{kij} = 1) = P(x_{kij} = 1, d_{ij} = 1)/P(x_{kij} = 1) \equiv a_k/b_k$$

a consistent estimator of p_k is obtained by

$$\hat{p}_k = \frac{\sum_{i=1}^{n}\sum_{j=1}^{m_i} x_{kij}d_{ij}}{\sum_{i=1}^{n}\sum_{j=1}^{m_i} x_{kij}} \equiv \frac{\hat{a}_k}{\hat{b}_k},$$

where $\hat{a}_k = M^{-1}\sum_{i=1}^{n}\sum_{j=1}^{m_i} x_{kij}d_{ij}$ and $\hat{b}_k = M^{-1}\sum_{i=1}^{n}\sum_{j=1}^{m_i} x_{kij}$.

We have

$$\hat{p}_k - p_k = \frac{\hat{a}_k b_k - a_k\hat{b}_k}{b_k\hat{b}_k} = \frac{b_k(\hat{a}_k - a_k) - a_k(\hat{b}_k - b_k)}{b_k^2} + o_p(n^{-1/2}),$$

where the ignorable error term $o_p(n^{-1/2})$ is added by replacing the consistent estimator $\hat{b}_k$ with b_k in the denominator. Then, for $a_{kij} = x_{kij}d_{ij}$ and $b_{kij} = x_{kij}$, we have

$$\sqrt{n}(\hat{p}_k - p_k) = \frac{\sqrt{n}}{M}\sum_{i=1}^{n}\sum_{j=1}^{m_i}\left\{\frac{1}{b_k}(a_{kij} - a_k) - \frac{a_k}{b_k^2}(b_{kij} - b_k)\right\} + o_p(1)$$

$$= \frac{\sqrt{n}}{M}\sum_{i=1}^{n}\epsilon_{ki} + o_p(1),$$

where, for $i = 1, ..., n$, $\epsilon_{ki} = b_k^{-1}\sum_{j=1}^{m_i}\{a_{kij} - a_k - p_k(b_{kij} - b_k)\}$ are independent random variables with mean 0. Hence, $\sqrt{n}(\hat{p}_k - p_k)$ is approximately normal with mean 0 and variance σ_k^2 that can be consistently estimated by

$$\hat{\sigma}_k^2 = \frac{n}{M^2}\sum_{i=1}^{n}\hat{\epsilon}_{ki}^2,$$

where $\hat{\epsilon}_{ki}$ is obtained from ϵ_{ki} by replacing a_k, b_k and p_k with their consistent estimators $\hat{a}_k$, $\hat{b}_k$ and $\hat{p}_k$, respectively, i.e., $\hat{\epsilon}_{ki} = \hat{b}_k^{-1}\sum_{j=1}^{m_i}\{a_{kij} - \hat{a}_k - \hat{p}_k(b_{kij} - \hat{b}_k)\}$.

Similarly, under $H_0 : p_1 = p_2$, we have

$$\hat{p}_1 - \hat{p}_2 = (\hat{p}_1 - p_1) - (\hat{p}_2 - p_2)$$
$$= M^{-1} \sum_{i=1}^{n} (\epsilon_{1i} - \epsilon_{2i}) + o_p(n^{-1/2}).$$

For $i = 1, ..., n$, we observe that $\epsilon_i = \epsilon_{1i} - \epsilon_{2i}$ are independent random variables with mean 0. Hence, under H_0, $\sqrt{n}(\hat{p}_1 - \hat{p}_2)$ is approximately normal with mean 0 and variance σ^2 that can be consistently estimated by

$$\hat{\sigma}^2 = \frac{n}{M^2} \sum_{i=1}^{n} (\hat{\epsilon}_{1i} - \hat{\epsilon}_{2i})^2.$$

The inference on NPV can be derived from that on PPV by replacing d_{ij} and x_{kij} with $1 - d_{ij}$ and $1 - x_{kij}$, respectively.

Simulations

Simulation studies are carried out to evaluate the finite sample properties of the discussed methods under a variety of conditions. At first, for sensitivity and specificity with single binary test outcome $m_i = 1$ per subject, we confirmed that our simple variance formulas yield the same numerical results as the lengthy and complicated formulas of Wang et al. (2006) that were derived by using the multivariate central limit theorem together and the delta method. So, we focused on comparing PPVs and NPVs between two binary tests with clustered paired outcomes. We specify the disease prevalence, the number of patients n, the positive predictive value, and the negative predictive value for both test $k(= 1, 2)$, PPV_k and NPV_k. In addition, we specify the variance (σ_c^2) for a subject-specific random effect that is used to induce the correlation among the multiple sites on the same subject and the variance (σ_u^2) for a site-specific random effect that is used to induce the correlation between the two test outcomes performed at each site.

Under each setting, we generate 5,000 simulation data sets and evaluate the empirical type I error rate under H_0 and power under H_1 for the discussed methods. Each simulated data set is generated as follows. First, we generate the number of sites (i.e., cluster sizes) m_i for patient i by generating a random number from $\{2, 4, 6, 8, 10\}$ with equal probabilities $1/5$. Given m_i, disease indicators $(d_{ij}, j = 1, ..., m_i)$ are randomly generated for each patient by first drawing a multivariate normal random vector and then dichotomizing each random variable for a binary indicator using a percentile corresponding to a specified disease prevalence. For each patient, independent random effects c_i and u_{ij} are generated from zero-mean normal distributions with variance σ_c^2 and σ_u^2 respectively, and binary test outcomes are generated using probit models with the parametrization $P(x_{kij} = 1 | d_{ij}, c_i, u_{ij}) = \Phi\{\alpha_k(1 - d_{ij}) +$

TABLE 18.1

Relationship between Kappa statistic and PPV values under different prevalences

Prevalence	PPV_1	PPV_2	Kappa
0.25	0.70	0.70	0.163
	0.70	0.75	0.169
	0.85	0.85	0.467
	0.85	0.90	0.515
0.50	0.70	0.70	0.284
	0.70	0.75	0.310
	0.85	0.85	0.506
	0.85	0.90	0.604
0.75	0.70	0.70	0.160
	0.70	0.75	0.188
	0.85	0.85	0.328
	0.85	0.90	0.426

$\beta_k d_{ij} + c_i + u_{ij}\}$ for medical test $k(=1, 2)$, where $\Phi(\cdot)$ is the cumulative distribution function of the standard normal distribution. The values of the parameters $(\alpha_1, \beta_1, \alpha_2, \beta_2)$ used in these probit models are chosen so that the true and false positivity rates are equal to those calculated and they in turn give the desired predictive values. By taking the expectation with respect to the random effects, we obtain the marginal rate for test k as a function of coefficients (α_k, β_k) and the variance of the random effects σ_c^2 and σ_u^2 by

$$P(x_k = 1|d) = \Phi\left\{\frac{\alpha_k(1-d) + \beta_k d}{\sqrt{1+\sigma_c^2+\sigma_u^2}}\right\}.$$

The empirical type I error rate and power for comparing PPVs or NPVs between two binary tests are examined. We assume a disease prevalence of 0.25, 0.5, or 0.7, and a sample size n of 100, 200, or 500. Table 18.1 lists the Kappa statistics as a measurement of correlation between the two test outcomes for each patient under the simulation settings of prevalence, PPV_1, and PPV_2. These are estimated from simulated data.

Table 18.2 reports the empirical type I error rate $\hat{\alpha}$ and power $1 - \hat{\beta}$ for testing the equality of two PPVs with two-sided $\alpha = 0.05$. We consider the null hypothesis that the two diagnostic tests have equal PPVs of 0.7 or 0.85. Under the alternative hypothesis, we set $\text{PPV}_1 = 0.7$ or 0.85 and $\text{PPV}_2 = \text{PPV}_1 + 0.05$. In these simulations, NPVs are fixed at 0.9. We observe that the empirical type I error rates are maintained closely to the nominal level of $\alpha = 0.05$ under the simulation settings. And, the empirical power increases in sample size and prevalence. Also, we have a larger power with $\text{PPV}_1 = 0.85$ than with 0.7 since the former has a larger odds ratio between the two prognostic tests and higher Kappa statistics as shown in Table 18.1.

TABLE 18.2

Empirical type I error rate $\hat{\alpha}$ under H_0 : $\text{PPV}_1 = \text{PPV}_2$ and power $1-\hat{\beta}$ under H_1 : $\text{PPV}_2 = \text{PPV}_1 + 0.05$ with $\text{PPV}_1 = 0.7$ or 0.85 for different n

		$\text{PPV}_1 = 0.7$		$\text{PPV}_1 = 0.85$	
Prevalence	n	$\hat{\alpha}$	$1-\hat{\beta}$	$\hat{\alpha}$	$1-\hat{\beta}$
0.25	50	0.059	0.095	0.065	0.152
	100	0.056	0.107	0.056	0.240
	200	0.053	0.156	0.052	0.412
	500	0.049	0.303	0.047	0.807
0.50	50	0.055	0.326	0.051	0.333
	100	0.056	0.531	0.055	0.554
	200	0.051	0.826	0.047	0.875
	500	0.054	0.996	0.050	0.997
0.75	50	0.057	0.652	0.061	0.674
	100	0.053	0.865	0.054	0.895
	200	0.052	0.937	0.055	0.995
	500	0.046	1.000	0.052	1.000

TABLE 18.3

Empirical power for H_1 : $\text{PPV}_1 = 0.85, \text{PPV}_2 = 0.75$ with $\text{NPV}_1 = \text{NPV}_2 = 0.85$ and $m_i = 1$. [1]: Weighted least square method by Wang et al. (2006); [2]: Generalized estimating equation method by Leisenring et al. (2000)

		Method		
Prevalence	n	**WLS[1]**	**GEE[2]**	**New**
0.25	100	0.040	0.063	0.073
	200	0.164	0.191	0.208
	500	0.386	0.399	0.404
0.50	100	0.346	0.367	0.390
	200	0.614	0.625	0.652
	500	0.954	0.954	0.966
0.70	100	0.781	0.791	0.821
	200	0.978	0.979	0.982
	500	1.000	1.000	1.000

We compare empirical test power of the new method discussed in this section with two previously proposed methods that allow only single site per subject, i.e., $m_i = 1$, based on 5,000 simulation samples. Empirical powers for H_1 : $\text{PPV}_1 = 0.85, \text{PPV}_2 = 0.75$ with the two NPVs fixed at 0.85 are calculated by weighted least square method by Wang et al. (2006), generalized estimating equation (GEE) method by Leisenring et al. (2000), and the proposed (New) method. We consider various scenarios with the disease prevalence of 0.25, 0.5, or 0.75 and the sample sizes of $n = 100$, 200, or 500. From Table

18.3, the proposed method seems to have similar or slightly higher power compared to the previously proposed methods.

We also conducted similar simulations on NPVs and observed almost the same results.

Example

For illustrative purpose, the testing methods investigated in this section are applied to real data from lung cancer diagnostic test introduced above (Um et al. 2015). Investigators are interested in comparing the performance of a new diagnostic test called EBUS with the standard mediastinoscopy. The patients with non-small cell lung cancer have come from a single-center prospective trial that is conducted to compare the diagnostic measures such as sensitivity, specificity, PPV and NPV of EBUS and those of mediastinoscopy to detect lymph node metastasis. Some lymph nodes are located in deeper place than others and it is important to confirm the presence of malignancy in differently located lymph nodes. Each examination was performed to evaluate multiple lymph nodes in various stations.

For each subject both diagnostic techniques look into several lymph nodes and determine positivity of cancer malignancy. Also, a gold standard involving lymph node dissection is available for each lymph node tested. Each test result is binary outcome. The number of lymph nodes tested per subject is widely varied from three to eighteen and the investigators agree to focus on five lymph nodes which are commonly used to make cancer staging. It is noted that not all five lymph nodes have gold standard test result and that even for the lymph node with gold standard result, some data were coded as missing in either diagnostic test outcome. In the latter case, the investigators agree to replace missing diagnostic test outcome with negativity since not being able to see a lymph node is deemed to imply that the unrecognizable lymph node is fine by the diagnostic test. This result in the number of lymph nodes to vary between two and five per patient, i.e., $m_i = 2 \sim 5$. A total of $n = 127$ patients with data of the two diagnostic tests and gold standard are included in the data analysis with a total of $M = 441$ lymph nodes.

For EBUS, we estimate PPV = 1 and NPV = 0.916. For mediastinoscopy, we estimate PPV = 1 and NPV = 0.901. Neither PPV nor NPV is significantly different between the two diagnostic tests. The 95% confidence interval for the difference is $(-0.048, 0.017)$ for NPVs, but not available for PPVs. Therefore, the two tests, EBUS and mediastinoscopy, do not seem to have a different PPV or NPV in diagnosing lymph node metastasis of lung cancer patients. The analysis results for sensitivity, specificity, accuracy, PPV, or NPV between EBUS and mediastinoscopy are presented in Table 18.4.

In this project, the investigators are actually interested in showing the non-inferiority of EBUS to mediastinoscopy in PPV and NPV. We formulate the null hypothesis stating that the PPV (or NPV) for EBUS is at least 10% worse

TABLE 18.4

Analysis of the lung cancer data for comparing the diagnostic performance between Mediastinoscopy (M) and EBUS (E)

Parameter	M	E	*p*-value*	95% CI**
Sens.	0.715	0.764	0.343	$(-0.150, 0.052)$
Spec.	1.000	1.000	1.000	NA
Accu.	0.921	0.934	0.343	$(-0.042, 0.015)$
PPV	1.000	1.000	1.000	NA
NPV	0.901	0.916	0.342	$(-0.048, 0.017)$

* two-sided p-value for $H_0 : p_M = p_E$
** 95% confidence interval for $p_M - p_E$

than the PPV (or NPV) of mediastinoscopy, whereas the alternative hypothesis that they want to prove is that the PPV (or NPV) for EBUS is not inferior. Following Silva et al. (2008), we obtain p-values of 0 and 1.27×10^{-7} for the noninferiority of PPVs and NPVs, respectively. One-sided lower confidence bound for the difference of PPVs and NPVs are 0 and -0.043, respectively. Since the both lower confidence bounds are larger than -0.1, the noninferiority margin, we conclude that EBUS is not inferior to mediastinoscopy in PPV and NPV.

Comparison of Paired ROC Curves

In this section, we consider biomarkers taking continuous values that are associated with a dichotomous disease status, called case and control. The performance of such a continuous biomarker is evaluated by the area under the curve (AUC) of its receiver operating characteristic (ROC) curve which plots the sensitivity against one minus the specificity calculated for all possible cutoff values of the biomarker observations.

Greenhouse and Mantel (1950) and Linnet (1987) considered the comparison of two sensitivities at a fixed specificity level of biomarkers with predetermined cutoff values. Hanley and McNeil (1982, 1983), McClish (1987), Delong et al. (1988), and Wieand et al. (1989) extend the testing methods to compare the whole or partial AUC of ROC curves of biomarkers.

Sample size calculation is one of the most important steps in the development of medical researches. Hwang and Su (2022) propose a sample size formula for the test statistic of Delong et al. (1988). Their variance formula of the difference of two AUCs include so many terms, even asymptotically negligible ones so that the number of design parameters to be specified for a sample size calculation is large, and they are not so intuitively interpretable that it is difficult to specify them at sample size calculations. This can limit the use of their sample size formula in designing real projects.

In this section, we discuss a simple non-parametric statistical test for comparing the AUC of ROC curves between two biomarkers. We show that our test statistic is asymptotically identical to that of Delong et al. (1988). While the statistical test is completely non-parametric, its power depends on the distributions of biomarkers. Biomarkers to be compared are correlated because they are collected from each subject. This results in additional problems in deriving a sample size formula. The power of our test statistic depends on the bivariate distributions between two biomarkers for controls and cases separately so that we need to specify two bivariate distributions for paired biomarker values, one for controls and the other for cases. We can calculate a sample size by specifying the two bivariate distributions of paired biomarkers. However, we can simplify the design parameters to be specified by noting that the AUC of an ROC curve is invariant to a monotone transformation of biomarker values. If there exists a transformation converting the marginal distributions of paired biomarkers to symmetric distributions with a location shift model and unit variances, then we can specify only the location parameter between controls and cases for each biomarker, which correspond to the AUCs, and the correlation coefficient between paired biomarkers after the transformation.

In the previous section, we have investigated statistical methods to compare the performance parameters of binary tests. Usually a binary test is developed by dichotomizing a continuous biomarker with respect to a cutoff value optimizing its performance. In this section, we are comparing the performance of different medical tests using the original continuous biomarker data before being dichotomized to create binary tests. Furthermore, each subject contributes paired biomaker values and disease status. In the next section, we will extend the results to the cases when clustered paired data are available from each subject.

A Statistical Test for Comparing Two Paired ROC Curves

Biomarkers 1 and 2 are collected from each subject. For biomarker $k(=1,2)$, let X_k and Y_k denote the random variables for observations from cases and controls, respectively. In a data set, we have copies of X_k, $x_{k1},...,x_{k,m}$ from m cases, and copies of Y_k, $y_{k1},...,y_{k,n}$ from n controls. For the total sample size $N(=m+n)$, $m/N \to \gamma \in (0,1)$ denote the prevalence of cases in the target population. Let $F_k(t)=P(X_k \le t)$ and $G_k(t)=P(Y_k \le t)$ denote the cumulative density function (CDF) of biomarker k for cases and controls, respectively, and $\hat{F}_k(t)=m^{-1}\sum_{i=1}^{m} I(x_{ki}\le t)$ and $\hat{G}_k(t)=n^{-1}\sum_{i'=1}^{n} I(y_{ki'}\le t)$ their empirical estimators.

Without loss of generality, we assume that a large biomarker is associated with a higher chance for case. As such, for a cutoff value t, $\bar{F}_k(t)=1-F_k(t)$ is called the sensitivity and $G_k(t)$ is called the specificity of biomarker k. For

$\bar{G}_k(t) = 1 - G_k(t)$, the ROC curve of biomarker k is the plot of $(\bar{G}_k(t), \bar{F}_k(t))$ with respect to all possible cutoff value t.

AUC of the ROC curve for biomarker k is $\theta_k = P(X_k \geq Y_k) = \int_0^\infty G_k(t) dF_k(t)$ that is estimated by

$$\hat{\theta}_k = \int_0^\infty \hat{G}_k(t) d\hat{F}_k(t) = \frac{1}{mn} \sum_{i=1}^{m} \sum_{i'=1}^{n} I(x_{ki} \geq y_{ki'}).$$

We want to test the null hypothesis $H_0 : \theta_1 = \theta_2$ against an alternative hypothesis $H_1 : \theta_1 \neq \theta_2$ by deriving a test statistic based on $\hat{\theta}_1 - \hat{\theta}_2$.

Note that

$$\hat{\theta}_k - \theta_k = \int_0^\infty G_k(t) d\{\hat{F}_k(t) - F_k(t)\} + \int_0^\infty \{\hat{G}_k(t) - G_k(t)\} dF_k$$
$$+ \int_0^\infty \{\hat{G}_k(t) - G_k(t)\} d\{\hat{F}_k(t) - F_k(t)\}. \tag{18.1}$$

Here, by Appendix of Emir et al. (2000), $\int_0^\infty (\hat{G}_k - G_k) d(\hat{F}_k - F_k) = o_p(N^{-1/2})$ so that we have

$$\hat{\theta}_k - \theta_k = m^{-1} \sum_{i=1}^{m} \epsilon_{ki} + n^{-1} \sum_{i'=1}^{n} e_{ki'} + o_p(N^{-1/2}),$$

where $\epsilon_{ki} = \int_0^\infty G_k(t) d\{I(x_{ki} \leq t) - F_k(t)\} = G_k(x_{ki}) - \theta_k$ and $e_{ki'} = \int_0^\infty \{I(y_{ki'} \leq t) - G_k(t)\} dF_k(t) = \bar{F}_k(y_{kj}) - \theta_k$. Hence, under H_0, we have

$$\hat{\theta}_1 - \hat{\theta}_2 = m^{-1} \sum_{i=1}^{m} (\epsilon_{1i} - \epsilon_{2i}) + n^{-1} \sum_{i'=1}^{n} (e_{1i'} - e_{2i'}) + o_p(N^{-1/2}) + o_p(N^{-1/2}). \tag{18.2}$$

While $(\epsilon_{1i}, \epsilon_{2i})$ and $(e_{1i'}, e_{2i'})$ are bivariate random vectors, $(\epsilon_{k1}, ..., \epsilon_{km})$ and $(e_{k1}, ..., e_{kn})$ are independent 0-mean random variables for each biomarker. So, by the central limit theorem, $(\hat{\theta}_1 - \hat{\theta}_2)/\hat{\sigma}$ converges to $N(0, 1)$, where

$$\hat{\sigma}^2 = m^{-2} \sum_{i=1}^{m} (\hat{\epsilon}_{1i} - \hat{\epsilon}_{2i})^2 + n^{-2} \sum_{i'=1}^{n} (\hat{e}_{1i'} - \hat{e}_{2i'})^2$$

and $\hat{\epsilon}_{ki}$ and $\hat{e}_{ki'}$ are obtained from ϵ_{ki} and $e_{ki'}$, respectively, by replacing F_k and G_k with their consistent estimators $\hat{F}_k$ and $\hat{G}_k$. That is,

$$\hat{\epsilon}_{ki} = \hat{G}_k(x_{ki}) - \hat{\theta}_k = \frac{1}{n} \sum_{i'=1}^{n} I(y_{ki'} \leq x_{ki}) - \hat{\theta}_k$$

and

$$\hat{e}_{ki'} = \hat{\bar{F}}(y_{ki'}) - \hat{\theta}_k = \frac{1}{m} \sum_{i=1}^{m} I(x_{ki} \geq y_{ki'}) - \hat{\theta}_k.$$

We reject H_0 if $|\hat{\theta}_1 - \hat{\theta}_2|/\hat{\sigma} > z_{1-\alpha/2}$. Appendix A shows that our variance estimator $\hat{\sigma}^2$ is asymptotically identical to that of DeLong et al. (1988). In this sense, our test statistic is asymptotically identical to that of DeLong et al. (1988), but our variance formula and its estimator are simpler.

In (18.2), we have $\epsilon_{1i} - \epsilon_{2i} = G_1(x_{1i}) - G_2(x_{2i})$ and $e_{1i'} - e_{2i'} = \bar{F}_1(y_{1i'}) - \bar{F}_2(y_{2i'}) = F_2(y_{2i'}) - F_1(y_{1i'})$ under H_0 so that we may use

$$\hat{\sigma}_0^2 = m^{-2}\sum_{i=1}^{m}\{\hat{G}_1(x_{1i}) - \hat{G}_2(x_{2i})\}^2 + n^{-2}\sum_{i'=1}^{n}\{\hat{F}_1(y_{1i'}) - \hat{F}_2(y_{2i'})\}^2$$

in place of $\hat{\sigma}^2$ for the test statistic of $H_0 : \theta_1 = \theta_2$.

Sample Size Calculation

Let $f(x_1, x_2)$ and $g(y_1, y_2)$ denote the bivariate probability density functions (PDFs) of (X_1, X_2) and (Y_1, Y_2), respectively. From (18.2), $\hat{\sigma}^2$ converges to $\sigma^2 = \text{var}(\hat{\theta}_1 - \hat{\theta}_2)$ that is expressed as

$$\sigma^2 = m^{-1}\{\sigma_1^2(\epsilon) + \sigma_2^2(\epsilon) - 2\sigma_{12}(\epsilon)\} + n^{-1}\{\sigma_1^2(e) + \sigma_2^2(e) - 2\sigma_{12}(e)\},$$

where

$$\sigma_k^2(\epsilon) = \text{var}\{G_k(X_k)\} = \int_0^\infty G_k^2 dF_k - \theta_k^2$$

$$\sigma_{12}^2(\epsilon) = \text{cov}\{G_1(X_1), G_2(X_2)\} = \int_0^\infty \int_0^\infty G_1(x_1)G_2(x_2)f(x_1, x_2)dx_1dx_2 - \theta_1\theta_2$$

$$\sigma_k^2(e) = \text{var}\{\bar{F}_k(Y_k)\} = \int_0^\infty \bar{F}_k^2 dG_k - \theta_k^2$$

and

$$\sigma_{12}^2(e) = \text{cov}\{\bar{F}_1(Y_1), \bar{F}_2(Y_2)\} = \int_0^\infty \int_0^\infty \bar{F}_1(y_1)\bar{F}_2(y_2)g(y_1, y_2)dy_1dy_2 - \theta_1\theta_2.$$

Note that $\text{var}(\hat{\theta}_k) = m^{-1}\sigma_k^2(\epsilon) + n^{-1}\sigma_k^2(e)$ and $\text{cov}(\hat{\theta}_1, \hat{\theta}_2) = m^{-1}\sigma_{12}(\epsilon) + n^{-1}\sigma_{12}(e)$. Further, the variance of $\sqrt{N}(\hat{\theta}_1 - \hat{\theta}_2)$, $v = N\sigma^2$, is given as

$$v = \gamma^{-1}\{\sigma_1^2(\epsilon) + \sigma_2^2(\epsilon) - 2\sigma_{12}(\epsilon)\} + \bar{\gamma}^{-1}\{\sigma_1^2(e) + \sigma_2^2(e) - 2\sigma_{12}(e)\}, \quad (18.3)$$

where $\bar{\gamma} = 1 - \gamma$. Hence, under $H_1 : \theta_1 - \theta_2 = \Delta(\neq 0)$, the power function for a given sample size N is

$$1 - \beta = P\left\{\frac{\hat{\theta}_1 - \hat{\theta}_2}{\hat{\sigma}} > z_{1-\alpha/2}\middle| H_1\right\}$$

$$= P\left\{\frac{\sqrt{N}(\hat{\theta}_1 - \hat{\theta}_2 - \Delta)}{\sqrt{v}} > z_{1-\alpha/2} - \frac{\Delta\sqrt{N}}{\sqrt{v}}\middle| H_1\right\}$$

$$= \bar{\Phi}\left(z_{1-\alpha/2} - \frac{\Delta\sqrt{N}}{\sqrt{v}}\right) \qquad (18.4)$$

where $\bar{\Phi}(z) = 1 - \Phi(z)$ and $\Phi(z)$ is the CDF of $N(0,1)$ distribution.

From (18.4), we have

$$-z_{1-\beta} = z_{1-\alpha/2} - \frac{\Delta\sqrt{N}}{\sqrt{v}}.$$

By solving this equation with respect to N, the required sample size is obtained as

$$N = \frac{v(z_{1-\alpha/2} + z_{1-\beta})^2}{\Delta^2}. \qquad (18.5)$$

Normally Distributed Biomarkers

Although the test statistic is completely non-parametric, the variance of our test statistic depends on the distributions of biomarkers for cases and controls through the variance of $\hat{\theta}_1 - \hat{\theta}_2$. So, we have to assume a parametric model for a sample size calculation.

Usually, the raw data of biomarkers take positive values. If we know the distributions of biomarkers, we may calculate a sample size based on the original distributions. For most bivariate positive distributions, however, their means, variances, and correlation coefficient are mutually associated so that it is not easy to specify the parameter values for a sample size calculation.

Note that AUC is invariant to a monotone transformation of X_k and Y_k. Oftentimes, we can find a transformation, such as logarithm, to change the distribution of a positive random variable to a (approximately) normal distribution, for which the parameter values are not associated and can be easily specified. Furthermore, such a transformation tends to stabilize the variance of random variables. So, we assume that, after a (log-)transformation, $X_k \sim N(EX_k, s_k^2)$ and $Y_k \sim N(EY_k, s_k^2)$ are independent.

We consider two steps of transformations that can be described as follows. Suppose that a log-transformation transforms the original biomarker data (X_k, Y_k) to normal random variables. Then, the data after the first transformation will be $(X'_k, Y'_k) = (\log X_k, \log Y_k)$. And, after the second transformation, the resulting data will be (X''_k, Y''_k), where $X''_k = (X'_k - EY'_k)/s_k$, $Y''_k = (Y'_k - EY'_k)/s_k$, and s_k is the standard deviation of X'_k and Y'_k. Note that, in the second transformation, both X'_k and Y'_k are subtracted by $E(Y'_k)$. Since $X''_k = (X'_k - EX'_k)/s_k + (EX'_k - EY'_k)/s_k$, X''_k is expressed as a sum of a $N(0,1)$ random variable plus $\delta_k = (EX'_k - EY'_k)/s_k$, the standardized effect size of biomarker k after the first transformation.

For notational simplicity, we assume that (X_k, Y_k) are the biomarker data after the two steps of transformations. Then, $X_k \sim N(\delta_k, 1)$ and $Y_k \sim N(0,1)$ are independent, and $\text{corr}(X_1, X_2) = \text{corr}(Y_1, Y_2) = \rho$. Let $\phi(t)$ denote the

PDF of $N(0,1)$ and $\phi_\rho(x,y)$ the PDF of bivariate normal distribution with 0 means, unit variances, and correlation coefficient ρ. Then, we have $F_k(x) = \Phi(x-\delta_k)$, $G_k(y) = \Phi(y)$, $f(x_1,x_2) = \phi_\rho(x_1-\delta_1, x_2-\delta_2)$, and $g(y_1,y_2) = \phi_\rho(y_1,y_2)$.

By Appendix B, we have $\sigma_k^2(\epsilon) = \sigma_k^2(e)$ and $\sigma_{12}(\epsilon) = \sigma_{12}(e)$. Hence, v in (18.3) is simplified to

$$v = (\gamma\bar{\gamma})^{-1}\{\sigma_1^2(\epsilon) + \sigma_2^2(\epsilon) - 2\sigma_{12}(\epsilon)\}, \tag{18.6}$$

where

$$\sigma_k^2(\epsilon) = \int_{-\infty}^{\infty} \phi(x-\delta_k)\Phi^2(x)dx - \theta_k^2$$

and

$$\sigma_{12}(\epsilon) = \int_{-\infty}^{\infty}\int_{-\infty}^{\infty} \Phi(x_1)\Phi(x_2)\phi(x_1-\delta_1, x_2-\delta_2)dx_1dx_2 - \theta_1\theta_2.$$

From (18.6), we find that the sample size depends on the prevalence of cases γ through $\gamma\bar{\gamma}$ and the required sample size will be unchanged between two γ values with an identical $|\gamma - 1/2|$ value. Furthermore, we have $\text{var}(\hat{\theta}_k) = (N\gamma\bar{\gamma})^{-1}\sigma_k^2(\epsilon)$ and $\text{cov}(\hat{\theta}_1, \hat{\theta}_2) = (N\gamma\bar{\gamma})^{-1}\sigma_{12}(\epsilon)$ so that $\text{corr}(\hat{\theta}_1, \hat{\theta}_2) = \sigma_{12}(\epsilon)/\{\sigma_1(\epsilon)\sigma_2(\epsilon)\}$ does not depend on γ.

A sample size calculation is conducted as follows. Suppose that biomarker data $\{(X_k, Y_k), k = 1,2\}$ marginally follow normal distributions after a log-transformation.

1. Specify:

   a. Type I error rate α and power $1-\beta$

   b. Prevalence of cases γ

   c. For biomarker $k(=1,2)$, effect size δ_k or AUC $\theta_k = \int_{-\infty}^{\infty}\phi(t-\delta_k)\Phi(t)dt$ under H_1

   d. $\rho = \text{corr}(X_1, X_2) = \text{corr}(Y_1, Y_2)$

2. Calculate v using (18.6).
3. Calculate the required sample size N using (18.5).

Numerical Studies

In the following numerical studies, we assume the bivariate normal distribution model with location shift as discussed above. Table 18.5 displays the values of θ_k and $\sigma_k^2(\epsilon)$ when $X_k \sim N(\delta_k, 1)$ and $Y_k \sim N(0,1)$. Note that, as δ_k increases, θ_k increases and $\sigma_k^2(\epsilon)$ decreases.

TABLE 18.5

Relationship between δ_k and $(\theta_k, \sigma_k^2(\epsilon))$ when $X_k \sim N(0, \delta_k)$ and $Y_k \sim N(0, 1)$

δ_k	0.2	0.4	0.6	0.8	1.0	1.2	1.4	1.6	1.8	2.0
θ_k	0.556	0.611	0.664	0.714	0.760	0.802	0.839	0.871	0.898	0.921
$\sigma_k^2(\epsilon)$	0.082	0.078	0.072	0.064	0.056	0.047	0.038	0.030	0.023	0.017

TABLE 18.6

Value of $\text{corr}(\hat{\theta}_1, \hat{\theta}_2)$ for given $(\rho, \delta_1, \delta_2)$ when $X_k \sim N(0, \delta_k)$, $Y_k \sim N(0, 1)$, and $\text{corr}(X_1, X_2) = \text{corr}(Y_1, Y_2) = \rho$

		ρ								
δ_1	δ_2	0.1	0.2	0.3	0.4	0.5	0.6	0.7	0.8	0.9
0.4	0.6	0.093	0.188	0.283	0.379	0.477	0.576	0.677	0.781	0.887
	0.8	0.092	0.185	0.280	0.375	0.472	0.570	0.671	0.774	0.879
	1.0	0.091	0.182	0.275	0.370	0.465	0.562	0.662	0.763	0.867
0.6	0.8	0.092	0.184	0.278	0.374	0.472	0.571	0.673	0.778	0.886
	1.0	0.090	0.182	0.275	0.369	0.466	0.565	0.666	0.770	0.877
	1.2	0.088	0.178	0.270	0.363	0.459	0.556	0.656	0.759	0.864
0.8	1.0	0.089	0.180	0.273	0.368	0.465	0.565	0.668	0.774	0.883
	1.2	0.087	0.177	0.268	0.362	0.459	0.558	0.660	0.766	0.875
	1.4	0.085	0.173	0.263	0.355	0.451	0.548	0.649	0.753	0.861
1.0	1.2	0.086	0.175	0.266	0.360	0.457	0.557	0.661	0.769	0.880
	1.4	0.084	0.171	0.261	0.354	0.450	0.550	0.653	0.760	0.872
	1.6	0.082	0.167	0.255	0.346	0.441	0.539	0.641	0.747	0.857
1.2	1.4	0.082	0.168	0.260	0.351	0.447	0.548	0.653	0.762	0.877
	1.6	0.080	0.164	0.252	0.344	0.440	0.539	0.644	0.753	0.867
	1.8	0.078	0.159	0.245	0.335	0.430	0.528	0.631	0.739	0.852
1.4	1.6	0.077	0.159	0.248	0.340	0.436	0.537	0.643	0.755	0.873
	1.8	0.076	0.157	0.242	0.331	0.427	0.528	0.633	0.744	0.862
	2.0	0.073	0.152	0.235	0.323	0.417	0.516	0.621	0.731	0.847
1.6	1.8	0.074	0.153	0.238	0.328	0.423	0.525	0.632	0.746	0.867
	2.0	0.072	0.149	0.231	0.320	0.414	0.515	0.622	0.736	0.857
	2.2	0.069	0.143	0.224	0.310	0.403	0.502	0.608	0.721	0.841
1.8	2.0	0.069	0.145	0.227	0.315	0.410	0.511	0.620	0.737	0.863
	2.2	0.067	0.140	0.220	0.306	0.400	0.501	0.609	0.726	0.851
	2.4	0.064	0.134	0.212	0.296	0.402	0.488	0.595	0.710	0.835
2.0	2.2	0.064	0.136	0.214	0.300	0.394	0.496	0.607	0.726	0.856
	2.4	0.062	0.130	0.207	0.291	0.383	0.485	0.595	0.714	0.845
	2.6	0.059	0.125	0.199	0.281	0.371	0.471	0.579	0.698	0.827

Table 18.6 displays values of $\text{corr}(\hat{\theta}_1, \hat{\theta}_2)$ for given $(\rho, \delta_1, \delta_2)$ when $X_k \sim N(0, \delta_k)$, $Y_k \sim N(0, 1)$, and $\text{corr}(X_1, X_2) = \text{corr}(Y_1, Y_2) = \rho$. In summary, $\text{corr}(\hat{\theta}_1, \hat{\theta}_2)$ increases in ρ, and decreases in δ_1 and $|\delta_1 - \delta_2|$. Note that

$\text{corr}(\hat{\theta}_1, \hat{\theta}_2)$ depends on (δ_1, δ_2), or (θ_1, θ_2), as well as ρ. In a sample size calculation, for given ρ and (δ_1, δ_2), we can obtain v by finding θ_k and $\sigma_k^2(\epsilon)$ from Table 18.5 and $\sigma_{12}(\epsilon)$ from Table 18.6.

Since there is a one-to-one relationship between AUC θ_k and location-shift parameter δ_k between X_k and Y_k, we may specify either (θ_1, θ_2) or (δ_1, δ_2) in sample size calculations. For the following sample size calculations, we specify $\theta_k(> 0.5)$ (and identify the corresponding location parameter θ_k) under H_1, together with the common correlation coefficient ρ for bivariate random vectors (X_1, X_2) and (Y_1, Y_2). We consider two-sided $\alpha = 0.05$. Given $(1-\beta, \gamma, \theta_1, \theta_2, \rho)$, we calculate the required sample size N, and generate $B = 10,000$ simulation samples of size N under H_0 and H_1 to calculate empirical type I error rate $\hat{\alpha}$ and power $1-\hat{\beta}$, respectively. Under H_0, we assume that both biomarkers have AUC θ_1. Table 18.7 reports the calculated sample sizes and simulation results. We find that sample size increases in $1-\beta$, and decreases in ρ, θ_1, $|\theta_1 - \theta_2|$, and $|\gamma - 1/2|$. From the simulation results, we find that our test statistic controls the type I error quite accurately and the calculated sample sizes are quite accurate in the sense that the empirical powers are close to the corresponding nominal power $1-\beta$ overall. If the calculated sample size is small and the allocation between cases and controls is much unbalanced (i.e., $\gamma = 0.1$), the empirical type I error rate can be slightly anti-conservative. However, the power is well maintained above the nominal level even in these cases.

Example: Suppose that we design a study to compare the performance of two biomarkers to detect a disease. The expected prevalence of the disease in the target population is $\gamma = 20\%$. After a log-transformation, the expected standardized effect size between disease group and non-disease group for biomarker 1 is $\delta_1 = 1$ with normal distributions, i.e., $X_1 \sim N(1,1)$ and $Y_1 \sim N(0,1)$, and that for biomarker 2 is $\delta_2 = 1.5$, i.e., $X_2 \sim N(1.5, 1)$ and $Y_2 \sim N(0,1)$. The correlation coefficient between X_1 and X_2 and that between Y_1 and Y_2 are expected to be commonly $\rho = 0.5$. For the given location parameters, the corresponding AUCs of ROC curves are $\theta_1 = 0.760$ and $\theta_2 = 0.856$ under H_1. We want to calculate the required sample size to detect a difference in AUC of $\Delta = \theta_1 - \theta_2 = 0.760 - 0.856 = -0.096$ with a power of $1 - \beta = 0.8$ by two-sided test with $\alpha = 0.05$. Under these assumptions, $z_{1-\alpha/2} = 1.960$, $z_{1-\beta} = 0.842$, $\sigma_1^2(\epsilon) = 5.572 \times 10^{-2}$, $\sigma_2^2(\epsilon) = 3.380 \times 10^{-2}$, and $\sigma_{12}(\epsilon) = 1.934 \times 10^{-2}$ so that

$$v = \frac{5.572 \times 10^{-2} + 3.380 \times 10^{-2} - 2 \times 1.934 \times 10^{-2}}{0.2 \times 0.8} = 0.318.$$

Hence, the required sample size is

$$N = \left\lceil \frac{0.318(1.960 + 0.842)^2}{(-0.096)^2} \right\rceil = 275$$

TABLE 18.7

Required sample size N (empirical type I error rate $\hat{\alpha}$ and power $1-\hat{\beta}$ in parenthesis) for given θ_k (and corresponding δ_k) for two-sided $\alpha = 0.05$ test

$1-\beta$	ρ	$\theta_1(\delta_1)$	$\theta_2(\delta_2)$	$\gamma = 0.1$	$\gamma = 0.3$	$\gamma = 0.5$
0.8	0.3	0.6(0.358)	0.7(0.742)	917(0.052, 0.806)	393(0.048, 0.794)	330(0.049, 0.795)
			0.75(0.953)	386(0.062, 0.785)	166(0.053, 0.795)	139(0.059, 0.793)
		0.7(0.742)	0.8(1.190)	731(0.057, 0.811)	313(0.054, 0.797)	263(0.054, 0.802)
			0.85(1.466)	298(0.064, 0.812)	128(0.054, 0.807)	107(0.054, 0.800)
		0.8(1.190)	0.9(1.812)	474(0.057, 0.823)	203(0.055, 0.813)	170(0.050, 0.812)
			0.95(2.326)	195(0.065, 0.879)	83(0.059, 0.864)	69(0.051, 0.858)
	0.6	0.6(0.358)	0.7(0.742)	548(0.060, 0.803)	235(0.051, 0.802)	198(0.051, 0.797)
			0.75(0.953)	236(0.062, 0.801)	101(0.053, 0.794)	85(0.051, 0.796)
		0.7(0.742)	0.8(1.190)	448(0.052, 0.804)	192(0.049, 0.799)	161(0.051, 0.802)
			0.85(1.466)	192(0.064, 0.827)	82(0.057, 0.811)	69(0.052, 0.809)
		0.8(1.190)	0.9(1.812)	314(0.057, 0.843)	134(0.048, 0.837)	112(0.050, 0.825)
			0.95(2.326)	153(0.072, 0.924)	65(0.053, 0.901)	53(0.048, 0.893)
	0.9	0.6(0.358)	0.7(0.742)	157(0.064, 0.814)	67(0.051, 0.783)	57(0.042, 0.779)
			0.75(0.953)	76(0.080, 0.818)	33(0.053, 0.757)	28(0.042, 0.762)
		0.7(0.742)	0.8(1.190)	140(0.065, 0.837)	60(0.046, 0.803)	51(0.041, 0.793)
			0.85(1.466)	76(0.074, 0.865)	33(0.047, 0.796)	28(0.038, 0.806)
		0.8(1.190)	0.9(1.812)	130(0.056, 0.916)	56(0.045, 0.864)	46(0.040, 0.849)
			0.95(2.326)	103(0.062, 0.969)	43(0.037, 0.927)	35(0.037, 0.907)
0.85	0.3	0.6(0.358)	0.7(0.742)	1049(0.054, 0.850)	450(0.050, 0.847)	378(0.052, 0.846)
			0.75(0.953)	442(0.055, 0.845)	190(0.050, 0.851)	159(0.050, 0.848)
		0.7(0.742)	0.8(1.190)	836(0.052, 0.851)	358(0.054, 0.842)	301(0.048, 0.846)
			0.85(1.466)	341(0.056, 0.860)	146(0.056, 0.858)	123(0.050, 0.855)
		0.8(1.190)	0.9(1.812)	542(0.054, 0.874)	232(0.055, 0.864)	194(0.051, 0.860)
			0.95(2.326)	223(0.063, 0.918)	95(0.053, 0.908)	79(0.053, 0.902)
	0.6	0.6(0.358)	0.7(0.742)	627(0.054, 0.854)	269(0.049, 0.850)	226(0.050, 0.847)
			0.75(0.953)	269(0.060, 0.852)	116(0.052, 0.848)	97(0.053, 0.852)
		0.7(0.742)	0.8(1.190)	512(0.054, 0.861)	220(0.055, 0.855)	185(0.049, 0.853)
			0.85(1.466)	219(0.066, 0.867)	94(0.050, 0.865)	79(0.045, 0.865)
		0.8(1.190)	0.9(1.812)	359(0.055, 0.882)	154(0.051, 0.875)	129(0.051, 0.874)
			0.95(2.326)	175(0.064, 0.949)	74(0.049, 0.939)	61(0.048, 0.927)
	0.9	0.6(0.358)	0.7(0.742)	179(0.058, 0.858)	77(0.048, 0.842)	65(0.045, 0.837)
			0.75(0.953)	87(0.079, 0.866)	38(0.047, 0.835)	32(0.039, 0.838)
		0.7(0.742)	0.8(1.190)	160(0.062, 0.890)	69(0.046, 0.855)	58(0.045, 0.851)
			0.85(1.466)	87(0.072, 0.909)	38(0.046, 0.881)	32(0.038, 0.873)
		0.8(1.190)	0.9(1.812)	149(0.061, 0.940)	63(0.041, 0.906)	53(0.036, 0.910)
			0.95(2.326)	118(0.063, 0.984)	49(0.042, 0.965)	40(0.035, 0.955)
0.9	0.3	0.6(0.358)	0.7(0.742)	1228(0.051, 0.899)	526(0.052, 0.896)	442(0.051, 0.897)
			0.75(0.953)	517(0.056, 0.891)	222(0.050, 0.900)	186(0.056, 0.902)
		0.7(0.742)	0.8(1.190)	978(0.054, 0.902)	419(0.052, 0.899)	352(0.052, 0.906)
			0.85(1.466)	399(0.057, 0.897)	171(0.054, 0.905)	144(0.053, 0.908)
		0.8(1.190)	0.9(1.812)	634(0.052, 0.914)	271(0.047, 0.913)	227(0.049, 0.912)
			0.95(2.326)	261(0.063, 0.953)	111(0.052, 0.944)	92(0.052, 0.944)
	0.6	0.6(0.358)	0.7(0.742)	733(0.058, 0.898)	315(0.055, 0.902)	264(0.050, 0.895)
			0.75(0.953)	315(0.061, 0.900)	135(0.054, 0.897)	114(0.053, 0.902)
		0.7(0.742)	0.8(1.190)	600(0.054, 0.915)	257(0.050, 0.902)	216(0.051, 0.906)
			0.85(1.466)	257(0.061, 0.912)	110(0.056, 0.914)	93(0.054, 0.912)
		0.8(1.190)	0.9(1.812)	420(0.059, 0.931)	180(0.053, 0.927)	150(0.048, 0.920)
			0.95(2.326)	205(0.061, 0.978)	86(0.053, 0.971)	71(0.049, 0.966)

(Continued)

TABLE 18.7 (Continued)

Required sample size N (empirical type I error rate $\hat{\alpha}$ and power $1-\hat{\beta}$ in parenthesis) for given θ_k (and corresponding δ_k) for two-sided $\alpha = 0.05$ test

$1-\beta$	ρ	$\theta_1(\delta_1)$	$\theta_2(\delta_2)$	$\gamma = 0.1$	$\gamma = 0.3$	$\gamma = 0.5$
	0.9	0.6(0.358)	0.7(0.742)	210(0.060, 0.915)	90(0.048, 0.895)	76(0.046, 0.896)
			0.75(0.953)	102(0.076, 0.922)	44(0.048, 0.902)	37(0.044, 0.893)
		0.7(0.742)	0.8(1.190)	188(0.061, 0.919)	81(0.049, 0.913)	68(0.048, 0.916)
			0.85(1.466)	102(0.065, 0.958)	44(0.045, 0.942)	37(0.038, 0.932)
		0.8(1.190)	0.9(1.812)	174(0.059, 0.971)	74(0.046, 0.961)	62(0.040, 0.958)
			0.95(2.326)	137(0.065, 0.996)	58(0.037, 0.989)	47(0.038, 0.984)

or $m = 0.2 \times 275 = 55$ and $n = 0.8 \times 275 = 220$, where $[x]$ denotes the round-up of x. In order to validate this sample size, we generated 10,000 samples of size $N = 275$ under the design setting, applied our test statistic to each sample using two-sided $\alpha = 0.05$, and obtained an empirical power of $1 - \hat{\beta} = 80.6\%$ as the proportion of the simulation samples that rejected the null hypothesis $H_0 : \theta_1 = \theta_2$. The empirical power is very close to the nominal level, $1 - \beta = 80\%$.

Comparison of Two ROC Curves with Clustered Pair Data

In the previous section, we assumed that each subject contribute only one site to study to collect a set of paired continuous biomarker values together with a gold standard outcome. Oftentimes, however, each subject may contribute multiple sites, each with a set of these observations. For example, Lim et al. (2012) investigate detection of liver metastases from various extrahepatic malignancies, including colorectal cancer, stomach cancer, duodenal cancer, and renal cell carcinoma. In their study, a total of 106 focal lesions (51 metastases and 55 benign) are found from $n = 36$ patients. They are interested in comparing two imaging biomarkers to detect liver metastases. In this section, we extend the testing method of paired ROC curves to that for clustered pair biomarker data as in Lim et al. (2012).

Suppose that there are N patients, and patient $i(= 1, ..., N)$ contribute m_i malignant sites (cases) and n_i benign sites (controls). For patient i and biomarker $k(= 1, 2)$, let x_{kij} denote the biomarker value from malignant site $j(= 1, ..., m_i)$ and $y_{kij'}$ the biomarker value from benign site $j'(= 1, ..., n_i)$. Let $m = \sum_{i=1}^{N} m_i$ and $n = \sum_{i=1}^{N} n_i$ denote the total numbers of malignant and benign sites, respectively.

Let $F_k(t) = P(X_k \leq t)$ and $G_k(t) = P(Y_k \leq t)$ denote the cumulative density function (CDF) of biomarker k for cases and controls, respectively, and $\hat{F}_k(t) = m^{-1} \sum_{i=1}^{N} \sum_{j=1}^{m_i} I(x_{kij} \leq t)$ and $\hat{G}_k(t) = n^{-1} \sum_{i=1}^{N} \sum_{j'=1}^{n_i} I(y_{kij'} \leq t)$ their empirical estimators based on the clustered data.

AUC of the ROC curve for biomarker k, $\theta_k = P(X_k \geq Y_k) = \int_0^\infty G_k(t)dF_k(t)$, is estimated by

$$\hat{\theta}_k = \int_0^\infty \hat{G}_k(t)d\hat{F}_k(t) = \frac{1}{mn}\sum_{i=1}^{N}\sum_{j=1}^{m_i}\sum_{j'=1}^{n_i} I(x_{kij} \geq y_{kij'}).$$

We want to test the null hypothesis $H_0 : \theta_1 = \theta_2$ against an alternative hypothesis $H_1 : \theta_1 \neq \theta_2$ by deriving a test statistic based on $\hat{\theta}_1 - \hat{\theta}_2$.

Note that

$$\hat{\theta}_k - \theta_k = \int_0^\infty G_k(t)d\{\hat{F}_k(t) - F_k(t)\} + \int_0^\infty \{\hat{G}_k(t) - G_k(t)\}dF_k$$

$$+ \int_0^\infty \{\hat{G}_k(t) - G_k(t)\}d\{\hat{F}_k(t) - F_k(t)\} \tag{18.7}$$

In (18.7), by Appendix of Emir et al. (2000), $\int_0^\infty (\hat{G}_k - G_k)d(\hat{F}_k - F_k) = o_p(N^{-1/2})$ so that we have

$$\hat{\theta}_k - \theta_k = m^{-1}\sum_{i=1}^{N}\sum_{j=1}^{m_i} \epsilon_{kij} + n^{-1}\sum_{i=1}^{N}\sum_{j'=1}^{n_i} e_{kij'} + o_p(N^{-1/2}),$$

where $\epsilon_{kij} = \int_0^\infty G_k(t)d\{I(x_{kij} \leq t) - F_k(t)\} = G_k(x_{kij}) - \theta_k$ and $e_{kij'} = \int_0^\infty \{I(y_{kij'} \leq t) - G_k(t)\}dF_k(t) = \bar{F}_k(y_{kij'}) - \theta_k$. Hence, under H_0, we have

$$\hat{\theta}_1 - \hat{\theta}_2 = \sum_{i=1}^{N}\{(\epsilon_{1i} - \epsilon_{2i}) + (e_{1i} - e_{2i})\} + o_p(N^{-1/2}), \tag{18.8}$$

where, for $k = 1, 2$,

$$\epsilon_{ki} = m^{-1}\sum_{j=1}^{m_i} \epsilon_{kij}$$

and

$$e_{ki} = n^{-1}\sum_{j'=1}^{n_i} e_{kij'}.$$

For paired data case that is discussed in the previous section, the cases and controls are independent because they are different patients. For the clustered pair data, however, some patients may contribute both benign and malignant sites so that cases and controls may be correlated. Hence, we have to derive a variance estimator of $\hat{\theta}_1 - \hat{\theta}_2$ differently.

Since $\{(\epsilon_{1i}-\epsilon_{2i})+(e_{1i}-e_{2i}), i=1,...,N\}$ are independent 0-mean random variables, by the central limit theorem for large N, $\hat{\theta}_1 - \hat{\theta}_2$ is approximately normal with mean 0 and variance σ^2 that can be consistently estimated by

$$\hat{\sigma}^2 = \sum_{i=1}^{N}\{(\hat{\epsilon}_{1i}-\hat{\epsilon}_{2i})+(\hat{e}_{1i}-\hat{e}_{2i})\}^2,$$

where $\hat{\epsilon}_{ki}$ and $\hat{e}_{ki}$ are obtained from ϵ_{ki} and e_{ki}, respectively, by replacing $F_k(t)$ and $G_k(t)$ by their consistently estimators $\hat{F}_k(t)$ and $\hat{G}_k(t)$.

In (18.8), we have

$$\epsilon_{1i}-\epsilon_{2i} = m^{-1}\sum_{j=1}^{m_i}\{G_1(x_{1ij})-G_2(x_{2ij})\}$$

and

$$e_{1i}-e_{2i} = n^{-1}\sum_{j'=1}^{n_i}\{\bar{F}_1(y_{1ij'})-\bar{F}_2(y_{2ij'})\} = -n^{-1}\sum_{j'=1}^{n_i}\{F_1(y_{1ij'})-F_2(y_{2ij'})\}$$

under H_0 so that we may use

$$\hat{\sigma}_0^2 = \sum_{i=1}^{N}\left[m^{-1}\sum_{j=1}^{m_i}\{\hat{G}_1(x_{1ij})-\hat{G}_2(x_{2ij})\} - n^{-1}\sum_{j'=1}^{n_i}\{\hat{F}_2(y_{2ij'})-\hat{F}_1(y_{1ij'})\}\right]^2$$

in place of $\hat{\sigma}^2$ for the test statistic of $H_0: \theta_1 = \theta_2$.

We can derive a sample size formula of this test statistic as in the paired ROC case discussed in the previous section. The power and sample size of this test statistic depends on the intracluster correlation coefficients among multiple sites for each biomarker as well as between two biomarkers.

Appendix A. Our variance formula for $\hat{\theta} - \hat{\theta}_2$ is asymptotically identical to that of DeLong et al. (1988)

By DeLong et al. (1988),

$$\mathrm{var}(\hat{\theta}_k) = \frac{(n-1)\xi_{10}+(m-1)\xi_{01}}{mn} + \frac{\xi_{11}}{mn}, \tag{18.A1}$$

where, for $i \neq i'$ and $j \neq j'$,

$$\xi_{10} = P(x_{ki} \geq y_{kj}, x_{ki} \geq y_{kj'}) - \theta_k^2$$

$$\xi_{01} = P(x_{ki} \geq y_{kj}, x_{ki'} \geq y_{kj}) - \theta_k^2$$

and

$$\xi_{11} = P(x_{ki} \geq y_{kj}) - \theta_k^2$$

On the other hand, from (18.1), we have

$$\hat{\theta}_k - \theta_k \approx \int_0^\infty G_k d(\hat{F}_k - F_k) + \int_0^\infty (\hat{G}_k - G_k) dF_k$$

$$= (\int_0^\infty G_k d\hat{F}_k - \theta_k) + (\int_0^\infty \hat{G}_k dF_k - \theta_k)$$

$$= \frac{1}{m}\sum_{i=1}^{m}\{G_k(x_{ki}) - \theta_k\} + \frac{1}{n}\sum_{j=1}^{n}\{\bar{F}_k(y_{kj}) - \theta_k\}$$

so that

$$\text{var}(\hat{\theta}_k) = \frac{1}{m^2}\sum_{i=1}^{m}\{G_k^2(x_{ki}) - \theta_k^2\} + \frac{1}{n^2}\sum_{j=1}^{n}\{\bar{F}_k^2(y_{kj}) - \theta_k^2\}$$

$$\approx \frac{1}{m^2}\sum_{i=1}^{m}\{\hat{G}_k^2(x_{ki}) - \theta_k^2\} + \frac{1}{n^2}\sum_{j=1}^{n}\{\hat{\bar{F}}_k^2(y_{kj}) - \theta_k^2\} \qquad (18.A2)$$

since $\hat{F}(t)$ and $\hat{G}(t)$ uniformly converge to $F(t)$ and $G(t)$, respectively.

Here,

$$\sum_{i=1}^{m}\hat{G}_k^2(x_{ki}) = \frac{1}{n^2}\sum_{i=1}^{m}\left\{\sum_{j=1}^{n} I(x_{ki} \geq y_{kj})\right\}^2$$

$$= \frac{1}{n^2}\sum_{i=1}^{m}\left\{\sum_{j=1}^{n} I(x_{ki} \geq y_{kj}) + \sum_{j\neq j'} I(x_{ki} \geq y_{kj}, x_{ki} \geq y_{kj'})\right\}$$

$$\approx \frac{m}{n}\{P(x_{ki} \geq y_{kj}) + (n-1)P(x_{ki} \geq y_{kj}, x_{ki} \geq y_{kj'})\}.$$

Similarly,

$$\sum_{j=1}^{n}\hat{\bar{F}}_k^2(y_{kj}) = \frac{1}{m^2}\sum_{j=1}^{n}\left\{\sum_{i=1}^{m} I(x_{ki} \geq y_{kj})\right\}^2$$

$$= \frac{1}{m^2}\sum_{j=1}^{n}\left\{\sum_{i=1}^{m} I(x_{ki} \geq y_{kj}) + \sum_{i\neq i'} I(x_{ki} \geq y_{kj}, x_{ki'} \geq y_{kj})\right\}$$

$$\approx \frac{n}{m}\{P(x_{ki} \geq y_{kj}) + (m-1)P(x_{ki} \geq y_{kj}, x_{ki'} \geq y_{kj})\}$$

Hence, from (18.A2), we have

$$\text{var}(\hat{\theta}_k) \approx \frac{\xi_{11} + (n-1)\xi_{10}}{mn} + \frac{\xi_{11} + (m-1)\xi_{01}}{mn}$$

$$= \frac{(n-1)\xi_{10} + (m-1)\xi_{01}}{mn} + \frac{2\xi_{11}}{mn}, \qquad (18.A3)$$

which is further simplified to $m^{-1}\sigma_k^2(\epsilon) + n^{-1}\sigma_k^2(e)$ as shown in the section 'Sample Size Calculation'. For large N, $\xi_{11}/(mn)$ in (18.A1) and $2\xi_{11}/(mn)$ in (18.A3) are negligible so that the two variances are asymptotically identical.

Also, by DeLong et al. (1988),

$$\text{cov}(\hat{\theta}_1, \hat{\theta}_2) = \frac{1}{n}\text{cov}\{\hat{G}_1(X_1), \hat{G}_2(X_2)\} + \frac{1}{m}\text{cov}\{\hat{\bar{F}}_1(Y_1), \hat{\bar{F}}_2(Y_2)\},$$

which is asymptotically identical to our covariance formula

$$\text{cov}(\hat{\theta}_1, \hat{\theta}_2) = \frac{1}{n}\text{cov}\{G_1(X_1), G_2(X_2)\} + \frac{1}{m}\text{cov}\{\bar{F}_1(Y_1), \bar{F}_2(Y_2)\}$$

as shown in the section 'Sample Size Calculation'. This completes the proof.

Appendix B. We have $\sigma_k^2(\epsilon) = \sigma_k^2(e)$ and $\sigma_{12}(\epsilon) = \sigma_{12}(e)$ if biomarkers have normal distributions

If (X_k, Y_k) are normally distributed and (X_1, X_2) and (Y_1, Y_2) are bivariate normal random variables, we have $F_k(x) = \Phi(x - \delta_k)$, $G_k(y) = \Phi(y)$, $f_k(x) = \partial F_k(x)/\partial x = \phi(x - \delta_k)$, $g_k(y) = \partial G_k(y)/\partial y = \phi(y)$, $f(x_1, x_2) = \phi_\rho(x_1 - \delta_1, x_2 - \delta_2)$, and $g(y_1, y_2) = \phi_\rho(y_1, y_2)$. So, we have

$$\sigma_k^2(\epsilon) = \int_{-\infty}^{\infty} \phi(x - \delta_k)\Phi^2(x)dx - \theta_k^2$$

$$= \int_{-\infty}^{\infty} \phi(y)\Phi^2(y + \delta_k)dy - \theta_k^2 \qquad \text{by substitution of } x = y + \delta_k$$

$$= \int_{-\infty}^{\infty} \phi(y)\bar{\Phi}^2(-y - \delta_k)dy - \theta_k^2 \qquad \text{since } \Phi(x) = \bar{\Phi}(-x)$$

$$= \int_{-\infty}^{\infty} \phi(-x)\bar{\Phi}^2(x - \delta_k)dx - \theta_k^2 \qquad \text{by substitution of } y = -x$$

$$= \int_{-\infty}^{\infty} \phi(x)\bar{\Phi}^2(x - \delta_k)dx - \theta_k^2 \qquad \text{since } \phi(x) = \phi(-x),$$

which is $\sigma_k^2(e)$.

Furthermore, we have

$$\sigma_{12}(\epsilon) = \int_{-\infty}^{\infty}\int_{-\infty}^{\infty} \Phi(x_1)\Phi(x_2)\phi(x_1 - \delta_1, x_2 - \delta_2)dx_1dx_2 - \theta_1\theta_2$$

$$= \int_{-\infty}^{\infty}\int_{-\infty}^{\infty} \bar{\Phi}(-x_1)\bar{\Phi}(-x_2)\phi(x_1 - \delta_1, x_2 - \delta_2)dx_1dx_2 - \theta_1\theta_2$$

since $\Phi(x) = \bar{\Phi}(-x)$

$$= \int_{-\infty}^{\infty}\int_{-\infty}^{\infty} \bar{\Phi}(-x_1)\bar{\Phi}(-x_2)\phi(-x_1 + \delta_1, -x_2 + \delta_2)dx_1dx_2 - \theta_1\theta_2$$

since $\phi(x_1, x_2) = \phi(-x_1, -x_2)$

$$= \int_{-\infty}^{\infty}\int_{-\infty}^{\infty} \bar{\Phi}(y_1 - \delta_1)\bar{\Phi}(y_2 - \delta_2)\phi(y_1, y_2)dy_1dy_2 - \theta_1\theta_2$$

by substitution of $y_k = -x_k + \delta_k$

which is $\sigma_{12}(e)$.

References

DeLong ER, Delong DM, (1988). and Clarke-Pearson DL. Comparing the areas under two or more correlated receiver operating characteristic curves: A nonparametric approach. Biometrics. 44: 837–845.

Emir B, Wieand S, Jung SH, Ying Z. Comparison of diagnostic markers with repeated measurements: a non-parametric ROC curve approach. Statics in Medicine 2000. 19: 511–523.

Greenhouse SW, Mantel N. The evaluation of diagnostic tests. Biometrics 1950; 6: 399–412.

Hanley JA, McNeil BJ. The meaning and use of the area under receiver operating characteristic (ROC) curve. Radiology 1982; 143: 29–36.

Hanley JA, McNeil BJ. Method for comparing the area under the ROC curves derived from the same cases. Radiology 1983; 148: 839–843.

Hu F, Schucany WR, Ahn C. Nonparametric sample size estimation for sensitivity and specificity with multiple observations per subject. Drug Information Journal 2010; 44(5): 609–616.

Hwang YT, Su NC. Sample size determination for comparing accuracies between two diagnostic tests under a paired design. Biometrical Journal 2022; 64: 771–804.

Jung SH, Kang SH, Ahn C. Sample size calculations for clustered binary data. Statistics in Medicine 2001; 20: 1971–1982.

Katsis, A. Sample size for testing homogeneity of two a priori dependent binomial populations using the Bayesian approach. Journal of Applied Mathematics and Decision Sciences 2004; 8(1): 33–42.

Kosinski AS. A weighted generalized score statistic for comparison of predictive values of diagnostic tests. Statistics in Medicine 2013; 32(6): 964–977.

Kwak M, Um SW, Jung SH. Comparison of operational characteristics for binary tests with clustered data. Statistics in Medicine 2015; 34(15): 2325–2333.

Leisenring W, Alonzo TA, Pepe MS. Comparisons of predictive values of binary medical diagnostic tests for paired designs. Biometrics 2000; 56: 345–351.

Linnet K. Comparison of quantitative diagnostic tests: type 1 error, power, and sample size. Statistics in Medicine 1987; 6: 147–158.

McClish DK. Comparing the areas under more than two ROC curves. Medical Decision Making 1987; 7: 149–155.

McNemar Q. Note on the sampling error of the difference between correlated proportions or percentages. Psychometrika 1947; 12: 153–157.

Moskowitz CS, Pepe MS. Comparing the predictive values of diagnostic tests: sample size and analysis for paired study designs. Clinical Trials 2006; 3: 272–279.

Porte H, Roumilhac D, Eraldi L, Cordonnier C, Puech P, Wurtz A. The role of mediastinoscopy in the diagnosis of mediastinal lymphadenopathy. European Journal of Cardio-Thoracic Surgery 1998; 13: 196–199.

Rao JNK, Scott AJ. A simple method for the analysis of clustered binary data. Biometrics 1992; 48: 577–585.

Silva, GT, Logan, BR, and Klein, JP. Methods for equivalence and noninferiority testing. Biology of Blood and Marrow Transplantation 2008; 15(1): 120–127.

Silvestri GA, Gonzalez AV, Jantz MA, et al. Methods for staging non-small cell lung cancer: Diagnosis and management of lung cancer, 3rd ed: American College of Chest Physicians evidence-based clinical practice guidelines. Chest 2013; 143(5): e211S–250S.

Um SW, Lee K, Kim HK, Jung SH, Han J, Lee KJ, Park HY, Choi YS, Shim YM, Ahn MJ, Park K, Ahn YC, Choi JY, Lee KS, Suh GY, Chung MP, Kwon OJ, Kim J, Kim H. Endobronchial Ultrasound versus Mediastinoscopy for Mediastinal Nodal Staging of Non-Small-Cell Lung Cancer. Journal of Thoracic Oncology 2015; 10(2): 331–337.

Wang W, Davis CS, Soong SJ. Comparison of predictive values of two diagnostic tests from the same sample of subjects using weighted least squares. Statistics in Medicine 2006; 25: 2215–2229.

Wieand S, Gail MH, James BR, and James KL. A family of nonparametric statistics for comparing diagnostic markers with paired or unpaired data. Biometrika 1989; 76: 585–592.

Index

Kolibri 360 GmbH
Ferdinand-Jühlke-Straße 7
99095 Erfurt, Deutschland
produktsicherheit@kolibri360.de